# Swimming Medicine IV

# International Series on Sport Sciences

Series Editors: **Richard C. Nelson and Chauncey A. Morehouse**

The principal focus of this series is on reference works primarily from international congress and symposium proceedings. These should be of particular interest to researchers, clinicians, students, physical educators, and coaches involved in the growing field of sport science. The Series Editors are Professors Richard C. Nelson and Chauncey A. Morehouse of The Pennsylvania State University. The series includes the eight major divisions of sport science: biomechanics, history, medicine, pedagogy, philosophy, physiology, psychology, and sociology.

Each volume in the series is published in English but is written by authors of several countries. The series, therefore, is truly international in scope and because many of the authors normally publish their work in languages other than English, the series volumes are a resource for information often difficult if not impossible to obtain elsewhere. Organizers of international congresses in the sport sciences desiring detailed information concerning the use of this series for publication and distribution of official proceedings are requested to contact the Series Editors. Manuscripts prepared by several authors from various countries consisting of information of international interest will also be considered for publication.

The *International Series on Sport Sciences* serves not only as a valuable source of authoritative up-to-date information but also helps to foster better understanding among sports scientists on an international level. It provides an effective medium through which researchers, teachers, and coaches may develop better communications with individuals in countries throughout the world who have similar professional interests.

Volume 1
Nelson and Morehouse. **BIOMECHANICS IV** (Fourth International Seminar on Biomechanics)

Volume 2
Lewillie and Clarys. **SWIMMING II** (Second International Seminar on Biomechanics of Swimming)

Volume 3
Albinson and Andrew. **CHILD IN SPORT AND PHYSICAL ACTIVITY** (First International Symposium on the Participation of Children in Sport)

Volume 4
Haag. **SPORT PEDAGOGY: Content and Methodology** (First International Symposium on Sport Pedagogy)

Volume 5
Figueras. **SKIING SAFETY II** (Second International Conference on Ski Trauma and Skiing Safety)

Volume 6
Eriksson and Furberg. **SWIMMING MEDICINE IV** (Fourth International Congress on Swimming Medicine)

Volume 7
Pařízková and Rogozkin. **NUTRITION, PHYSICAL FITNESS, AND HEALTH**

International Series
on Sport Sciences, Volume 6

# SWIMMING MEDICINE IV

Proceedings of the Fourth International Congress on Swimming Medicine, Stockholm, Sweden

Edited by: **Bengt Eriksson, M.D.**
University of Göteborg
Göteborg, Sweden
and
**Bengt Furberg, M.D.**
Umeå, Sweden
Series Editors: **Richard C. Nelson, Ph.D.**
and
**Chauncey A. Morehouse, Ph.D.**
The Pennsylvania State University



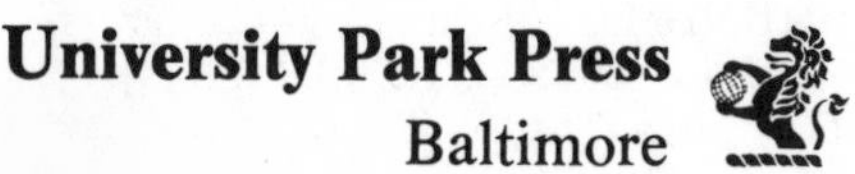
University Park Press
Baltimore

**UNIVERSITY PARK PRESS**
International Publishers in Science and Medicine
233 East Redwood Street
Baltimore, Maryland 21202



Typeset by Everybodys Press

Manufactured in the United States of America by
The Maple Press Company.



Selected publications and reports given at the Fourth International Congress on Swimming Medicine, held June 5–10, 1977, in Stockholm, Sweden.

**Library of Congress Cataloging in Publication Data**
International Congress on Swimming Medicine, 4th,
Stockholm, Sweden, 1977.
Swimming Medicine IV.
(International series on sport sciences; v. 6)
1. Swimming—Physiological aspects—Congresses. 2. Swimming—Therapeutic use—Congresses. 3. Sports medicine—Congresses. I. Furberg, Bengt. II. Eriksson, Bengt. III. Title. IV. Series. [DNLM: 1. Swimming—Congresses. 2. Sport medicine—Congresses. W3 IN662M 4th 1977s / QT260 I56 1977s]
RC1220.S8I57 1977 612'.044 78-5971
ISBN 0-8391-1214-9

# Contents

## PHYSIOLOGY



## METABOLISM

## THERMOREGULATION



## BIOMECHANICS

# Contributors

**J. Alloway** Department of Human Movement Studies, University of Queensland, Brisbane, Q 4067 Australia

**P. Apor** Research Institut of the Hungarian University of Physical Education, TFKI, H-1123, Alkotas u 44, Budapest XII, Hungary

**C. G. S. Araújo** Laboratório de Performance Humana, Universidade gama Filho, Rua Manoel Vitorino, 625 Piedade, Rio de Janeiro, Brazil, 20.000

**J. L. Ardisson** Laboratoire de Physiologie, U.E. R. de Médecine, Université de Nice, Avenue de Vallombrose, F-06034 Nice, France

**P.-O. Åstrand** Department of Physiology III, Karolinska Institutet, Lidingövägen 1, S-114 33 Stockholm, Sweden

**R. R. Bechbache** Department of Physiology, Medical Sciences Bldg., University of Toronto, Toronto, Ontario, Canada

**A. N. Belcastro** Human Performance Research Laboratory, School of Physical Education, Dalhousie University, Halifax, Nova Scotia, Canada B3H 3J5

**K. Berg** Department of Pediatrics, University of Göteborg, Östra Sjukhuset, S-416 85 Göteborg, Sweden

**U. Bergh** Department of Physiology III, Karolinska Institutet, Lidingövägen 1, S-114 33 Stockholm, Sweden

**T. Bober** Academy of Physical Education, Biomechanics Laboratory, A1. Olimpijska 35, 51-612 Wroclaw, Poland

**A. Bonen** Human Performance Research Laboratory, School of Physical Education, Dalhousie University, Halifax, Nova Scotia, Canada B3H 3J5

**B. Carlmark** Department of Internal Medicine, Karolinska Sjukhuset, S-104 01 Stockholm, Sweden

**N. J. Christensen** Second Clinic of Internal Medicine, Kommunehospitalet, Aarhus, Denmark

**J. P. Clarys** Vrye Universiteit Brussel-Campus Sette, Instituut voor Morfologie, Bosstraat B-1090, Brussel, Belgium

**D. L. Costill** Human Performance Laboratory, Departments of Physical Education and Biology, Ball State University, Muncie, Indiana 47306 USA

**A. B. Craig, Jr.** Department of Physiology, School of Medicine, University of Rochester, Rochester, New York, USA

**D. A. Cunningham** Department of Physiology, University of Western Ontario, London, Ontario, Canada

**J. V. Daniel** University of Toronto, 121 St. Joseph Street, Toronto, Ontario, Canada

**P. E. di Prampero** Centro Studi de Fishiologia del Lavoro Muscolare, C.N.R., Milian, Italy

**R. H. Dominguez** Wheaton Orthopaedics, 393 Schmale Rd.,Wheaton, Illinois 60187 USA

**B. L. Drinkwater** Institute of Environmental Stress, University of California, Sanata Barbara, California 93106

**J. Duffin** Department of Physiology, University of Toronto, Toronto, Ontario, Canada

**L. Ehn** Department of Internal Medicine, Karolinska Sjukhuset, S-104 01 Stockholm, Sweden

**B. Ekblom** Department of Physiology III, Karolinska Institutet, Lidingövägen 1, S-114 33 Stockholm, Sweden

**B. O. Eriksson** Department of Pediatrics, University of Göteborg, Östra Sjukhuset, S-416 85 Göteborg, Sweden

**U. Ersson** Sjukgymnastikavdelningen, Akademiska Sjukhuset, Fack, S-750 14 Uppsala, 14, Sweden

**Z. Firsov**, Skaternyi Pereulok 4, Moscow 69, USSR

**K. Fitch** Department of Physical Education and Recreation, The University of Western Australia, Nedlands, Western Australia 6009

**D. E. FitzGerald** Angiology Research Group, Irish Foundation for Human Development, Dublin, Ireland

**M. Foyer** Sjukgymnastikavdelningen, Akademiska Sjukhuset, Fack, S-750 14 Uppsala 14, Sweden

**H. Galbo** Institute of Medical Physiology B., University of Copenhagen, Copenhagen, Denmark

**M. Gastaud** Laboratoire de Physiologie, U.E.R., de Médecine, Universite de Nice, Avenue de Vallombrose, F-06034 Nice, France

**R. C. Goode** Department of Physiology, University of Toronto, Toronto, Ontario, Canada

**L. Gullstrand** Department of Physiology, GiH. Lidingövägen 1, S-114 33 Stockholm, Sweden

**K. Haaland** Childrens' Asthma and Allergy Institute, Voksentoppen, Oslo 3, Norway

**S. Haglund** Stenberg-Flygt Co., Fack, S-171 20 Solna, Sweden

**S. Höglund** LHC, Drottninggat. 56, S-105 33 Stockholm, Sweden

**I. Holmér** Department of Work Physiology, Arbetarskyddsstyrelsen, Fack, S-100 26 Stockholm, Sweden

**J. J. Holst** Department of Surgery A, Bispebjerg Hospital, Copenhagen, Denmark

**S. M. Horvath** Institute of Environmental Stress, University of California, Santa Barbara, California 93106 USA

**M. E. Houston** Department of Kinesiology, University of Waterloo, Waterloo, Ontario N2L 3G1, Canada

**L. W. Jankowski** Department d'Education Physique, Universite de Montreal, CEPSUM, 2100 Edouard-Montpetit, Montreal, P.Q., Canada H3T 1J3

**F. W. Kasch** San Diego State University, San Diego, California 92182 USA

**W. R. Keatinge** Department of Physiology, London Hospital Medical College, Turner Street, London, E 1-2 AD, England

**M. Kendall** Childrens' Asthma and Allergy Institute, Voksentoppen, Oslo 3, Norway

**J. C. Kennedy** Head of Division of Orthopedics, 312-111 Waterloo Street, Western Ontario, London N6B 2MG, Canada

**L. Kipke** Physical Culture and Sports Research Institute, Friedrich-Ludwig-Jahn-Allee 59, 701 Leipzig, German Democratic Republic

**V. Klissouras** Ergophysiology Laboratory, McGill University, Montreal, Canada

**K. Kočnar** Institute of Sports Medicine, J. E. Purknyjés University, Pekarska st. 53, 600 00 Brno, Czechoslovakia

**S. Kornecki** Academy of Physical Education, Biomechanics Laboratory, A1. Olimpijska 35, 56-612 Wroclaw, Poland

**R. B. Larsen** Childrens' Asthma and Allergy Institute, Voksentoppen, Oslo 3, Norway

**W. Ling** Endocrine Laboratory, Department of Obstetrics and Gynecology, Dalhousie University, Halifax, Nova Scotia, Canada B3H 3J5

**M. Llobet** Department of Orthopaedic Surgery, Hospital Cruz Roja, Barcelona, Spain

**A. Lundin** Department of Physiology, G1H. Lindingövägen 1, Gymnastikoch Idrottshögskolan, S-114 23 Stockholm, Sweden

**P. Marconnet** Service Bio-Medical, Parc des Sports de l'Ouest, 181 route de Grenoble, F, 06200 Nice, France

**W. B. McCafferty** Department of Physical Education, University of Redlands, Redlands, California 92373 USA

**J. A. Merino** Department of Orthopaedic Surgery, Hospital Cruz Roja, Barcelona, Spain

**M. Miyashita** Laboratory for Exercise Physiology and Biomechanics, Faculty of Education, University of Tokyo, Hongo 7-3-1- Bunkyo-ku, Tokyo, Japan

**Y. Mutoh** Department of Orthopedic Surgery, Nagoya University School of Medicine, 65 Tsuruma-Cho, Showa-ku, Nagoya, Japan

**R. C. Nelson** Biomechanics Laboratory, The Pennsylvania State University, University Park, Pennsylvania 16802 USA

**B. Nielsen** August Krogh Institute, The University of Copenhagen, 13 Universitetsparken, DK-2100 Copenhagen, Denmark

**E. Neilsen** August Krogh Institute, University of Copenhagen, 13 Universitetsparken, DK-2100 Copenhagen, Denmark

**E. Nygaard** August Krogh Institute, University of Copenhagen, 13 Universitetsparken, DK-2100 Copenhagen, Denmark

**M. O'Brien** Department of Anatomy, Royal College of Surgeons in Ireland, Dublin, Ireland

**W. O'Hara** Defense and Civil Institute of Environmental Medicine, Ontario, Canada

**S. Oseid** Childrens' Asthma and Allergy Institute, Voksentoppen, Oslo 3, Norway

**D. R. Pendergast** Department of Physiology, 120 Sherman Hall, State University of New York at Buffalo, Buffalo, New York 14214, USA

**N. L. Pike** Biomechanics Laboratory, The Pennsylvania State University, University Park, Pennsylvania 16802 USA

**K. Reischle** Institut für Sport and Sportwissenschaft, der Universität Heidelberg, Im Neuenheimer Feld 700, 6900 Heidelberg, Federal Republic of Germany

**D. W. Rennie** Departments of Physiology and Physical Education, State University of New York at Buffalo, Buffalo, New York 14214 USA

**R. D. Rochelle** Institute of Environmental Stress, University of California, Santa Barbara, California 93106 USA

**T. T. Romet** Department of Physiology, University of Toronto, Toronto, Canada

**J. Rouš** Institute of Sports Medicin, J. E. Purkynje University, Pekarska st. 53, 600 00 Brno, Czechoslovakia

**L. E. Roy** Unite des Soins a Domicile, Centre Hospitalier Maisonneuve Rosemont, 5415 Boul. de l'Assomption, Montreal, P. Q. Canada H1T 2M4

**N. Roydhouse** Middlemore Hospital, Auckland, New Zealand

**B. Saltin** August Krogh Institute, University of Copenhagen, 13 Universitetsparken, DK-2100 Copenhagen, Denmark

**R. Selbekk** Childrens' Asthma and Allergy Institute, Voksentoppen, Oslo 3, Norway

**J. Shaw** Department of Human Movement Studies, University of Queensland, Brisbane, Q. 4067, Australia

**A. A. Simpson** Endocrine Laboratory, Department of Obstetrics and Gynecology, Dalhousie University, Halifax, Nova Scotia, Canada B3H 3J5

**W. S. Sinning** Applied Physiology Research Laboratory, Kent State University, Kent, Ohio 44240 USA

**I. Sjöberg** Sjukgymnastikavdelningen, Akademiska Sjukhuset, Fack S-750 14 Uppsala 14, Sweden

**W. Spinel** Laboratoire de Physiologie, U.E.R. de Medecine, Universite de Nice, Avenue de Vallombrose, F-06034 Nice, France

**G. Szekely** Institute for Medicine of Physical Education and Sports, Hungarian Ministry of Public Health, Alkotas u. 48, 1123 Budapest, Hungary

**J. Taranger** Department of Pediatrics, University of Göteborg, Östra Sjukhuset, S-416 85 Göteborg, Sweden

**C. Thorén** Department of Pediatrics and Karolinska Institutet, St. Göran's Children's Hospital, Box 12500 S-112 81 Stockholm, Sweden

**Z. D. Torma** Institute for Medicine of Physical Education and Sports, Hungarian Ministry of Public Health, Alkotas u. 48, 1123 Budapest, Hungary

**R. J. Treffene** Department of Physics, Queensland Institute of Technology, Box 246, P. O. North Quay, Q. 4000, Australia

**M. J. Tropea** University of Toronto, 121 St. Joseph Street, Toronto, Ontario, Canada

**T. Tsunoda** Laboratory for Exercise Physiology and Biomechanics, Faculty of Education, University of Tokyo, Hongo 7-3-1, Bunkyo-ku, Tokyo, Japan

**D. W. Wilson** Department of Physiology, State University of New York at Buffalo, Buffalo, New York 14214 USA

**J. Zeigler** The Canadian Red Cross Society, Safety Services Division, Jarvis and Wellesley Streets, Toronto, Ontario, Canada

# Organizing Committee of the Fourth International Congress on Swimming Medicine


**Bengt O. Eriksson, M.D.** chairman
*Department of Pediatrics,*
*University of Göteborg,*
*Östra Sjukhuset,*
*S-416 85 Göteborg,*
*Sweden*

**Ejnar Eriksson, M.D.**
*Department of Surgery,*
*Karolinska Hospital,*
*S-104 01 Stockholm,*
*Sweden*

**Bengt Furberg, M.D.**
*Ringvägen 22B,*
*S-902 54 Umeå,*
*Sweden*

**Ingvar Holmér, Ph.D.**
*Department of Work Physiology*
*Arbetarskyddstyrelsen*
*Fock, S-100*
*26 Stockholm, Sweden*

**Curt Broquist, B.A.**
*Svenska Simförbundet,*
*Box 6506,*
*S-113 83 Stockholm,*
*Sweden*


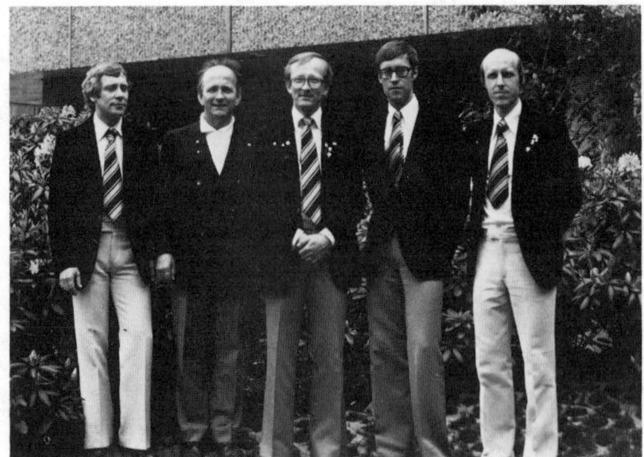

Organizing Committee of the Fourth International Congress on Swimming Medicine. From the left: Curt Broquist, Ejnar Eriksson, Bengt O. Eriksson, Bengt Furberg, and Ingvar Holmér.

# Sponsors, Fourth International Congress on Swimming Medicine

FISONS, Sweden AB
Förenade Liv
Riksförbundet mot Allergi
Riksidrottsförbundet
Scandinavian Airline System, SAS
Stenberg & Flygt AB
Svenska Livräddningssällskapet—Simfrämjandet, SLS
Svenska Renault AB
The Council of the County of Stockholm
The Council of the City of Stockholm
Trygg-Hansa

## FINA International Sports Medicine Committee

**Dr. Z. Firsov,** Chairman
*Skaternyi Pereulok 4,*
*Moscow 69 USSR*
*Phone: 290-24-71, 290-24-90 Cable:*
*Moscow 69*
*SPORTKOMITET USSR*

**J. A. Merino,** Vice Chairman
*Madrazo 84, Barcelona 6 SPAIN*

**Dr. A. J. dePape,** Secretary
*128 Lawndale Avenue, Winnipeg,*
*Manitoba CANADA R2H 1T3*

**Dr. H. N. Bleasdale,**
*25 Newlyn Road, Meols, Hoylake,*
*Merseyside England L47 7AR*
*Phone: 051-632-2012*

**Dr. Ioan Dragan,**
*15A Et. 4-Ap. 10 Boul Ana Ipatescu,*
*Sector 1 Rumania*
*Phone: 505153 Telex: 11180*

**Dr. Bengt O. Eriksson,**
*Tranvägen 5,*
*S-433 00 Partille,*
*Sweden*
*Phone: 031-26-65-00*

**Dr. Raul Gamboa,**
*Av. Arequipa 2450 Of. 708 Lima,*
*Peru*
*Phone: 223914*

**Dr. Chester Jastremski,**
*424 Meadowbrook,*
*Bloomington, Indiana 47401, USA*
*Phone: (812) 339-7342*

**Dr. Lothar Kipke,**
*Deutscher Schwimmsport-Verband*
*der DDR,*
*Storkower Str. 118,*
*1055 Berlin, German Democratic*
*Republic*

**Dr. Mohamed Kouidri,**
*Antares 7 Chemin de la Madeleine,*
*Hydra-Alger, Algeria*

**Dr. Jiri Rous,**
*Vrchlickeho Sad 4,*
*Brno, Czechoslovakia 6000*

**Dr. I. Zurita,**
*Playa Langosta No. 103,*
*Mexico 13 D.F.,*
*Mexico*

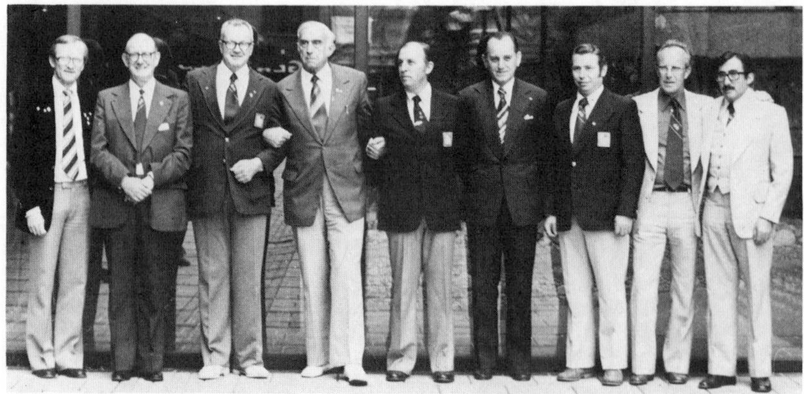

FINA International Sports Medicine Committee. From the left: Bengt O. Eriksson, H. Noel Bleasdale, Bert De Pape, Z. Firsov, J. A. Merino, Ioan Dragan, Lothar Kipke, Jiri Rous, and Ismael Zurita. Not present: Raul Gamboa, Chester Jastremski and Mohamed Kouidri.

# Preface

Swimming medicine is a broad field involving almost all medical disciplines as well as psychology, pedagogy, sociology, and coaching. It is almost impossible to cover the entire field of swimming medicine, and that is not our intention in presenting this volume. Instead, we would like to shed some light on six important fields: medicine, orthopaedics, physiology, metabolism, thermoregulation, and biomechanics.

We hope that this book will reach all people interested in the field of swimming medicine. We especially hope that the existing distance separating medical doctors, scientists, and coaches can be overcome to some extent by means of this book. We believe that the only way to get these three groups to understand each other is through communication. This was also the main reason that the Swedish Swimming Federation to the Fédération Internationale de Natation Amateur (FINA) for sponsorship of the Fourth International Congress on Swimming Medicine.

All the articles in this book are based on presentations at the Fourth International Congress on Swimming Medicine, which was held in Stockholm, Sweden in June, 1977. The First Congress was held in London, England, in 1969 (Chairman, H. N. Bleasdale), the Second Congress in Dublin, Ireland, in 1971 (Chairman, Desmond Carney), and the Third Congress in Barcelona, Spain, 1974 (Chairman, J. Merino). As mentioned above, six themes were chosen for this Congress. For each theme, two or three well known and outstanding scientists were invited as review speakers. All but one of these reviews are presented in this book. In addition to these reviews, 45 free communications were presented at the Fourth Congress. However, they are not all included in this volume. We are very glad that *Swimming Medicine IV* will be presented in this way. It is our intention that future FINA swimming medicine congresses will appear as proceedings in the International Series on Sport Sciences. We are deeply obliged to University Park Press and Co-editors Professor Richard C. Nelson and Chauncey A. Morehouse for their help.

To all sponsors in Sweden, without whose generosity neither this Congress nor these Proceedings would be possible, we would like to express our deep gratitude.

Finally, we hope that readers of this book will be stimulated to do scientific work in the field of swimming medicine. We also hope that they will be interested in participating in future Congresses on swimming medicine.

Bengt Eriksson
Bengt Furberg

# Introduction

The role of medicine in swimming is expanding from year to year. Twenty-five delegates attended the First International Congress on Swimming Medicine in 1969, 32 delegates participated in the Second International Congress in Dublin in 1971, 46 foreign delegates were present at the Third International Congress in Barcelona in 1974. At the Fourth International Congress, held in Stockholm June 5–10, 1977, there were about 100 foreign delegates from all continents. This growth is not difficult to explain: swimming as a sport is a great source of human fitness and it has gained popularity with people the world over.

Supplementing the numerous rivers, seas, and lakes already available, about one million swimming pools have been constructed during the last half-century. Many countries have started year-round training in swimming for school children. Millions of fathers and mothers start to teach their babies to swim in home baths soon after birth, long before the babies begin to walk.

Recent progress in swimming records is fantastic. The Swedish swimmer, Arne Borg, is well known from half a century ago as the first in the world to swim 1,500 meters in less than 20 min. More than 10 years passed before his world's record of 19.07 min was broken, a quarter of a century before his European record was beaten. Today, thousands of swimmers can beat this time and the world's record approaches 15 min. About 55 years ago, a well known American swimmer, Johnny Weissmüller, swam the 100-m freestyle in less than 1.00 min. Today, thousands of children, including girls, swim at such a speed. At the Olympic Games in Montreal in 1976, the Russian schoolgirl Marina Koshevaia won the gold medal in the 200-m breast stroke with a new world's record of 2:33.35 min, and a 17 year old girl from the German Democratic Republic swam the 200-m butterfly in a time approaching 2.10 min. Twenty-five years ago, male swimmers could not swim with such speed.

Preparation for top records, struggles for Olympic medals, and victories at world championships require that coaches begin training their athletes at the ages of 8–10 years. Young swimmers must train 4–5 hr a day and close to the limits of their physical capabilities. As a result, some of them start to regress, and many times leave the sport at the age of 15 or 16 years. The above-mentioned examples indicate the need for and an increasing role of a doctor who can protect the swimmers' health. Our duty is to follow the motto proclaimed at the Second International Congress on Swimming Medicine in Dublin: "To swim for health from birth to the age of 100 years."

The Fourth International Congress was conducted on a highly organized and methodical level. The well planned arrangements for the Congress, the diverse program, and the cordial attention to the Congress paid by the County and City Councils of Stockholm, the Swedish Swimming Federation, the Trygg-Hansa Insurance Company, and all the others should be noted. The hospitality offered at the reception in the City Hall of Stockholm given by the President of the City Council, Mr. Rutger Palme, was much appreciated.

On behalf of the FINA Bureau and all the delegates to the Congress, we express our gratitude to the Organizing Committee and especially to our friend, Dr. Bengt Eriksson, for the excellent organization. The FINA Medical Commitee has decided to apply to the FINA Bureau to reward Dr. Eriksson with the Honorary FINA Diploma. I would also like to point out the up-to-date content of most presentations, the interesting illustrations with slides, photos, and motion pictures, combined with good senses of humor. There is no doubt that each of the papers contributes to further improvements of training methods for swimming and to prevention of the unhealthy consequences of improper and overloaded training.

Most of the Congress presentations will be used in the FINA Medical Committee's recommendation to all the FINA affiliated countries as well as in the FINA Charter and Rules.

While making these positive statements, I would also like to present some critical remarks. It seems to me that the primary research work of doctors and scientists is directed toward swimming. We should not forget diving, water polo, and synchronized swimming, because, as you know, FINA also has jurisdiction over these sporting events. This fact should be taken into account in future work. In my opinion, the predominant trend of the papers and the communications was theoretical. As a whole this wasn't bad; however, I believe that scientists must provide more practical recommendations to coaches and swimmers concerning how to increase competitive speeds. We need to find new ways of increasing velocity and of carrying out research in 50-m swimming pools, and not just in swimming flumes or by use of other more artificial methods. Only scientists and doctors are able to instruct coaches about when 5 hr training per day in 13–14 year old girls and boys increases their fitness and when it is unhealthy. The coaches are waiting for your recommendations on how the athletes can swim 100 m at the same speed at which they can now swim 50 m, as well as on how they can swim 200 m at a 100 m speed.

At the end of May 1977, the FINA Bureau approved the new 100 m freestyle world record of Skinner: 49.44. It means that athletes can theoretically swim 200 m in approximately 1.40, 10 sec faster than today's world's record. The question is: How can this be done? Scientists must provide the answer.

The Fifth International Congress of the FINA Medical Committee, which will be held at the end of 1979, should adopt the motto: "Drawing near to the practical."

Z. Firsov
*President of the FINA Medical Committee*

# Swimming Medicine IV

# Medicine

# Training Girls for Swimming from Medical and Physiological Points of View, with Special Reference to Growth

**B. O. Eriksson and C. Thorén**

For the last 15 years, various studies have been made of the influence on girls of strenuous training for swimming. This chapter is a review of both published and unpublished studies, the results of worthwhile teamwork among various specialists.

The first study began in 1961 with 30 girls aged 12–16 years representing the top swimmers in four different clubs in Stockholm. The girls were investigated with special reference to respiratory and circulatory adaptation and to gynecological and psychiatric aspects. The results were published in the article "Girl Swimmers," (Åstrand et al., 1963).

## OBSERVATIONS

The evaluation of the girls' physical and mental health and development, and of their social and family backgrounds, revealed special features. Most of the girls came from the upper social groups. Most of their parents had once been active athletes and were extremely interested in the girls' progress in sports, which the parents greatly encouraged and facilitated in various ways. The girls were advanced in growth, expressed in greater than average height in relation to age and a somewhat early menarche. They also had good to superior intelligence and were extroverted and energetic.

The gynecological examination disclosed no signs of menstrual disturbance. However, the presence of pathogenic organisms in the vaginas of 12 of the 30 girls indicated a risk of infection in connection with swimming during menstruation, though no cases of salpingitis were reported in this series.

The physiological studies showed that the girl swimmers as a group were advanced in functional development. The functional dimensions—lung volume, total amount of hemoglobin (THb), blood volume (BV), and heart volume (HV)—as well as the functional capacity determined by maximal oxygen uptake ($\dot{V}_{O_2}$ max) were significantly higher than average in relation to body size. There was, however, considerable variation. The largest deviation noted was in heart volume, which in some cases was greater by 50–60% (Figure 1). In two girls, the maximal oxygen uptake was higher than the highest values previously reported in bicycle ergometer tests in women (Figure 2). There was a high coefficient of correlation (r = 0.90), between $\dot{V}_{O_2}$ max

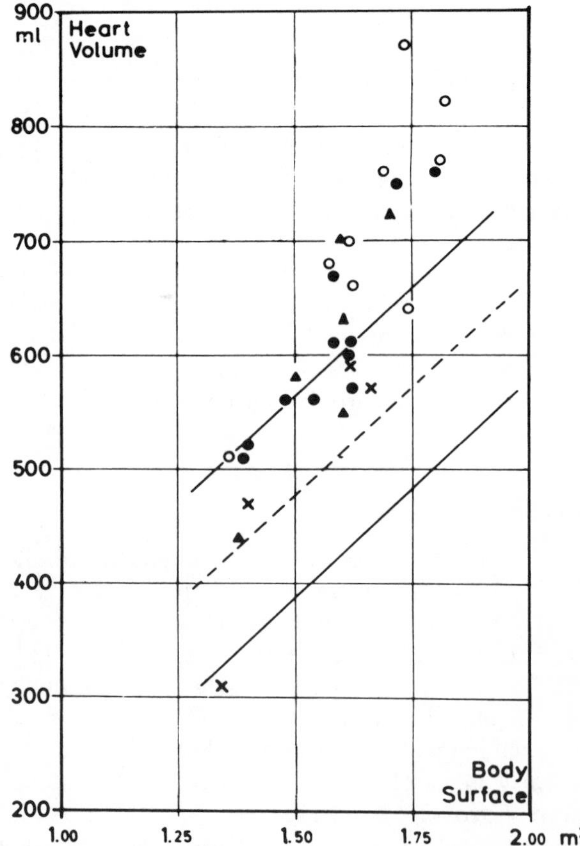


Figure 1. This graph illustrates individual values for heart volume in relation to body surface in girl swimmers (Åstrand et al., 1963). The different symbols denote the four different clubs to which the girls belonged.

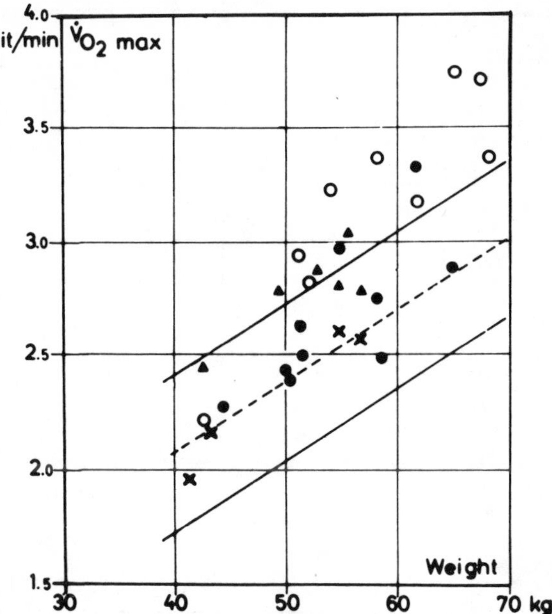


Figure 2. Individual values are given for maximal oxygen uptake in relation to body weight in girl swimmers (Åstrand et al., 1963). The different symbols denote the four different clubs to which the girls belonged.

and HV and the relation between HV and THb was within normal limits. Both vital capacity (VC) and total lung capacity (TLC) were found to be great in relation to height. Both showed good correlation to $\dot{V}_{O_2}$ max.

Functional development was closely related to the amount and intensity of training. It should be noted that intensive physical training during this rapid growth phase could explain the changes observed.

Physiological studies made during swimming activity showed that swimming at competitive speeds requires maximal or near maximal involvement of both aerobic and anaerobic energy-producing processes. This finding was also supported by the high correlation between the best results achieved in competitions, expressed in points according to an international scale, and the maximal oxygen uptake during the bicycle ergometer test (Figure 3).

## LONG-TERM FOLLOW-UP

The subsequent development of the girls was followed and new studies of the same girls were made that included the same physiological measurements at 2, 4, 7 (Eriksson et al., 1971), and 10 years (Eriksson et al., in press) after the original study. At the last examination in 1971,

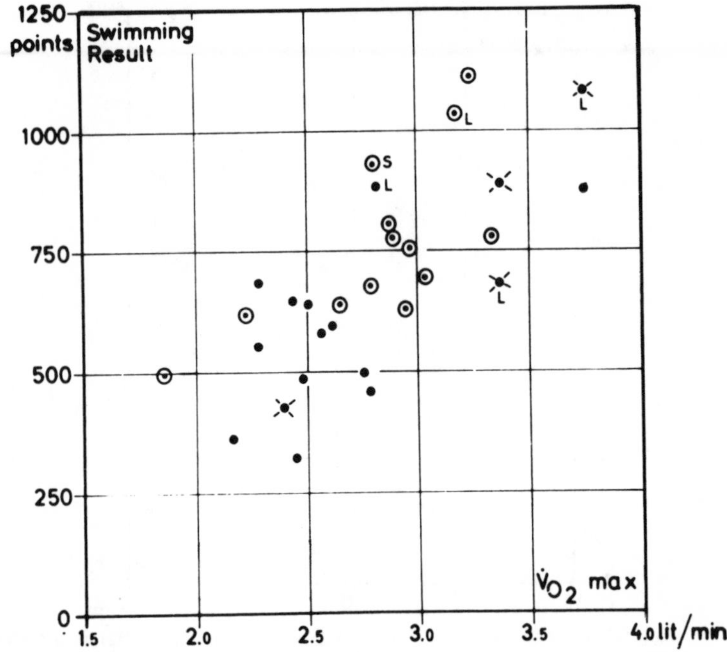


Figure 3. Performance in swimming competition is related to maximal oxygen uptake in girl swimmers (Åstrand et al., 1963).

the average age of the 30 girls was 23.9 years (range: 21.4–26.3 years). The average interval since the girls had stopped training for swimming was 7.5 years prior to the 1971 study, the average age at cessation of training was 16.6 years (range: 13.3–20.7). One girl had continued to train until the Olympic games in Mexico City in 1968. In the 1965 study, only five of the 30 girls were still training; by the time the 1968 and 1971 studies were made, all had stopped training for competition (Figure 4).

After the training ended, most of the girls became sedentary. From a sociological point of view, it is interesting to note that in 1971, 11 of the 30 girls were married. Nine of them had had a total of 12 children. Almost all of them were involved in professions. Six of the girls were teachers, five were nurses, four were secretaries, three were airline stewardesses, and four were still studying at universities. Only one girl, who had married abroad, was not involved in a profession.

Six of the girls had had some medical problems. Three had suffered from mental depression. One of these had experienced mental disturbances that were thought to be related to the swimming training and competition; this girl had been the first to stop training. A fourth girl had developed petit mal epilepsy, a fifth knee arthritis, and a sixth an arterial hypertension of a slight degree. None of these last three disor-

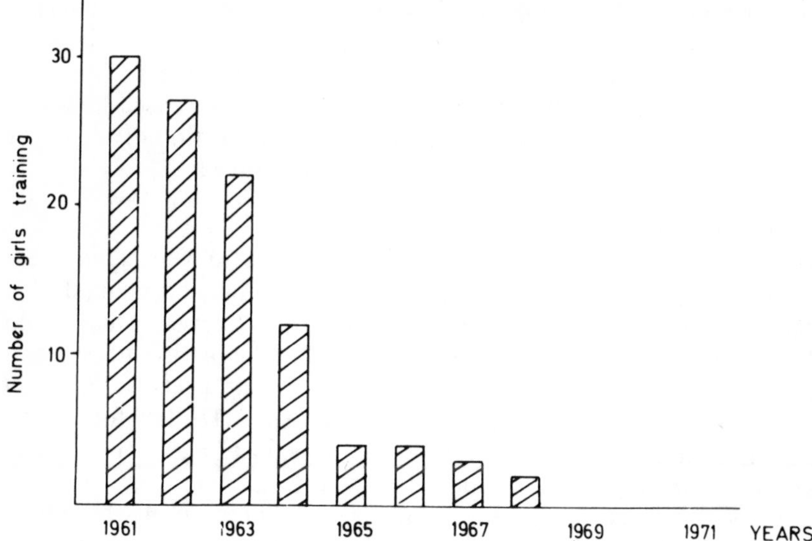


Figure 4. Shown here is the number of girls still training for swimming year by year in the follow-up of former girl swimmers (Eriksson et al., 1978).

ders were attributed to the girl's swimming. No gynecological problems were noted. In general, no future detrimental effect, physical or mental, was revealed.

## Growth

At the time of the first study in 1961, these 30 girls as a group were taller than average by Swedish growth standards (Åstrand et al., 1963). This greater mean height could be ascribed to early puberty (Eriksson et al., in press). Thus, the heights they had attained by the 1971 study could be predicted from their body heights at the age of 7 years. Body weights had not increased more than could be predicted from heights. A few girls had experienced an increased relative weight gain during the first years after cessation of training; however, their weights later returned to normal.

These 30 girls differed markedly among themselves in the amount and intensity of training and in swim performances as early as in the 1961 study. Therefore, the nine most strenuously trained of the girls from that club were analyzed separately and compared with the other 21 girls. Vital capacity in these nine girls was greater in relation to the height-standard in the 1961 study. A further increase in absolute values was obtained through the years; this increase, however, was directly related to the increase in body size. On the other hand, residual volume (RV) and thus FRC and TLC increased more than could be ascribed to normal growth, but within + 1 SD when compared with

Swedish norms. During the follow-up period of 10 years, no changes were found in either the different lung volumes per height cubed or the relative differences between the best girls and the others. Thus, the open question of whether the training caused the increased lung volumes measured in 1961, or whether the girls with constitutionally larger lungs became the top swimmers, remains unresolved.

**Lung Volume**

In another longitudinal study on 29 girls followed from 10–12 years to 16 years of age, it was found that girls who continued training during the entire period had increased in lung volume (VC) greater than could be anticipated from growth alone (Figure 5), while girls who stopped training early did not show such an increase (Engström et al., 1971). On the other hand, Eriksson, Berg, and Taranger (pp. 147–160) found lung volumes already increased in 18 boys 10 years of age who had just started swimming training, indicating that large lungs may be a requirement for becoming a top swimmer. The question of what effect this training has on lung volume remains unanswered.

**Heart Volume**

In marked contrast to lung volume, THb decreased an average of 16% and BV decreased by 14% in the 1971 follow-up study of 30 girls. It was

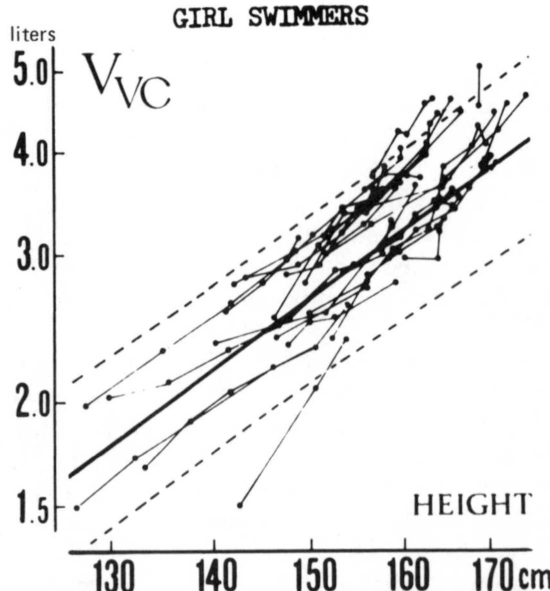


Figure 5. This graph depicts vital capacity ($V_{VC}$) in relation to height for 29 girls in training for swimming (Engström et al., 1978).

further observed that the girls who had had the highest values for THb and BV in 1961 experienced greater decreases of these values than did the others. The significant difference between the nine best swimmers and the other 21 girls thus almost disappeared. Heart volume (HV) was, on the average, 21.5% greater than the value predicted in the 1961 study. More or less unchanged absolute values were found in the follow-up period (Figure 6). A slight but insignificant decrease was thus achieved when the correction for the increase in body size was made.

It is well known that former top athletes also have enlarged HV (Holmgren and Strandell, 1959; Saltin and Grimby, 1968). In older athletes who are still active, the stroke volume during exercise is related to heart volume (Grimby, Nilsson and Saltin, 1966). In these 30 girls, however, no such relationship could be found in a separate study by Eriksson, Lundin, and Saltin (1975). This discrepancy between heart and stroke volumes could indicate a change in heart performance. However, no other signs of impaired heart function were found, and an increased heart volume per se does not necessarily mean an abnormal heart. In 1961, a significant difference was found between the heart volumes of the nine most strenuously trained girls (150.7 ml/m³) and the other 21 girls (133.3 ml/m³). This difference had disappeared by the 1971 study, when almost identical values were found: 135.6 and 134.7 ml/m³,

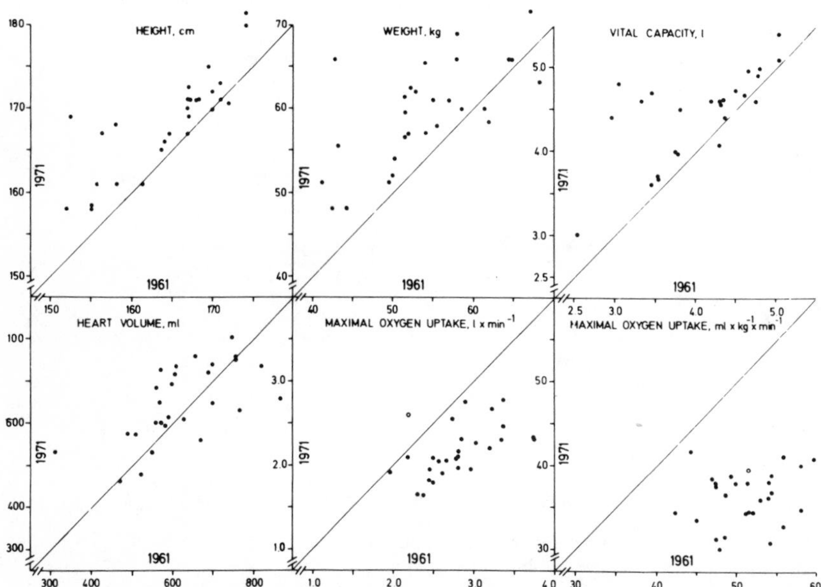


Figure 6. Individual values for height, weight, vital capacity, heart volume and maximal oxygen uptake in 30 former girl swimmers 10 years after the first study are shown here (Eriksson et al., 1978).

respectively (Figure 7). Thus, the biggest heart volumes decreased while the others were unchanged. The decrease in HV obtained for the nine top athletes indicates a partial adaptation to a nontraining situation relatively less pronounced than for THb, for BV, and for the aerobic power. A long-term follow-up over a period of 30-50 years seems necessary to decide whether or not these larger than average hearts may lead to any impaired heart function.

## Aerobic Power

The remarkable decrease in aerobic power that was found exceeds what was previously reported (Åstrand and Rodahl, 1970). Only the decrease found after several weeks of bedrest is comparable (Saltin et al., 1968). The decrease in absolute values averaged 2.80 to 2.18 liters/min (22%), but as the girls increased in body size, the decrease in $\dot{V}_{O2}$ max per kg of body weight was almost 30%. Thus, the 1961 value of 51.4 ml/kg × min (range: 43–58) had decreased to 36.4 ml/kg × min

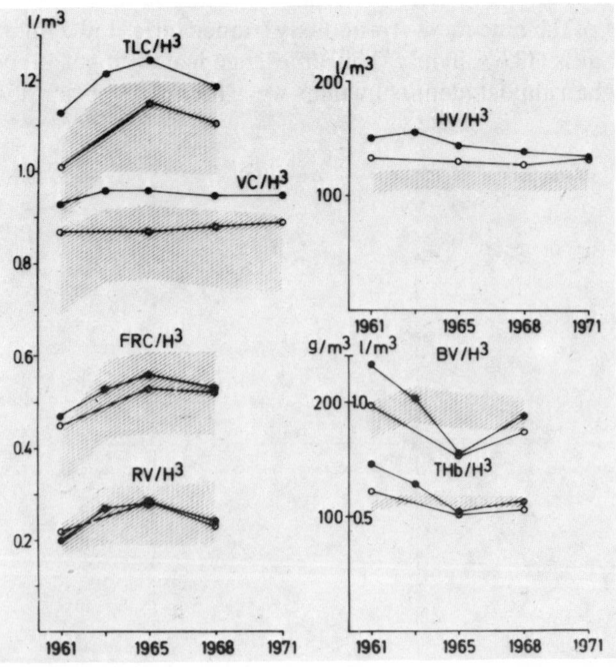


Figure 7. Mean values are given here for lung volumes, heart volumes, blood volumes, and total amount of hemoglobin in former girl swimmers during a 10 year follow-up period (Eriksson et al., in press). All values are corrected for the influence of growth. Filled symbols denote the nine girls in the best club in the original study (Åstrand et al., 1963); unfilled symbols denote the other 21 girls. Shadowed areas denote normal values for Swedish women (Eriksson et al., 1978).

(range: 30–42) (Figure 6). In 1976, when the girls were 30 years old, five of the nine best girl swimmers were reexamined; the mean value of $\dot{V}_{O_2}$ max was then 36.8 ml/kg × min (34–40) (Eriksson, Lundin, and Thorén, in preparation).

In the 1961 study, a very high correlation was found between the heart volume and the $\dot{V}_{O_2}$ max (r = 0.90). Gradually this correlation decreased: in 1965, r = 0.68; in 1968, r = 0.76; and in 1971, r = 0.56 (Figure 8). The correlation between heart volume and the aerobic power thus became less strong. If a high correlation between these two variables is a criterion for normality, the situation in 1971 must then be regarded as less normal. However, no certain statements can be made from these results. To answer fully the question of what effects intensive physical training may have on a growing subject, further studies of these girls during another 10–30 years would be necessary.

Another longitudinal study followed 29 girls selected at ages 8.6–13.7 years for rigorous training for swimming (Engström et. al., 1971; Eriksson et al., in press). They have been followed up annually to 16

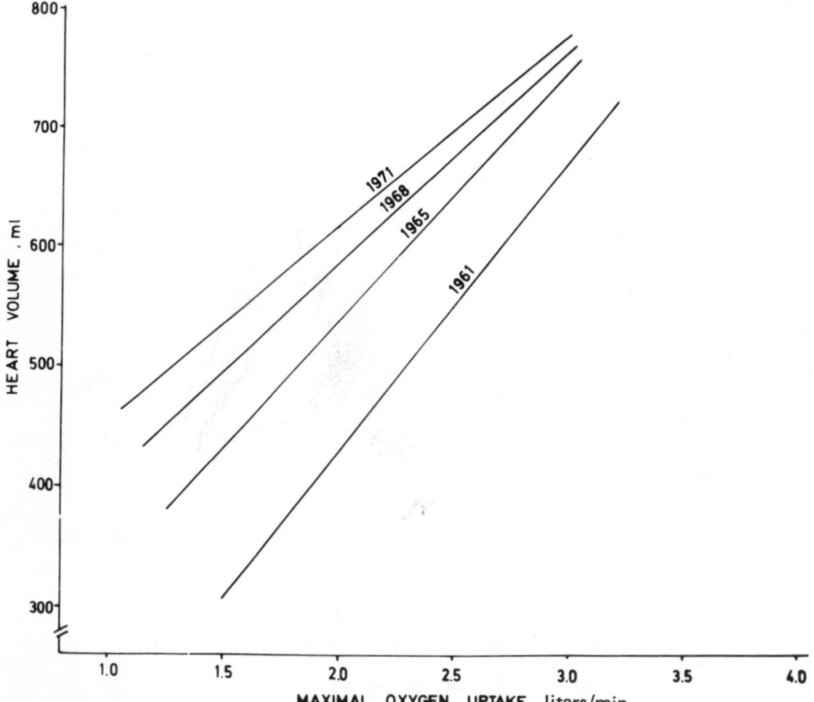


Figure 8. Regression lines for heart volume are shown in relation to maximal oxygen uptake in girl swimmers as measured in four different examinations (Eriksson et al., 1978).

years of age. Half of the girls dropped successively out of training; thus only 15 were still training at the age of 15 years. They were trained in the same swim club and were selected by the coach.

These girls showed an increase in heart volume (Figure 9). When the girls who continued to train were separated from the girls who did not, a difference was found that indicated that the training performed had an influence on the heart volume. However, most of the increase in heart volume could be attributed to growth, whether the girls were training or not.

Maximal oxygen uptakes also increased in absolute value (liters/min). However, when the values were corrected to accommodate the influence of growth, the girls in training showed a small increase (Figure 10). Maximal oxygen uptake per kg of body weight is often used as a measure of aerobic capacity. One reason for this is that values per kg of body weight should allow valid comparisons among individuals. However, body weight increases more rapidly in girls than does maximal oxygen uptake during these years. This is true even for girls undergoing intensive training. This means, in fact, that $\dot{V}_{O_2}$ max/kg drops (Figure 11). However, this does not mean a decrease in aerobic power;

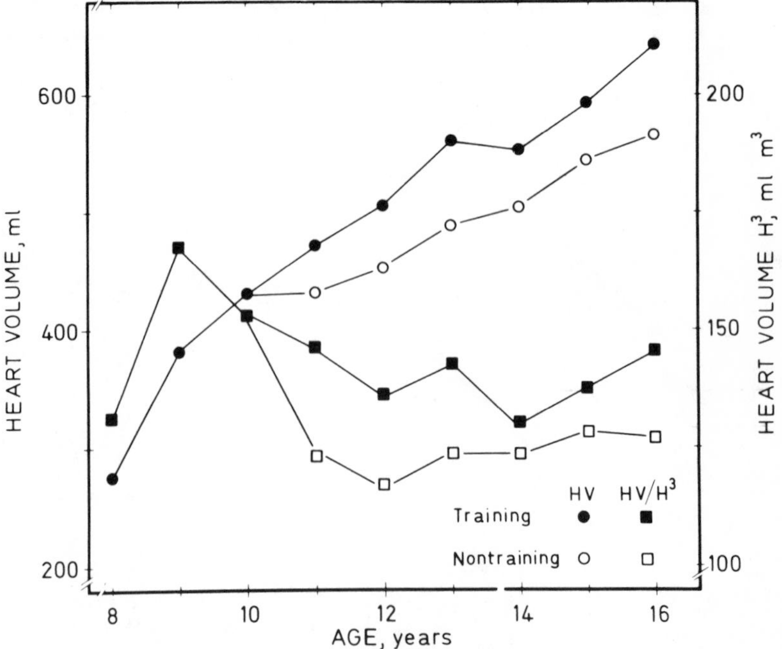


Figure 9. This figure depicts mean values for heart volume and heart volume per height cubed in 29 girls originally involved in training for swimming and followed in a longitudinal study (Eriksson et al., unpublished results).

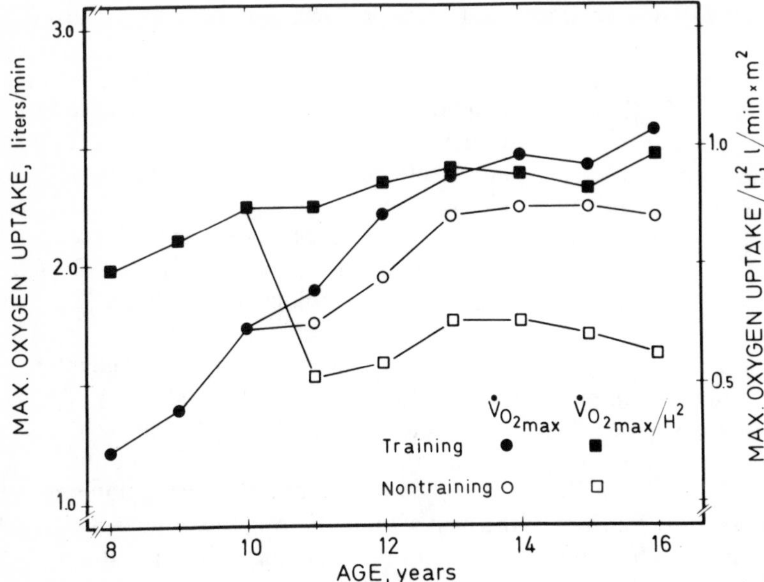


Figure 10. Shown here are mean values for maximal oxygen uptake and maximal oxygen uptake per height squared in 29 girls originally involved in training for swimming and followed in a longitudinal study (Eriksson et al., unpublished results).

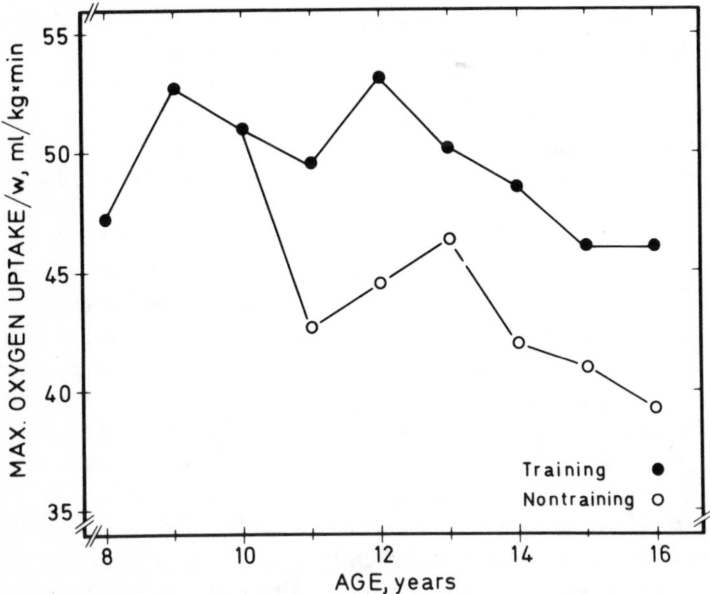


Figure 11. This graph illustrates mean values for maximal oxygen uptake per kg of body weight in 29 girls originally involved in training for swimming and followed in a longitudinal study (Eriksson et al., unpublished results).

it actually demonstrates that using $\dot{V}_{O_2}$ max/kg provides an erroneous estimate of aerobic power.

Sixteen of the 30 female former swimmers took part in a retraining study in 1971 (Eriksson, Lundin, and Saltin, 1975). The aim of the study was to analyze the relationship between different cardiorespiratory dimensions and $\dot{V}_{O_2}$ max and the effect of 12 weeks of swimming training, 2–3 times a week. The average increase of $V_{O_2}$ max was 13.8% (from 2.17 to 2.47 liters/min) and $\dot{V}_{O_2}$ max/kg of body weight increased to 41.2 ml/kg × min. The increase obtained was similar to the results found when 20 year old men were trained (Ekblom et al., 1968). The same increase was also found when training middle-aged sedentary men (Saltin et al., 1969). Thus, high aerobic capacity achieved through intensive training in swimming and later lost because of a sedentary life style cannot easily be regained. Therefore, there does not seem to be a great advantage in this respect to having been very fit earlier in life.

To complete the retraining study, another investigation was performed in 1976. Four of the best swimmers from the original study took part in the later study. Along with these subjects, four girl friends who had never taken part in any regular physical training outside the school's physical education program also trained for swimming. Before training, former swimmers had a mean $\dot{V}_{O_2}$ max of 2.32 liters/min, corresponding to 36 ml/kg × min (range: 34–39), the control girls 1.91 liters/min or 33 ml/kg × min (range: 26–38). On the bicycle ergometer, all had the same rate of perceived exertion on submaximal to maximal levels when scored according to Borg (1973). No differences were obtained regarding maximal heart rate and maximal blood lactate concentration between the two groups of girls. The eight girls trained together in swimming three times a week for 4 months, ending with a training camp of a week's intensive daily training. The most striking difference between the groups was the lovely, smooth swimming performed by the former swimmers; swimming for them was easy and enjoyable. The former swimmers increased their aerobic capacities somewhat more than did the controls. The increase averaged 16% compared with a 12% increase for the control women. With very energetic training, one of the former girl swimmers increased her $\dot{V}_{O_2}$ max by 25% or 28% in relation to body weight, i.e., from 39 to 50 ml/kg × min. On the other hand, one subject in each group showed no increase at all in maximal oxygen uptake. Despite this attempt using more intensive training than that in the earlier retraining study (Eriksson, Lundin, and Saltin, 1975), the increase in aerobic power was slightly, but not significantly greater for the former swimmers than for the controls (Eriksson, Lundin, and Thorén, in preparation).

## REFERENCES

Åstrand, P-O., Engström, L., Eriksson, B. O., Karlberg, P., Nylander, I., Saltin, B., and Thorén, C. 1963. Girl swimmers. Acta Paediatr. Scand. (suppl. 147):1–75.

Åstrand, P.-O., and Rodahl, K. 1970. Textbook of Work Physiology. McGraw-Hill Book Company, New York.

Borg, C. 1973. Perceived exertion: A note on history and methods. Med. Sci. Sports 5:90–93.

Ekblom, B., Åstrand, P.-O., Saltin, B., Stenberg, J. and Wallström, B. 1968. Effect of training on circulatory response to exercise. J. Appl. Physiol. 24:518–528.

Engström, I., Eriksson, B. O., Karlberg, P., Saltin, B., and Thorén, C. 1971. Preliminary report on the development of lung volumes in young girl swimmers. Acta Paediatr. Scand. 60(suppl. 217):73–76.

Eriksson, B. O., Engström, I., Karlberg, P., Lundin, A., Saltin B., and Thorén, C. 1978. Long-term effect of intensive swim training in girls. A 10-year follow-up of the girl swimmers. Acta Paediatr. Scand.

Eriksson, B. O., Engström, I., Karlberg, P., Saltin, B., and Thorén, C. 1971. A physical analysis of former girl swimmers. Acta Paediatr. Scand. 60(suppl. 217):68–72.

Eriksson, B. O., Engström, I., Karlberg, P., Saltin, B., and Thorén, C. Longitudinal study of the effect of intensive swim-training in young girls. In preparation.

Eriksson, B. O., Lundin, A., and Saltin, B. 1975. Cardiopulmonary function in former girl swimmers and the effects of physical training. Scand. J. Clin. Lab. Invest. 35:135–145.

Eriksson, B. O., Lundin, A., and Thorén, C. Intensive retraining of former girl swimmers. In preparation.

Grimby, G., Nilsson, N. J., and Saltin, B. 1966. Cardiac output during submaximal and maximal exercise in active middle-aged athletes. J. Appl. Physiol. 21:1150–1156.

Holmgren, A., and Strandell, T. 1959. The relationship between heart volume, total hemoglobin and physical working capacity in former athletes. Acta Med. Scand. 163:149–160.

Saltin, B., Blomqvist, G., Mitchell, J. H., Johansson, R. L., Jr., Wildenthal, K., and Chapman, C. P. 1968. Response to exercise after bed rest and training. Circulation 38(suppl. 7).

Saltin, B. and Grimby, G. 1968. Physiological analysis of middle-aged and old former athletes. Comparison with still active athletes of the same age. Circulation 38:1104–1115.

Saltin, B., Hartley, L. H., Kilbom, Å., and Åstrand, I. 1969. Physical training in sedentary middle-aged and older men. II. Oxygen uptake, heart rate, and blood lactate concentrations at submaximal and maximal exercise. Scand. J. Clin. Lab. Invest. 24:323–334.

# Swimming Medicine and Asthma

K. Fitch

The interaction of swimming and clinical medicine is divisible into two fundamental components—the application of clinical medicine to swimming, and the application of swimming to clinical medicine. This chapter briefly reviews these areas and provides an in-depth examination of pertinent aspects from the point of view of a sports physician who is both responsible for an Olympic swimming team and involved in researching the role of exercise in the lives of asthmatics. Finally, some overlap of these two concepts of swimming and medicine is revealed in a discussion of Olympians with asthma.

## APPLICATION OF CLINICAL MEDICINE TO SWIMMING

A physician for an elite or national team must be familiar with the physiological and biomechanical requirements of swimmers who, at peak training, may swim 65–110 km per week. A comprehensive physical examination including cardiorespiratory and hematological investigations is mandatory, either before the season or at the time the athlete is selected for training. The immersion of the external ear and upper air passages in chlorinated water for up to 25 hr per week is inevitably associated with otorhinological problems (Roydhouse, 1976) that tend to be further increased by adding as many as 250 daily tumble turns to the training routine. The performance of perhaps 50,000 strokes with each shoulder each week predisposes swimmers to certain overuse syndrome injuries of the musculotendinous structures. These physical medicine conditions are discussed later in this volume in the section on swimming orthopaedics.

The dietary and nutritional requirements for such large daily calorie expenditures, the need to manipulate menstruation to avoid its clashing with major competition, and a variety of medical problems commonly encountered in the normal practices of family physicians are significant aspects of swimming medicine for team medical officers. Two important features that demand more detailed consideration are training while the swimmer is suffering from a viral infection and the use of vitamin, mineral, and especially iron supplements.

### Training and Viral Infections

One contentious issue is the necessity for and the duration of exclusion from training during an acute viral illness. At one extreme are the swimming coaches who tolerate no absences from training for any reason whatsoever. Such coaches seem to believe that the training loads accomplished by their swimmers afford immunity from all illness and that every omitted training session causes irretrievable loss of fitness and, eventually, of performance. Perhaps this attitude is in part a consequence of the contrasting view by which prolonged and often unnecessary exclusion of squad members with minor ailments is recommended by physicians with no knowledge of or interest in sports medicine.

It has been reported that the severity of some viral infections is apparently increased by strenuous physical activity during the prodromal phase. Vigorous activity in the pre-icteric stages of hepatitis seemed to increase the severity of this condition and the liability to acute hepatic necrosis (Krikler and Zilberg, 1966). Intraperitoneal inoculation of a cardiotropic strain of Coxsackie A9 virus into mice was followed by isolation of the virus in significantly higher titers from myocardial tissue of mice that were exercised vigorously by daily swimming than found in control mice that were not exercised after virus inoculation (Tilles et al., 1964). The association of Coxsackie B virus myocarditis with exercise in the prodromal phase was also noted in humans (Smith, 1970).

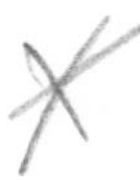

In addition to potential fatalities from viral hepatitis and viral myocarditis, extensive clinical experience confirms the aggravating effect of training or competition during the acute and febrile phases of upper respiratory infections and mononucleosis. It is doubtful that training during a febrile illness will be physiologically beneficial in any case; feverish squad members would do far better to rest at home and not spread the infection to other team members. However, while lavage of infected upper air passages with pool water may predispose a swimmer to secondary complications of sinusitis and otitis media, the practice of excluding athletes from training should not differentiate between swimmers and nonaquatic sports participants. Once the acute febrile phase has resolved, a graduated return to full training should be permitted.

## Vitamin and Mineral Supplements

Without contesting the dubious honor already claimed by United States athletes (Hanley, 1972) of excreting the most expensive urine in the world, it is sad to restate that the level of vitaminuria in Australian swimmers remains grossly elevated and shamefully wasteful (Fitch, 1975a). This vitaminophagy is also potentially unhealthy. It has been widely recognized that excessive intake of fat-soluble vitamins has been associated with clinical syndromes of hypervitaminosis A and D (Davidson, Passmore, and Brock, 1972). Recently, however, doubts have also been cast upon the safety and freedom from side effects of prolonged ingestion of excessive quantities of ascorbic acid. The possible destruction of Vitamin $B_{12}$ by concomitant ingestion of Vitamin C (Rhead and Schrauzer, 1971) and the potential hazard of becoming scorbutic upon cessation of an habitual oversupply of Vitamin C (Herbert and Jacob, 1974) have been described. Table 1 lists every agent that 26 of the 28 members of the 1976 Australian Olympic swimming team admitted taking; one male and one female swimmer took no supplements. (It must be stated that close personal inquiry and association revealed that no swimmer took or had ever taken any doping or banned agent.)

Evidence demonstrating that any ergogenic effect results from excessive dosing with any listed agent is totally lacking. Each swimmer was provided with a sufficient amount of home-cooked food to satisfy the large daily energy expenditure required for twice daily training. The diet also contained an abundance of all vitamins and minerals; previous investigation had documented the adequacy of essential nutrients in the diets of Australian Olympic athletes (Steel, 1970).

The recommendation to ingest such volumes of expensive, urine-discoloring placebos is made predominantly by each swimmer's personal coach and reflects the powerful influence that coaches exert on their adolescent charges and on parents, who must purchase these unnecessary additives. The coaches' reasoning is obscure, but is

Table 1. Vitamin and mineral supplements taken by 1976 Australian Olympic swimmers

| | | |
|---|---|---|
| Vitamins A, $B_1$, $B_2$, $B_6$, $B_{12}$, C, D, and E | Iron | Sodium chloride |
| Nicotinamide | Calcium | Wheat germ oil |
| Panthenol | Potassium | Kelp |
| Biotin | Magnesium | Gelatin |
| Folic acid | Manganese | Lecithin |
| | Phosphorus | |

perhaps based upon the erroneous premise that because vitamin and mineral deficiencies may impair performance, a superabundance will enhance the same. It is noteworthy that the pharmacological vitamin and mineral intake of Australian swimmers greatly exceeded that of the competitors in all 17 other sports in which Australia participated at Montreal. This is in marked contrast to the intake of the 16 silver medallists of the field hockey team, who took no supplements whatsoever.

### Iron Ingestion and Iron Stores

Can prolonged, excessive intake of oral iron supplements lead to the development of hemosiderosis in swimmers? Recent development of a sensitive immunoradiometric assay that quantifies serum levels of ferritin permitted the investigation of this possibility (Fitch, 1975a). Ferritin, the major iron storage protein in the body, is present in small quantities of 10–200 μg/liter in normal serum. These levels reflect body iron storage, and each μg/1 of ferritin in the serum represents about 8 mg of storage iron (Walters, Miller, and Worwood, 1973). The mean level in adult males (about 70 μg/1 liter) is twice that of females.

Iron must be in its ferrous state for absorption from the jejunum, and probably less than 10% of dietary iron is absorbed. The recommended daily iron requirement in food is around 12 mg (Davidson, Passmore, and Brock, 1972). Ascorbic acid facilitates iron absorption, seemingly by reduction of ferric to ferrous ions. The mechanism by which iron intake is regulated remains uncertain but is thought to correlate with body iron stores and bone marrow activity. Nevertheless, nutritional siderosis is recognized in the Bantu (Bothwell, 1964) and has been reported in the USA and France (Davidson, Passmore, and Brock, 1972), as well as in Manchuria (Bothwell, 1964). In the first three instances, high dietary iron intakes were associated with excessive ethanol ingestion, the hepatotoxic effects of which may assist in iron deposition in the liver.

In June 1976, within a week of the team's departure for Montreal and coincident with maximal training duration and intensity, blood was drawn from 27 of the 28 members of the Australian Olympic Swimming Team for hematological investigation, including estimation of serum ferritin. Detailed personal interrogation revealed that the swimmers were divisible into two groups: those who did and those who did not take oral iron tablets. Fourteen team members took such supplements (most took a multivitamin preparation in addition). The remaining 13 swimmers took no iron, although 10 did take multivitamins, the majority of which contained 5 mg elemental iron as well as 1 g ascorbic acid.

The serum ferritin levels and concurrent hematological parameters of hemoglobin, the percentage of reticulocytes, the serum iron, and the total iron-binding capacity are shown in Figures 1 and 2. Significant differences were noted only in ferritin levels and thus body iron stores. In particular, the ingestion of iron tablets in addition to the very adequate iron content of the provided food afforded no hematological advantage whatsoever.

Three swimmers recorded serum ferritin levels in excess of 200 $\mu$g/liter. A 22 year old male with a level of 216 $\mu$g/liter had been on

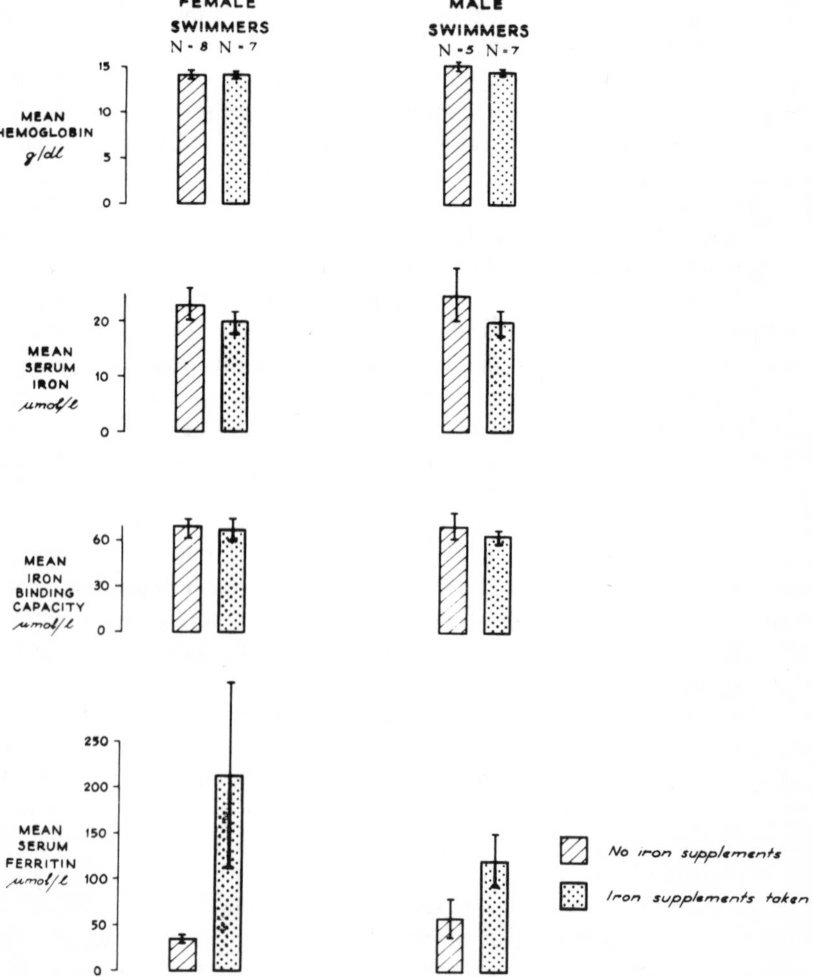


Figure 1. This figure depicts the mean values (±SEM) of hemoglobin, serum iron, iron-binding capacity, and serum ferritin of the 1976 Australian Olympic Swimming Team grouped by use or nonuse of iron supplements.

continuous daily supplements of 105 mg of elemental iron for 7 years. One 15 year old female who had been given 315 mg of elemental iron in sustained release tablets each day for 3 years had a ferritin level of 283 μg/liter, reflecting iron stores of approximately eight times the amount expected. The highest serum ferritin level 800 μg/liter, was observed in an 18 year old female swimmer who had been taking four capsules of ferrous succinate (providing a daily total of 140 mg of elemental iron) for 5 years. Her iron stores, around 6.4 g, were more than 20 times the normal value. It is noteworthy that each of these three competitors was taking at least 1 g of ascorbic acid daily. If each of the 14 swimmers taking iron supplements has a mean annual nondietary iron intake of 45 g of elemental iron, with such iron-enriched and discolored excreta, is it any wonder that Australia is one of the world's largest sources of iron ore?

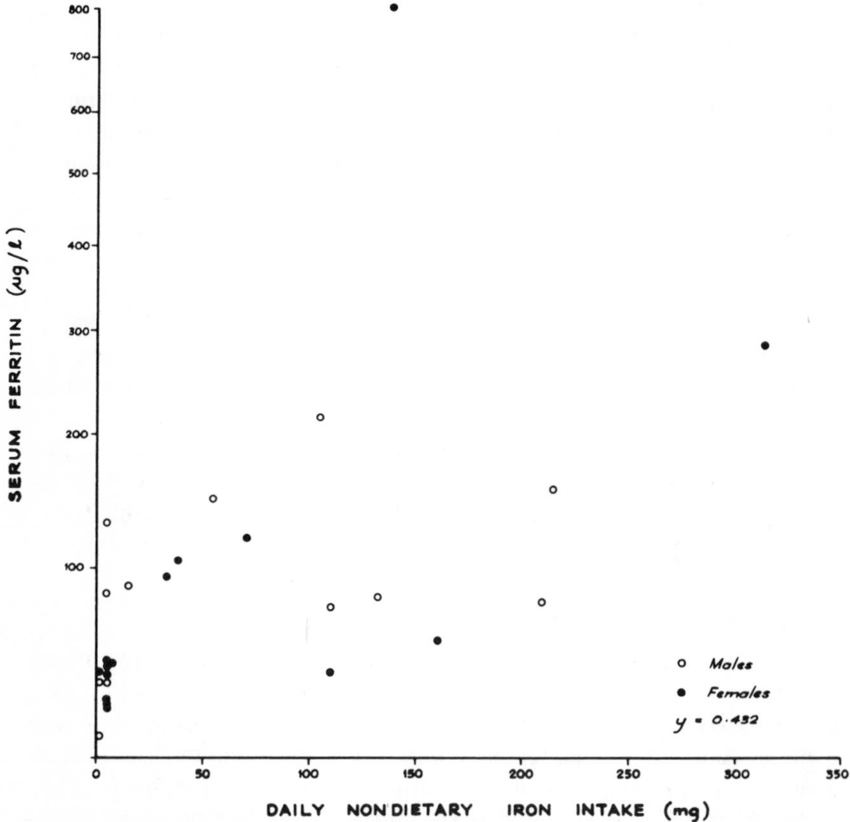


Figure 2. Shown here is the relationship between serum ferritin levels and daily nondietary iron intake of the 1976 Australian Olympic Swimming Team. Note semi-logarithmic plot of ferritin values.

To determine whether the heavy training schedules might provoke hemosideruria, a consequence of exercise hemoglobinuria (De Gruchy, 1970), urine was obtained from every swimmer immediately after a 2-hr strenuous training session. No iron was detected in the centrifuged deposits of the urine of any competitor. Reticulocyte counts ranged from 0.7–2.8% (mean: 1.6%), and hemoglobin values were unchanged from those recorded in the same laboratory at the commencement of Olympic team training. These facts make it most unlikely that traumatic intravascular hemolysis occurs in swimming, in contrast to the incidence of this condition reported in running, marching, squash (De Gruchy, 1970), and karate (Streeton, 1967).

## APPLICATION OF SWIMMING TO CLINICAL MEDICINE

### Swimming as Therapy

During the last decade, swimming has been used increasingly in the physical rehabilitation of and recreation therapy for a wide variety of medical conditions. Recreational swimming is organized for a number of groups handicapped by conditions such as arthritis (degenerative and rheumatoid), blindness, cerebral palsy, diabetes mellitus, epilepsy, mental retardation, muscular dystrophy, multiple sclerosis, and multiple handicaps. Swimming is an excellent exercise to restore or maintain fitness in patients with chronic obstructive pulmonary disease, ischemic heart disease (including myocardial infarction), obesity, poliomyelitis, and sports injuries. There is a third category of disorders in which swimming is beneficial both as physical rehabilitation and for long-term physical recreation and sport. These disorders include: amputations; a heterogenous group of spinal conditions such as ankylosing spondylitis, intervertebral disc disease, juvenile discogenic disease (Scheuermann's), scoliosis and kyphoscoliosis, spondylolysis and spondylolisthesis, spina bifida, traumatic paraplegia and tetraplegia, and asthma.

### Swimming and Asthma

Among the tests selected for the 1968 Australian Olympic Swimming Team was a 60-sec maximal effort on a bicycle ergometer as part of a modified Hyman test (Hyman, 1966). This exertion provoked severe exercise-induced asthma (EIA) in one 18 year old swimmer. Less than 3 months later, this competitor performed a maximal effort for 65.5 sec in the Mexico City Olympic pool and won the 100-meter women's butterfly event. No wheezing followed this exertion. Why should two maximal efforts of similar duration provoke such markedly different respiratory responses?

Inquiry disclosed that the specificity of exercise in the provocation of EIA had been recognized as long ago as the seventeenth century. Floyer (1698), an English physician who had asthma, wrote:

> All violent exercise makes the asthmatic to breathe short . . . . Walking is more vehement than riding but not so great as the others: those exercises that move the arms, exercise the lungs most.''

Floyer also noted that running provoked more obstruction to the passage of air than other forms of exercise.

Further inquiry revealed that swimming, which was not mentioned by Floyer, had been recommended as an appropriate exercise for children with asthma, although the origins of such advice and the justification for its implementation could not be discovered. The earliest prescription of swimming for asthma that could be located was for Theodore Roosevelt (later President of the USA), almost 110 years ago (Szanton, 1969).

Asthmatics, who possess an inherited condition of overresponsiveness of the bronchial airways to a variety of factors, initially react to the physical challenge of exercise by mild bronchodilatation and then by moderate or severe bronchoconstriction (Figure 3). The severity of the EIA does not always reflect the clinical features of the condition; it is not uncommon to encounter incapacitatingly severe EIA occurring in persons with mild clinical asthma.

Standard submaximal exercise challenge has confirmed that running causes the greatest frequency and severity of EIA and is thus the preferred exercise challenge (Fitch and Morton, 1971). Swimming is the least asthmagenic and is therefore an exercise eminently suitable for asthmatics (Figure 4). The variable severity of asthma induced by other types of exercise has also been investigated (Fitch, 1975b; Fitch and Godfrey, 1976). Despite many theories, the mechanism by which EIA develops remains fascinatingly obscure (Anderson et al., 1975b).

Equally perplexing is the reason for the low asthmagenicity of swimming. The use of the upper limbs as the major source of propelling force in swimming does not appear to be a factor because kayaking (Fitch and Morton, 1974) and arm cranking exercises (Anderson, 1972; Strauss et al., 1976) have not been accompanied by similar reductions in EIA. The horizontal position of swimming seems irrelevant because supine (Poppius et al., 1970) and erect (Pierson, Bierman, and Stamm, 1969) cycling have produced similar postexercise responses. The suggestion that body vibration is an etiological factor in the high incidence of running-induced asthma has not been substantiated. Subjecting asthmatics to whole body vibration (Anderson et al., 1975b) and bouncing heavy medicine balls off the chests of asthmatic boys and prepubertal (of course) girls (Fitch, 1974) had no effect on lung volumes.

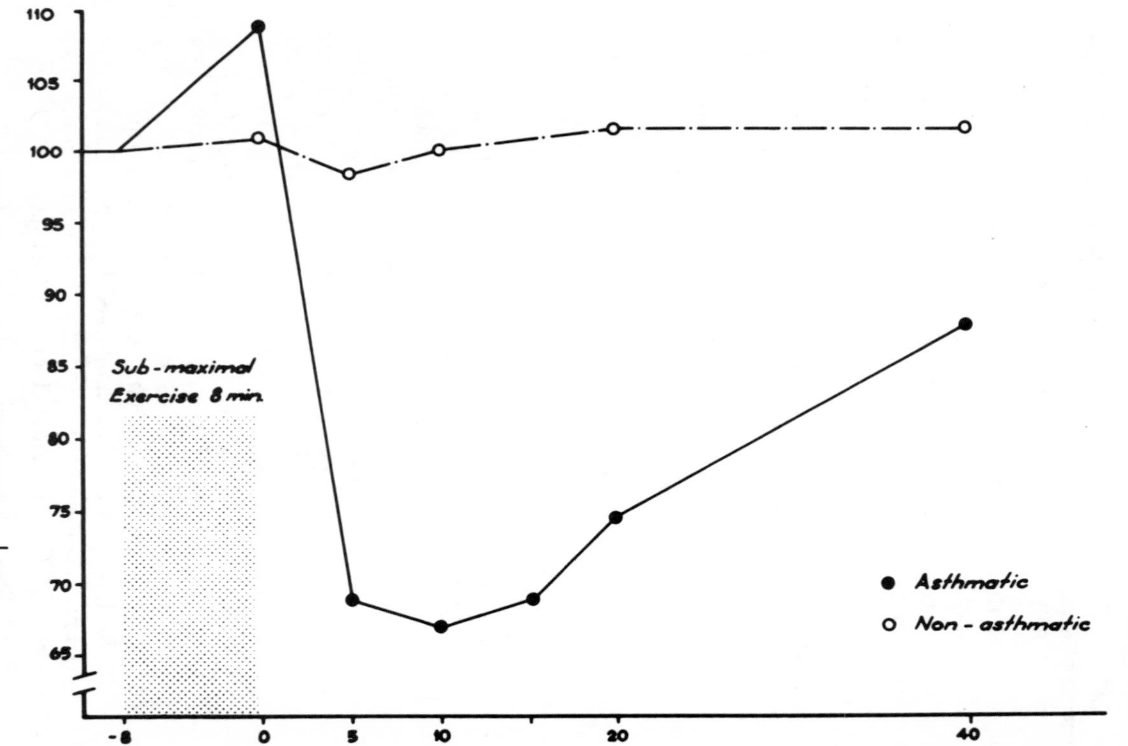


Figure 3. Typical ventilatory responses are expressed here as percent of change from the pre-exercise forced expiratory volume in the first second ($FEV_1$) of two 12 year old boys, one asthmatic and one nonasthmatic, to 8 min of submaximal treadmill running.

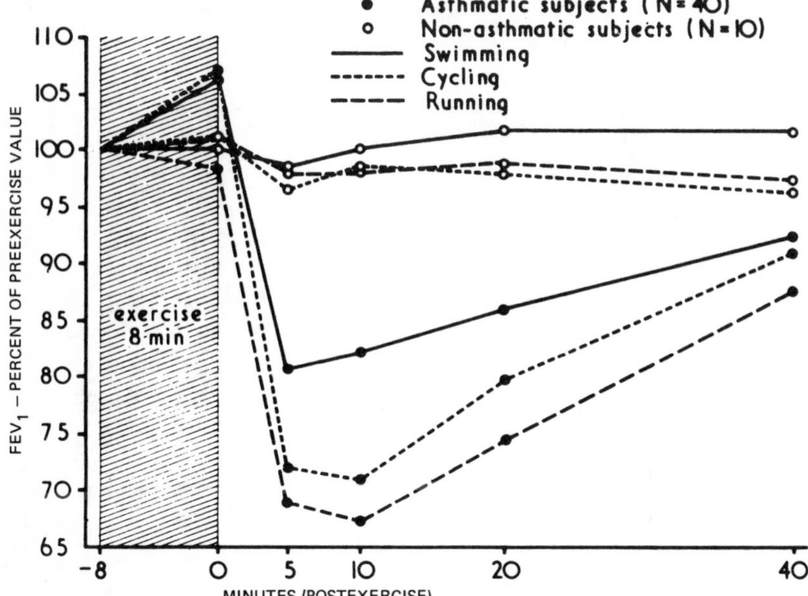


Figure 4. Percent change in mean $FEV_1$ after 8 min of submaximal running, cycling, and swimming in asthmatic and nonasthmatic subjects is shown here (reproduced from Fitch and Morton (1971), with permission of the editor of the *British Medical Journal*).

The relative hypoventilation of submaximal swimming when compared with running (Holmér et al., 1974) is not comparable to the difference in EIA. One seemingly logical explanation for reduced EIA in swimming is the controlled breathing pattern of conventional stroking, including expiration against resistance while the face is immersed. This is not valid, however, because the reduction of postswimming asthma is unrelated to either swimming ability or style (Fitch and Morton, 1971), a fact that any experienced coach of asthmatics can confirm. Because breathing cold air will provoke bronchoconstriction (Millar et al., 1965), the lowered temperature gradient between the inspired air and the bronchial wall mechanoreceptors is a possible factor yet to be examined. Recent studies in Israel (Bar-or, Newman, and Dotan, 1976) demonstrated that the humidification of inspired air can reduce running-induced bronchoconstriction and therefore provides evidence that the higher humidity of air inspired during swimming may be responsible for the decreased EIA.

Judicious medication before exercise can greatly assist the majority of asthmatics in reducing or inhibiting their attacks of EIA. Sodium cromoglycate, a unique drug that is taken by inhalation and has never been classed as a doping agent, has been shown to be an effective

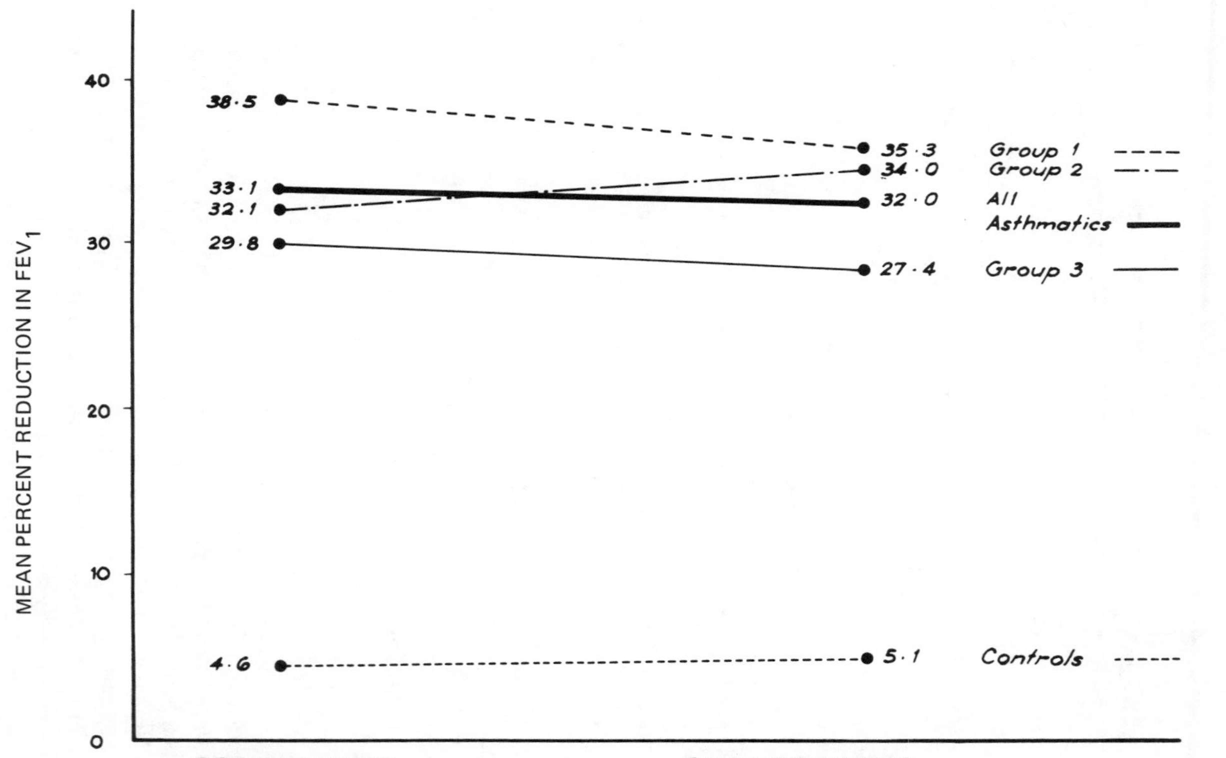


Figure 5. This figure shows the effect of 5 months of swimming training on mean maximum percentage reduction of $FEV_1$ after 9 min of submaximal treadmill running to attain and maintain heart rates of 170 beats per minute. Grouping of asthmatic swimmers was based on achieved swimming distance. Group 1 (N = 14) swam less than 50 km; Group 2 (N = 16) swam 50–100 km; Group 3 (N = 16) swam more than 100 km; Control Group (N = 10) were nonasthmatics and swam more than 100 km.

agent, and regular therapy is not necessary to achieve this response (Morton and Fitch, 1974). Salbutamol (Godfrey and König, 1976) and terbutaline (Anderson, personal communication), selective $\beta_2$-adrenergic receptor stimulants, are excellent agents to prevent or ameliorate EIA, and, in addition, they will rapidly reverse EIA should it occur. Aerosol administration of these preparations is preferred (Anderson et al., 1975a). Because of the relatively brief duration of maximum protection, either the modification of regular medication or an additional dose before exercise is essential to achieve the optimum benefit.

Regular swimming training of 46 children and adolescents with moderate or severe asthma has confirmed that swimming is an excellent exercise prescription for asthmatics (Fitch, Morton, and Blanksby, 1976). Improved posture and fitness, reduced fat folds, and enhanced swimming ability were noted after a 5-month training program during which these asthmatics (mean age: 12 years) swam a total distance of 3,600 km. Both the asthma experienced and the drugs taken declined during the program, and this decrease was related to training volume. Physical and emotional benefits to the swimmers were recognized by the majority of parents, and the attitudes of many parents towards their asthmatic children appeared to be modified.

Another noteworthy feature was that the frequency and severity of EIA, determined by a running challenge at the conclusion of the study, were unchanged from pretraining levels (Figure 5). This was a little surprising in view of the impressive physiological and conditioning effects observed in many subjects. Nevertheless, this finding reinforces the concept demonstrated by the asthmatic gold medal winner at the 1968 Olympic Games: no amount of swimming training and fitness is guaranteed to obliterate exercise bronchial hyperreactivity.

As a consequence of these studies, it is recommended that every child with asthma be taught to swim with due regard for their specific difficulties. These include intolerance to cold, because breathing cold air can provoke wheezing (Millar et al., 1965). Furthermore, many asthmatic children possess scanty body fat, affording poor insulation against cold water and poolside conditions. This paucity of body fat may result in poor buoyancy, although a counter-balancing effect is present in some severe asthmatics because of an increased total lung capacity due to air-trapping in their barrel-shaped chests.

Fear of the water and reluctance to immerse the face are commonly encountered and arise from previous episodes of dyspnea from wheezing. Reduced self-confidence in attempting exertional sports and parental overanxiety contribute to the tendency of the asthmatic child to require a longer period of time to achieve basic swimming competence. The psychological boost of acquiring the ability to swim (exhibited by all children) is particularly valuable in children with asthma. They soon discover that they do not exercise or compete with the same respiratory disadvantage in water that they have on land. After the acquisition of swimming competence with customary controlled breathing techniques, asthmatics should be encouraged to join swimming training squads supervised by capable coaches and should not be managed differently from nonasthmatic squad members.

Classes specifically intended to teach asthmatic children to swim have been conducted extensively in Australia during the last 15 years. The conventional methods are employed to achieve the students' water confidence and stroke development through in-pool instruction from experienced and patient teachers. Experiences from this program have confirmed the infrequency of asthma induced by swimming (especially if medication before the exercise is utilized). The beneficial effect of exercise-induced bronchodilatation by which mild wheezing or chest "tightness" is relieved through the exertion of swimming, the benefits afforded both child and parents, and the rarity of unfavorable consequences of participation are features that are evident from close observation of this asthma swimming program.

During 1976, a 3-month program of classes commenced at three heated indoor pools. The program involved 30 asthmatic adults ages 18–70 years, with a mean age of 40 years. A high degree of acceptance and enthusiasm was noted in almost all subjects, who reported considerable pride and pleasure at the gains achieved. Improved control of breathing, less medication, fewer asthmatic attacks, and encouragingly positive psychological attitudes were acknowledged. Unfavorable comments were restricted to the intolerance of cold conditions.

Confirmation that swimming is a positive activity for asthmatics and that they compete without respiratory disadvantage in the pool is readily available from the examination of Olympic swimming results. Dawn Fraser, who won gold medals at the 1956, 1960, and 1964 Olympic Games, originally began swimming "to lick her asthma." Her 1964 100-m freestyle victory was achieved despite an asthmatic attack on the day of the final race requiring oral and aerosol medication (Fraser, 1965).

To complete the sequence of five consecutive Olympic swimming victories by asthmatics, a 16 year old American high school student who suffered from asthma and an allergic diathesis (Thomas, personal communication), won the 400-m men's freestyle event at the Munich

Olympics. He was disqualified, however, when ephedrine was detected in significant quantities in routine postrace urinalysis (Beckett, personal communication). (Sadly, he had probably not benefited from the drug because of the low asthmagenicity of swimming and because ephedrine is a relatively ineffective agent.)

The promotion of swimming as rehabilitation and recreation for asthma is proving highly successful. This is evident from the medical records of the 1976 Australian Olympic Swimming Team. No less than five of the 13 males and three of the 15 female members have or had asthma. Four of the eight asthmatic Olympians had become swimmers to relieve their asthmatic conditions. This group of eight, representing 28.6% of the nation's swimming team, had an impressive swimming record: five were national title holders, four won gold medals at the 1974 Commonwealth Games, and two held or had held world freestyle records.

It is regrettable that the international athlete with asthma, who must undertake doping control procedures, is still subjected to unnecessary and discriminatory restrictions. In a decision seemingly based upon pharmacological ignorance, the selective $\beta_2$-adrenergic receptor stimulants were banned on the evening before the commencement of the 1972 Olympic Games (Beckett, personal communication). This action was reversed by the International Olympic Committee Medical Commission in May 1975. However, they added a demand that on every occasion on which an asthmatic required salbutamol or terbutaline, written notification to the Commission must be made of the name of the drug, the dosage, the route of administration, and the time it was administered to the competitor. With a disease as capricious as asthma, this is an onerous task for a team physician with 21 asthmatics (11.8% of all competitors), as Australia had in Montreal. Because these agents have negligible cardiac and vasopressor effects (Nayler, 1971), there is scant pharmacological justification to introduce such a rider. A bronchodilating aerosol dosage of 200–250 $\mu$g-represents about one-twentieth of one oral tablet, and it is virtually impossible to detect residues through urinalysis (Paterson, personal communication). Because the fundamental reason for approving salbutamol and terbutaline should have been to permit athletes with asthma to compete without respiratory disadvantage, this unwarranted rider should be rescinded by the I.O.C. Medical Commission.

## REFERENCES

Anderson, S. D. 1972. Physiological Aspects of Exercise-Induced Bronchoconstriction. Doctoral thesis, University of London.

Anderson, S. D., Rozea, P. J., Dolton, R., and Lindsay, D. A. 1975a. Inhaled and oral bronchodilator therapy in exercise induced asthma. Aust. N. Z. J. Med. 5:544–550.

Anderson, S. D., Silverman, M., König, P., and Godfrey, S. 1975b. Exercise-induced asthma—a review. Br. J. Dis. Chest 69:1–39.

Bar-or, O., Newman, I., and Dotan, R. 1976. The effects of humid and dry climates on exercise-induced asthma in children. Paper presented at the Eighth European Symposium on Pediatric Work Physiology, September 21–24, Bisham Abbey, England.

Bothwell, T. H. 1964. Iron overload in the Bantu. In: F. Gross (ed.), Iron Metabolism, pp. 362–373. Springer-Verlag, Berlin.

Davidson, S., Passmore, R., and Brock, J. F. 1972. Human Nutrition and Dietetics. 5th Ed. Churchill Livingstone, Edinburgh.

De Gruchy, G. C. 1970. Clinical Haemotology in Medical Practice. 3rd Ed. Blackwell, Oxford. p. 339.

Fitch, K. D. 1974. Effects of Exercise on Asthma. MD thesis, University of Western Australia.

Fitch, K. D. 1975a. The ethics of artificial aids and the sportsman. N. Z. J. Sports Med. 3(2):7–13.

Fitch, K. D. 1975b. Comparative aspects of available exercise systems. Pediatrics 56(suppl.):904–907.

Fitch, K. D., and Godfrey, S. 1976. Asthma and athletic performance. JAMA 236:152–157.

Fitch, K. D., and Morton, A. R. 1971. Specificity of exercise in exercise-induced asthma. Br. Med. J. 4:577–581.

Fitch, K. D., and Morton, A. R. 1974. Differences in ventilatory responses in asthmatic subjects following work involving arm muscles and work involving leg muscles. Aust. J. Sports Med. 6(2):4–11.

Fitch, K. D., Morton, A. R., and Blanksby, B. A. 1976. Effects of swimming training on children with asthma. Arch. Dis. Child. 51:190–194.

Floyer, J. 1698. A Treatise of the Asthma. R. Wilkin and W. Innis, London.

Fraser, D. 1965. Gold Medal Girl. Lansdowne, Melbourne.

Godfrey, S., and König, P. 1976. Inhibition of exercise-induced asthma by different pharmacological pathways. Thorax 31:137–143.

Hanley, D. F. 1972. Health problems at the Olympic Games. JAMA 221:987–990.

Herbert, V., and Jacob, E. 1974. Destruction of vitamin $B_{12}$ by ascorbic acid. JAMA 230:241–242.

Holmér, I., Stein, E. M., Saltin, B., Ekblom, B., and Åstrand, P.-O. 1974. Hemodynamic and respiratory responses compared in swimming and running. J. Appl. Physiol. 37:149–154.

Hyman, A. S. 1966. The estimation of cardiovascular physical fitness. R. I. Med. J. 49:723–726.

Krikler, D. M., and Zilberg, B. 1966. Activity and hepatitis. Lancet 2:1046–1047.

Millar, J. S., Nairn, J. R., Unkles, R. D., and McNeill, R. S. 1965. Cold air and ventilatory function. Br. J. Dis. Chest 59:23–27.

Morton, A. R., and Fitch, K. D. 1974. Sodium cromoglycate in the prevention of exercise-induced asthma. Med. J. Aust. 2:158–162.

Nayler, W. G. 1971. Some observations on the pharmacological effects of salbutamol with particular reference to cardiovascular system. Postgrad. Med. J. 47 (suppl.):16–21.

Pierson, W. E., Bierman, C. W., and Stamm, S. J. 1969. Cyclo-ergometer-induced bronchospasm. J. Allergy 43:136–144.

Poppius, H., Muittari, A., Kreus, K-E., Korhonen, O., and Viljanen, A. 1970. Exercise asthma and disodium cromoglycate. Br. Med. J. 4:337–339.

Rhead, W. J., and Schrauzer, G. N. 1971. Risks of long term ascorbic acid overdosage. Nutr. Rev. 29:262–263.

Roydhouse, N. 1976. Ear and nose problems in sports medicine. In: J. G. P. Williams and P. N. Sperryn (eds.), Sports Medicine, pp. 341–351. Edward Arnold, London.

Smith, W. G. 1970. Coxsackie B myopericarditis in adults. Am. Heart J. 80:34–46.

Steel, J. E. 1970. A nutritional study of Australian Olympic athletes. Med. J. Aust. 2:119–123.

Strauss, R. H., Haynes, R., Ingram, R. H., and McFadden, E. R. 1976. Comparison of arm versus leg work in exercise-induced asthma. Am. Rev. Resp. Dis. 113(suppl.):251.

Streeton, J. A. 1967. Traumatic haemoglobinuria caused by karate exercises. Lancet 2:191–192.

Szanton, V. L. 1969. Theodore Roosevelt, the asthmatic. Ann. Allergy 27:485–489.

Tilles, J. G., Elson, S. H., Shaka, J. A., Abelmann, W. H., Lerner, A. M., and Finland, M. 1964. Effects of exercise on Coxsackie A9 myocarditis in adult mice. Proc. Soc. Exp. Biol. Med. 117:777–782.

Walters, G. O., Miller, F. M., and Worwood, M. 1973. Serum ferritin concentration and iron stores in normal subjects. J. Clin. Pathol. 26:770–772.

# Exercise Studies on Asthmatic Children Before and After Regular Physical Training

**S. Oseid and K. Haaland**

Strenuous exercise may induce bronchoconstriction in asthmatic subjects. In some cases wheezing after exercise is the patient's main complaint. For young asthmatic children this represents a severe handicap in daily life and restricts normal physical and psychological development.

The effect of exercise on asthmatics' pulmonary function depends largely on the duration of the exercise (Jones, Buston, and Wharton, 1962; Silverman and Anderson, 1972), but also depends on the intensity of effort (Katz et al., 1971; Silverman and Anderson, 1972). Physical exercise of short duration (1–2 min) increases the ventilatory capacity through rises in peak expiratory flow rate (PEFR) and in forced expiratory volume (FEV) in both normal and asthmatic subjects (Lefcoe, 1969). Exercise of longer duration (6–8 min) causes post-exercise bronchoconstriction in most asthmatic patients (Jones, Buston, and Wharton, 1962; Jones, 1966; Lefcoe, Carter, and Ahmad, 1971; Anderson, 1972; Cropp, 1975). Godfrey (1974) has proposed that this is caused by a pronounced bronchial lability, calculated by an index that takes into account both the early bronchodilation and any subsequent increase of airway resistance in asthmatic subjects.

The fall in pulmonary function usually appears within 3–5 min of ceasing exercise and is most marked 5–12 min posteffort (Jones, Buston, and Wharton, 1962; Perison and Bierman, 1975). Normal function generally returns spontaneously within 40–60 min. However, great individual variations are found.

The purposes of this chapter are to present patient material from Voksentoppen Asthma and Allergy Institute and, particularly, to describe the medication and physical activity programs being used to help asthmatic children overcome the tendency to experience exercise-induced bronchoconstriction.

## PATIENT MATERIAL AND PROCEDURES

The patients included 86 asthmatic children (52 boys and 34 girls, 7–16 years of age) with multifactorial "extrinsic" bronchial asthma and histories suggestive of exercise-induced bronchoconstriction. These individuals were tested on a mechanically braked bicycle ergometer, described by von Döbeln (1954), performing submaximal work of 6 min duration. The heart rate in steady-state exercise was determined with a cardiometer. Pulmonary function studies were performed before, immediately after, and 5, 10, 15, 20, 25, 30, and 45 min after the ergometer test with a Wright's peak flow meter and a Bernstein spirometer. The minimum individual response for a diagnosis of exercise-induced bronchoconstriction was set at a 20% reduction of both PEFR and $FEV_1$ (forced expiratory volume during one second).

Thirty-four patients (21 boys and 13 girls) were tested on the same individual workload level after administration of disodium cromoglycate (Intal).

Maximal oxygen uptake was tested, by the Douglas bag method, in 10 patients before and after a 14-day period of intensive training. All direct determinations of maximal oxygen uptake were performed on a motor-driven treadmill. The patients were running uphill (3° or 5–25% incline) at a speed that caused exhaustion within 4–6 min.

In another group of asthmatic children, dynamic muscle strength was tested before and after a 3-month training period that included muscle-strengthening exercises. The evaluation was done by a point scoring system. The children were tested for strength of arm flexors, arm extensors, back extensors, abdominal muscles, knee extensors, and hip flexors and for vertical jump performance.

The same group of children was also tested on a bicycle ergometer before and after 3 months of regular physical activity (endurance training of the short-interval type), two to three times weekly, with administration of Intal before each activity. This program was followed by 14 days in a training camp in the mountains where the children performed three training sessions daily. The group was compared with a control group of 10 comparably asthmatic children of the same age and sex distribution. The control group was not subjected to any physical activity programs.

## RESULTS

Table 1 shows the results of submaximal bicycle exercise. Sixty-eight patients (79%) developed exercise-induced bronchoconstriction, 63 of them after the cessation of work, while 18 patients (21%) showed a negative exercise test. Most of the changes in pulmonary function de-

Table 1. Results of submaximal bicycle exercise in 86 asthmatic children (7–16 years)[a]

| | | | |
|---|---|---|---|
| Number of boys tested | : | 52 | |
| Number of girls tested | : | 34 | |
| Number of children with exercise-induced asthma | : | 68 | (79%) |
| Elicited during exercise | : | 5 | |
| Elicited after work stop | : | 63 | |
| Negative exercise test | : | 18 | (21%) |

[a] Twenty-four patients (16 boys and 8 girls) were tested on the same work load after administration of disodium cromoglycate. All showed improvement on exercise testing with reduction of exercise-induced asthma and only minor changes in PEFR and $FEV_1$.

veloped after work stopped, with minimum values for PEFR and $FEV_1$ 5–10 min after completion of the ergometer test.

All the patients who were tested against the same individual workload after administration of Intal showed improvement, with only minor changes in PEFR and $FEV_1$ occurring following exercise. This was even more pronounced when Intal was administered 10–15 min before exercise. The effect lasted for at least 1 hr, and, in most instances, up to 2 hr. However, as shown in Figure 1 the effect on the postexercise PEFR value was very pronounced in some cases, although the Intal had been administered 30 min before the submaximal workload occurred.

Table 2 shows the increase in $\dot{V}_{O_2}$ max in 10 patients who were tested directly by conventional methods on a motor-driven treadmill. There was great variation within the group, but it should be noted that all subjects showed values well below the expected maximum $\dot{V}_{O_2}$ for age and sex. Two of the girls were not retested because of asthmatic attacks when they returned to the test laboratory. One of the boys would not participate in the test before the training period, but was motivated to take the test after the activity programs had been completed.

Table 3 shows heart rates at submaximal workloads in 10 patients before and after a 3-month training program, and compared with the control group. It is noticeable that all the children in the test group showed substantial decreases in heart rate in steady-state exercise after the training period when retested at the same individual workload level. In the control group, there was no difference in heart rates before and after the 3-month interval.

The results indicate that the test groups improved their aerobic capacity as a result of the physical activity program and that these

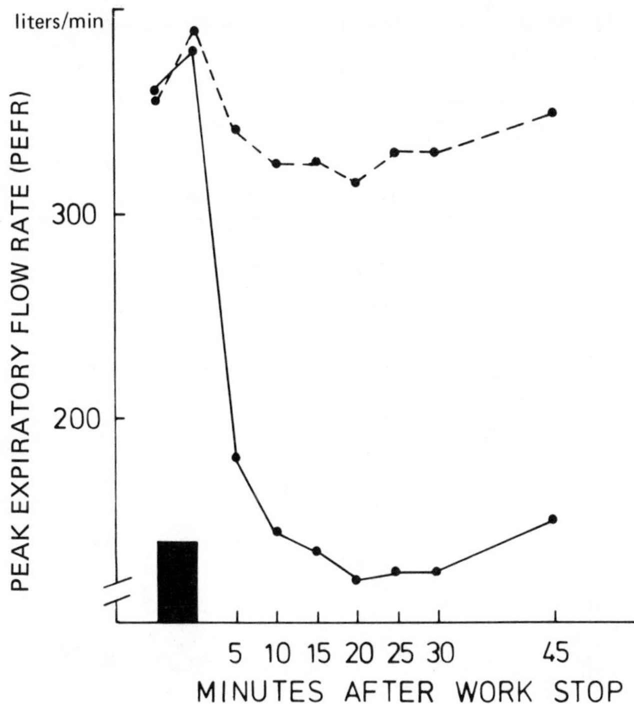


Figure 1. Peak expiratory flow rates (PEFR) are shown before and after a 6-min submaximal workload, with *(dotted line)* and without *(solid line)* premedication of Intal.

Table 2. Maximal oxygen uptake (max $V_{O_2}$) in asthmatic children (treadmill exercise) before and after a 14-day conditioning program

| Age (years) | Sex | $\dot{V}_{O2}$ max (ml/kg × min) before | $\dot{V}_{O2}$ max (ml/kg × min) after | Percent rise | Expected $\dot{V}_{O_2}$ max (ml/kg × min) |
|---|---|---|---|---|---|
| 11 | F | 36 | 42 | 16.5 | 53 |
| 11 | F | 31 | 42 | 36 | 53 |
| 13.5 | F | 47 | 49 | 4 | 50 |
| 13.5 | F | 39 | | | 50 |
| 13.5 | F | 37 | | | 50 |
| 14 | F | 32 | 37 | 16 | 50 |
| 10.5 | M | | 46 | | 58 |
| 11.5 | M | 48 | 56 | 16.5 | 59 |
| 12.5 | M | 47 | 52 | 10.5 | 62 |
| 13 | M | 47 | 53 | 12.5 | 63 |

Table 3. Heart rate at submaximal workloads (bicycle ergometer) in asthmatic children, before (upper number) and after (lower number) a 3-month conditioning program, compared with a control group

| Training group | | | | Control group | | | |
|---|---|---|---|---|---|---|---|
| Age (years) | Sex | Workload (kpm/min) | Heart rate | Age (years) | Sex | Workload (kpm/min) | Heart rate |
| 11.5 | F | 375 | 174<br>158 | 11 | F | 375 | 188<br>185 |
| 12 | F | 450 | 166<br>161 | 11.5 | F | 450 | 164<br>161 |
| 12.5 | F | 300 | 160<br>148 | 13 | F | 375 | 178<br>not tested |
| 14 | F | 600 | 168<br>146 | 13.5 | F | 525 | 167<br>165 |
| 16 | F | 600 | 171<br>157 | 14 | F | 450 | 157<br>148 |
| 16.5 | F | 525 | 177<br>not tested | 17 | F | 600 | 164<br>172 |
| 11 | M | 375 | 152<br>144 | 11 | M | 375 | 174<br>174 |
| 11.5 | M | 525 | 163<br>155 | 11 | M | 375 | 175<br>185 |
| 12.5 | M | 525 | 178<br>165 | 11.5 | M | 450 | 180<br>184 |
| 16.5 | M | 600 | 180<br>150 | 11.5 | M | 525 | 176<br>167 |

asthmatic children were able to work at the same load with less energy expenditure than before.

Table 4 shows the differences in dynamic muscle strength between the test group and the control group. The test group showed an overall increase of 34% in the point system, while the control group exhibited a minor reduction in muscle strength. These increases in aerobic capacity and muscle strength enable asthmatic children to take part more freely in play activities and recreational games, including those also involving nonasthmatic children. It is expected that increased physical capability would also influence the degree of bronchoconstriction in the postexercise period.

This is demonstrated in Figure 2. The decrease in PEFR values in the postexercise period in this asthmatic girl was much smaller after the training period than before. There was only a minor increase in pulmonary function immediately after exercise, the main effect being an increase in aerobic capacity that enabled the child to undergo exercise of similar intensity and duration more efficiently, and with consequently

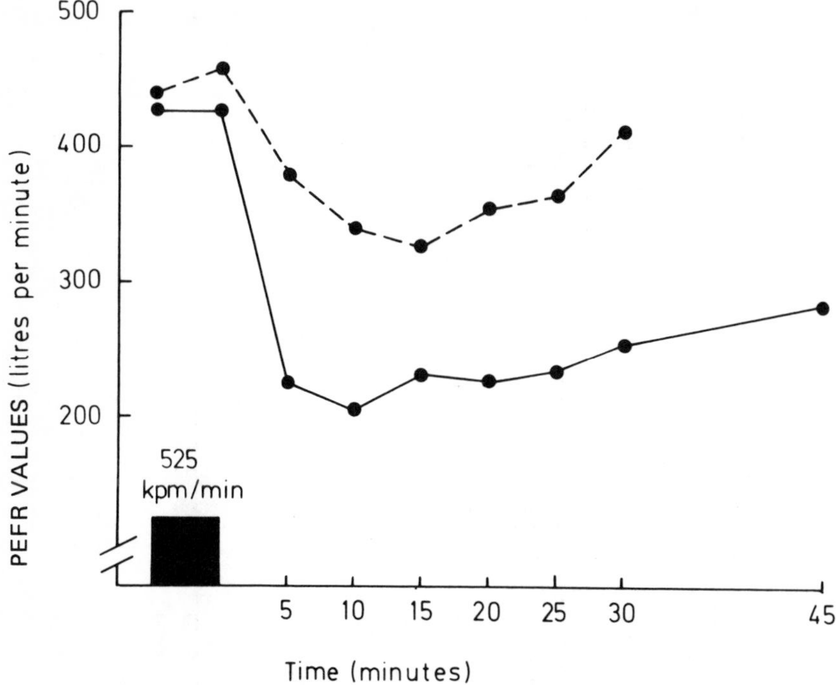


Figure 2. Peak expiratory flow rate (PEFR) in a 13½ year old girl given ergometer exercise before *(solid line)* and after *(dotted line)* a 14-day conditioning program is shown here.

reduced use of oxygen. Thus the tolerance threshold was higher and the fall in pulmonary function in the postexercise period was considerably smaller. Similar improvement of pulmonary function in the post-exercise period has been demonstrated in most asthmatic children taking part in regular physical training programs (Oseid, in preparation).

## DISCUSSION

Nearly 80% of the asthmatic children at Voksentoppen develop exercise-induced bronchoconstriction. This is a higher prevalence than previously reported on a bicycle ergometer (Poppius et al., 1970; Bevegaard et al., 1971), but this can be explained by the fact that most patients admitted to this Institute suffer from severe and multifactorial asthmatic conditions. The prevalence is actually even greater than 80%, because the minimum individual response for a diagnosis of exercise-induced bronchoconstriction in this study is set at a 20% reduction in pulmonary function in contrast to the 15% reduction set by others (Bierman, Kawabori, and Perison, 1975; Fitch, 1975a). Furth-

Table 4. Dynamic muscle strength in 7 different tests in 10 asthmatic children, before and after a 3-month conditioning program, compared with a control group

| | Arm flexors | Arm extensors | Back extensors | Abdominal muscles | Knee extensors | Hip flexors | Vertical jump | Total score |
|---|---|---|---|---|---|---|---|---|
| Training group | | | | | | | | |
| Before | 76 | 147 | 262 | 211 | 100 | 135 | 125 | 1056 |
| After | 155 | 162 | 309 | 270 | 162 | 207 | 152 | 1417 |
| Progress/Decline | +79 | +15 | +47 | +59 | +62 | +72 | +27 | +361 (+34%) |
| Control group | | | | | | | | |
| Before | 59 | 112 | 180 | 192 | 58 | 126 | 115 | 842 |
| After | 46 | 90 | 155 | 217 | 53 | 136 | 124 | 821 |
| Progress/Decline | −13 | −22 | −25 | +25 | −5 | +10 | +9 | −21 (−2.5%) |

ermore, an additional 40 children have been tested at Voksentoppen since this study was completed, bringing the incidence of exercise-induced bronchoconstriction near 85%.

The incidence of exercise-induced bronchoconstriction also depends upon the mode of exercise (Anderson, Connolly, and Godfrey, 1971; Fitch and Morton, 1971). Running induces somewhat more bronchospasm than does the performance of equivalent work on a bicycle ergometer (Jones, Wharten, and Buston, 1963; Anderson, 1972), and the incidence of bronchospasm is least marked following swimming (Godfrey, Silverman, and Anderson, 1973). Using the most evocative exercise stimulus—free running—Jones, Buston, and Wharton (1962) found that 90% of asthmatic children developed exercise-induced bronchoconstriction, even if they required a 25% functional loss before diagnosis.

Why different types of exercise do not produce comparable effects remains unexplained. A recent review (Shephard, 1977) discussed several factors. The origin is probably multifactorial, with reflex stimulation of tracheal receptors (Simonsson, Jacobs, and Nadel, 1967), altered sympathetic neural discharge (Sly et al., 1967), release of prostaglandins (Piper and Vane, 1971), and cell sensitization being involved on different occassions. The prophylactic effect of Intal (Davies, 1968; Silverman and Andrea, 1972; Godfrey et al., 1974) indicates that the mast cell and biochemical mediators play an important role in the pathogenesis. This was also confirmed in this study (Table 1 and Figure 1).

Asthmatic children generally have a very low physical work capacity. They have lost the natural increase in oxygen uptake that active play induces in normal children. Table 2 shows that all the children had aerobic capacities well below the expected values for age and sex, even after intensive training. However, the increase was substantial in most patients and facilitated participation in play and games with other children.

A 3-month conditioning program resulted in a pronounced increase not only in endurance and muscle strength (Tables 3 and 4), but also in general physical performance that was of great help to all the children in their everyday activities. Afterwards, the majority of these children were able to participate in a full physical education program at school with a minimum of restriction, provided they used prophylactic medication (Intal) regularly and also made use of a longer than usual warm-up period (10–15 min). Some of them showed such progress that they were able to take up competitive sports, as previously reported by Fitch (1975b).

However, the most important effect of training that the children experienced was a much slighter fall in pulmonary function following exercise, provided the workload was identical. Figure 2 illustrates this, and the increase in ventilatory function makes it possible for asthmatic children to integrate with other children in play activities with less discomfort, less bronchospasm, and less use of symptomatic medication.

Positive psychological effects were also recorded. All the children showed a significant increase in self-confidence, they became more motivated for physical activity, and they were able to use their bodies in different physical activities, an experience that considerably influenced their understanding of body function. After the training programs, many of them admitted spontaneously that they were able to mobilize enough energy and strength to take part in various activities of which they had never thought themselves capable. This effect was perhaps the most convincing one, and follow-up studies have shown that the psychological and social effects are long-lasting.

## REFERENCES

Anderson, S. D. 1972. Physiological aspects of exercise-induced bronchoconstriction. Doctoral thesis, University of London.

Anderson, S. D., Connolly, N. M., and Godfrey, S. 1971. Comparison of bronchoconstriction induced by cycling and running. Thorax 26: 396–401.

Bevegaard, S., Eriksson, B. O., Graff-Lonnevig, V., Kraepelien, S., and Saltin, B. 1971. Circulatory and respiratory dimensions and functional capacity in boys aged 8–13 years with bronchial asthma. Acta Paediatr. Scand. 217 suppl.: 86–89.

Bierman, C. W., Kawabori, I., and Perison, W. E., 1975. Incidence of exercise-induced asthma in children. Pediatrics 56 suppl.: 847–850.

Cropp, G. J. A. 1975. Grading, time course, and incidence of exercise-induced airway obstruction and hyperinflation in asthmatic children. Pediatrics 56 suppl: 868–879.

Davies, S. E. 1968. Effect of disodium cromoglycate on exercise-induced asthma. Br. Med. J. 3: 593–594.

von Döbeln, W. 1954. A simple bicycle ergometer. J. Appl. Physiol. 7: 222–226.

Fitch, K. D. 1975a. Comparative aspects of available exercise systems. Pediatrics 56 suppl.: 904–907.

Fitch, K. D. 1975b. Exercise-induced asthma and competitive athletics. Pediatrics 56 suppl.: 942–943.

Fitch, K. D., and Morton, A. R. 1971. Specificity of exercise in exercise-induced asthma. Br. Med. J. 4: 577–581.

Godfrey, S. 1974. Problems peculiar to the diagnosis and management of childhood asthma. BTTA Rev. 4:1.

Godfrey, S., Silverman, M., and Anderson, S. D. 1973. Problems of interpreting exercise-induced asthma. J. Allergy 52: 199–209.

Godfrey, S., Zeidifard, E., Brown, K., and Bell, J. H. 1974. The possible site of action of sodium cromoglycate assessed by exercise challenge. Clin. Sci. Mol. Med. 46:265–272.

Jones, R. S. 1966. Assessment of respiratory function in the asthmatic child. Br. Med. J. II:972–975.

Jones, R. S., Buston, M. H., and Wharton, M. J. 1962. The effect of exercise on ventilatory function in children with asthma. Br. J. Dis. Chest 56:78–86.

Jones, R. S., Wharton, M. J., and Buston, M. H. 1963. The place of physical exercise and bronchodilator drugs in the assessment of the asthmatic child. Arch. Dis. Child. 38:539–545.

Katz, R. M., Whipp, B. J., Heimlich, E. M., and Wasserman, K. 1971. Exercise-induced bronchospasm, ventilation and blood gases in asthmatic children. J. Allergy 47:148–158.

Lefcoe, N. M. 1969. The time course of maximum ventilatory performance during and after moderately heavy exercise. Clin. Sci. 36: 47–52.

Lefcoe, N. M., Carter, R. P., and Ahmad, D. 1971. Post-exercise bronchoconstriction in normal subjects and asthmatics. Am. Rev. Resp. Dis. 104:562–567.

Perison, W. E., and Bierman, C. W. 1975. Free running test for exercise-induced bronchospasm. Pediatrics 56 suppl.:890–892.

Piper, P., and Vane, J. R. 1971. The release of prostaglandins from lung and other tissues. Ann. NY Acad. Sci. 180:363–385.

Poppius, H., Muittari, A., Kreus, K. E., Korhonen, O., and Viljanen, A. 1970. Exercise, asthma and disodium cromoglycate. Br. Med. J. 4:337–339.

Shephard, R. J. 1977. Exercise-induced bronchospasm—A review. Med. Sci Sports 9:1–10.

Silverman, M., and Anderson, S. D. 1972. Standardization of exercise tests in asthmatic children. Arch. Dis. Child. 47:882–889.

Silverman, M., and Andrea, T. 1972. Time course of effect of disodium cromoglycate on exercise—induced asthma. Arch. Dis. Child. 47:419–422.

Simonsson, B. G., Jacobs, F. M., and Nadel, J. A. 1967. Role of autonomic nervous system and the cough reflex in the increased responsiveness of airways in patients with obstructive airway disease. J. Clin. Invest. 46:1812–1818.

Sly, R. M., Heimlich, E. M., Busser, R. J., and Strick, L. 1967. Exercise-induced bronchospasm: Effect of adrenergic or cholinergic blockage. J. Allergy 40:93–99.

# Physical Activity Programs for Children with Exercise-Induced Asthma

S. Oseid, M. Kendall, R. B. Larsen, and R. Selbekk

Most exercise studies on asthmatic children deal with the acute effect of exercise on the posteffort pulmonary function. Little is known about the long-term effects of regular physical activity on the total rehabilitation of asthmatic children. For the last 5 years, the Voksentoppen Children's Asthma and Allergy Institute has tried to work out and organize exercise programs that generally can be used in the rehabilitation process for children with severe bronchial asthma. The purpose of this chapter is to present these experiences with such physical activity programs.

## GOALS

Traditional physical treatment of asthmatic children has been oriented toward coping with attacks (by breath control and resting positions), postural drainage, and isolated exercises to correct chest deformities.

It is important to offer asthmatic children some form of treatment beyond the acute stage. These children must be enabled *to enjoy* physical activity and be given the confidence and enthusiasm to take part in activities beyond the treatment program. They must be shown that this is possible *despite* their asthma.

Many people feel that isolated breathing exercises are, in contrast, of little value and often burdensome to the child, the parents, and the physiotherapist. Isolated thorax-mobilizing exercises are also unnecessary, if they can be incorporated into other activities that are more enjoyable and natural.

Treatment of the child with asthma through physical training programs, with the emphasis on group treatment, has played a major role in the total rehabilitation of the Institute's patients. It must be remembered that this approach involves treatment of the more severe asthmatics. Not all asthmatic children have the problems mentioned here, since, as in other illnesses, there are many degrees of disability.

Why are physical training programs relevant for the child with asthma?

Asthmatic children need regular physical activity, as do all children. In fact, asthmatics need to be *more physically fit* than healthy children in order to have something to fall back on in periods of regression. Children with asthma are often in poor states of general fitness; even small amounts of exercise can prove to be difficult and will often promote wheeziness. Those who have thoracic deformities profit from a general physical training, making isolated thorax exercises unnecessary. Children with exercise-induced asthma benefit from a systematic program of endurance and muscle-strengthening exercises. Their exercise tolerance levels are thus increased, allowing them to take part more freely in physical activities with less asthmatic repercussions.

It is important that a child with asthma develop a positive attitude toward physical activity. The restrictions placed upon the child and the often overprotective parental attitude can result in social isolation. Physical activity is often associated with wheeziness, distress, and defeat. The child eventually withdraws from any form of exercise that makes physical demands upon him and looks upon himself as physically inferior. The child is assigned to the category of a "sick" person. The psychological implications of the disease can be demonstrated schematically:

The need to feel that one belongs to a group is very important, especially to children. Asthmatic children are often onlookers wanting to join in but unable to do so because of their disability. Because they are often exempt from physical education at school, a physical training program can be used as a springboard giving them the necessary encouragement to take part in school physical education classes.

Before taking part in these group activities, however, they must be given the opportunity to test their own limits under secure medical supervision. An exercise tolerance test (an ergometer bicycle test, a treadmill test, or an ordinary step test) is a valuable and objective method by which both child and leader can assess progress. Cooperation between doctor and group leader is therefore advantageous whenever possible. A physical activity program also allows the children to discover how much they can tolerate before becoming wheezy.

How well a child functions physically depends upon his confidence in his own capabilities. Therefore, one of the aims of the

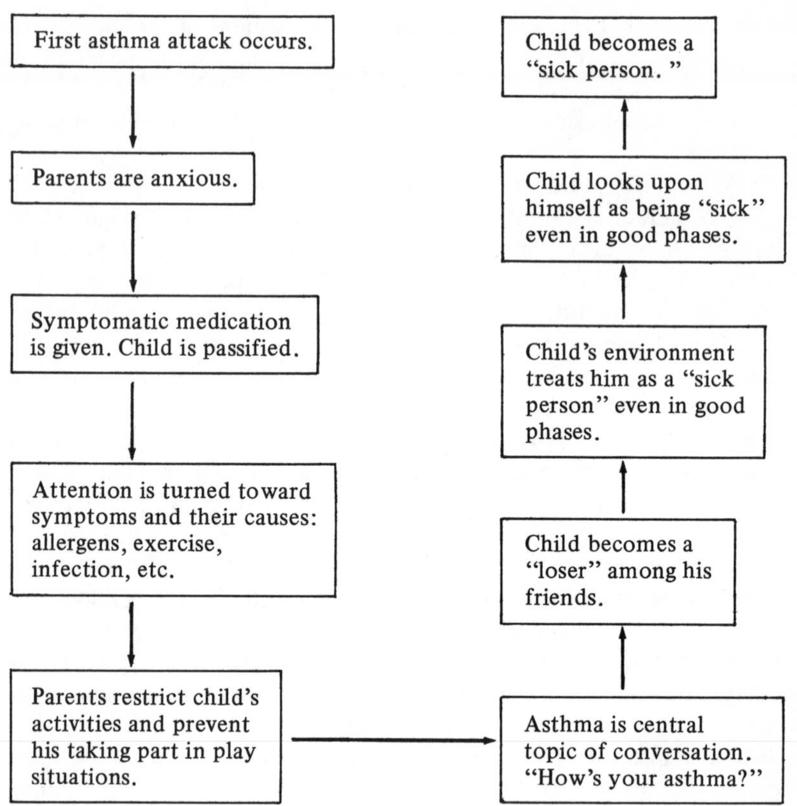


physical training program is to help the child realize that "I can take part despite my asthma."

## PROCEDURES

1. Before participating in any physical activity, premedication with Intal is essential for the majority of patients with exercise-induced asthma. This should be administered 5–10 min before starting an activity. If a child is wheezy, $\beta$-adrenergic medication should be administered before Intal is taken, to facilitate the distribution of Intal to peripheral airways.
2. In order to prevent wheeziness, it is essential to have a longer (10–15 min) and less strenuous warm-up period than usual. This is especially important for children with exercise-induced asthma, because beginning a training session with activities that put strong demands upon the cardiorespiratory system results invariably in

bronchial obstructions despite premedication. The warm-up period should include activities in which the patient can control the intensity himself and thereby discover his own exercise tolerance level and its limits. Interval training principles should also be used in this warm-up period.

3. It is generally accepted that interval training is especially useful for developing endurance. When working with asthmatic individuals, it is important that the work periods not exceed 3–4 min if bronchial obstruction is to be prevented. This does not mean that an activity should be stopped suddenly (this is both artificial and unnecessary), but that less strenuous work periods should be alternated with more strenuous ones. Games containing natural interval training can be utilized. Ball games such as football, handball, basketball, or water polo are ideal. The training programs should be as natural as possible to avoid reminding the child continually of his asthma. Interspersing breathing exercises in a physical activity program serves only to remind the child of his illness in what is otherwise an enjoyable situation. Above all, group treatment should be enjoyable. Apart from teaching the child breath control during an attack, which is both important and necessary, breathing exercises have been found to be of little value.
4. Asthmatics should train with a submaximal load. To ensure that the work load is not too great, a physical training program should try to attain a pulse rate of 160–170 in children from 10–15 years old. If the pulse rate exceeds this limit, the child works anaerobically, and the danger of inducing asthma is therefore considerably increased.
5. To a child, physical training is play, and play is part of his natural development; play activities should therefore be consciously incorporated into the training program. The word "training" is traditionally associated with competition and with blood, sweat, and tears. Acceptance of the idea that play is a form of training will result in a program that offers the asthmatic child a more enjoyable approach to physical conditioning. This is especially important for asthma patients who are reluctant to take part in physical activities. They must be motivated by stimulating and enjoyable training programs that they can master—and that motivate them in turn to participate in further training, even at home. This does not mean that play reduces the demands put on the child. Learning correct swimming techniques, for example, makes pool activities more effective and more fun.

## SAMPLE TRAINING SESSION

It must be emphasized that this patient group does not require specially designed exercises; a "recipe" is therefore undesirable because it would tend to create a rigid attitude towards the "expert's" model. All exercises and activities taken out of context can seem meaningless, and it is sincerely hoped that each therapist, in conjunction with his or her patients, will work toward a model that feels right for the group involved.

### Warming Up

***Foot Tag*** The group joins hands in a circle. One member tries to tag another using his foot, and this second child in turn tries to tag another. This type of exercise is useful in bringing the group closer together from the beginning of the training program.

***In Time to Music*** Jog around the room, walk around the room, and run around the room. Jog/walk/run many times.

***Standing/sitting*** Perform exercises for shoulder girdle and arms (using small equipment, e.g., balls, jump ropes, hoops, etc.).

***Walking Activities*** Walk like a rag doll. Walk like a soldier. Walk tall, small, quietly, noisily, etc.

***Standing*** Free movement to music. Move arms only. Move legs only. Move whole body.

***Moving Freely to Music*** When the music is turned off, everyone follows the leader's instructions to "lie on your tummy," "lie on your back," "go to the top of the wall bars," etc.

***Monkey Tag (for Smaller Children)*** Everyone has a tail (jump rope, band, etc.), and the aim is to acquire as many "tails" as possible while retaining one's own tail. (Older children can play normal tag if they feel that this is too childish.)

### Circuit Training

The following circuit contains both endurance and muscle-strengthening exercises. A circuit can be set up that contains whatever exercises the group requires, e.g., for balance, mobility, coordination, etc.

1. Sit-ups (abdominal exercise)
2. Step test
3. Back extension exercises
4. Jogging on a very thick, soft mattress
5. Press-ups/pull-ups
6. Skipping

## Partnership and Trust Exercises

1. *A* makes a bridge with his body and *B* finds all possible ways of going under and over it.
2. *A* and *B* sit back to back, arms linked, and both try to stand up.
3. "How many ways can you balance each other?"
4. Roll each other, with and without resistance.

## Relay Races

Many activities can be incorporated in relay races of differing degrees of difficulty, in slalom races, in ball races, and in obstacle races. These games are greatly appreciated.

## Team Games

Team games and ball games—football, basketball, indoor hockey, etc.—provide a natural form of interval training. These games increase endurance and are excellent for developing coordination and teamwork. They are best introduced at the end of a session and should last for at least 15 min in order to produce any training effect.

## Other Recreational Activities

Mime, body movement, and free dance provide excellent opportunities for self-expression and make the individual more body-conscious. These activities are exciting and challenging and often give a sense of freedom. Because of the asthmatics' inhibitions and lack of self-confidence in physical activity, it may take these children a little longer than others to loosen up. The aim is to make the child feel more secure in expressing himself, both individually and in a group. The results are very positive both mentally and physically, and, in addition, contribute the benefits of increased self-confidence.

## Swimming

Swimming is an extremely good activity for asthmatic children because it rarely induces an asthmatic attack, as do other forms of exercise of comparable intensity. Nonasthmatics often experience an increase in lung volume with regular swimming, and similar results can also be achieved in asthmatic subjects. The increase in lung volume is only one of the advantages of swimming. The psychologically beneficial effect of being equal to healthy children in the swimming pool is very important, giving the child more self-confidence and a feeling of belonging. The swimming pool is useful for individual or group treatments, depending upon technical skills. Relay races and water polo are excellent pool activities for asthmatic children.

Many complain that chlorine provokes asthma, but, in the Institute's experience, this is very rare. Chlorine often causes irritation of the eyes and nose, even in nonasthmatics. This disappears quickly, however, and should not prevent the use of pool therapy. Swimming is an excellent and often enjoyable way of improving muscle power, posture, and general fitness.

Asthmatic children should be warned against diving, which can be dangerous. Because of an increased tendency toward air-trapping in the peripheral airways, asthmatics are in danger of bursting the small alveoli; this can result in segmental collapse. This caution does not include short underwater swimming but does refer to diving with or without special equipment.

## Outdoor Activities

It is important to stimulate asthmatic children to take part in outdoor activities, too. Outdoor pursuits should be encouraged for the family as a whole, because these children tend to be treated as "hothouse plants." The asthmatic child should be allowed to take part in family walks if this is a natural part of family life. The parents should *not* be given the task of training their child if this is unnatural for them, because it might add to the responsibilities of the already overburdened parents. The parents should, however, be encouraged to stimulate rather than to restrict the child's participation in outdoor activities.

## Walking and Rambling

***Nature Walks*** Nature walks can be used as a form of endurance training by jogging or running between various preset posts. A number of small tasks, such as finding leaves and stones or identifying birds or animals, gives the child the necessary rest periods between running—once again using the interval training principle.

## Orienteering

This is a progressively popular sport because the ability to find one's way through a wood or over hilly terrain is so rewarding. This is also good recreation for asthmatics including those allergic to pollen, provided that not too much grass pollen or tree pollen is in the area. Pine and spruce forests are ideal for those allergic to pollen, because few people react to pollen from these trees.

## Mountain Walking and Climbing

Mountain walking may seem too strenuous an activity for asthmatic children, but it is important that they be given the opportunity to get into the mountains. Experience has demonstrated that mountain pursuits are both well tolerated and enjoyed by this group of patients. Again, one must remember to stop often, and to refrain from starting out too rapidly. With stops at reasonable intervals (preferably in a natural way, by taking photographs, looking at plants, etc.), even asthmatics can climb mountains. A summer holiday in the mountains is often more beneficial for a patient allergic to pollen than a holiday at a sea level location, where the pollen count is much higher.

### Canoeing

Canoeing is a good method of building up arm and postural muscles and is therefore a good activity for asthmatics. It is a stimulating form of training, offering the opportunity to be out in the fresh air and to experience nature at her best.

### Bicycling

Bicycling can be used for physical training, provided the correct guidelines are followed. Premedication and a long warm-up period are, again, essential. A family bicycle trip out in the countryside is a good way of promoting fitness, and can also give the child a valuable psychological boost.

### Skiing

In countries where skiing is a natural activity, an ideal form of training is available to the child with asthma. Cross-country skiing offers both endurance and muscle training. Cold and windy weather, however, can induce bronchoconstriction.

## GROUP TREATMENT AS A REHABILITATION METHOD

Many considerations must be taken into account when setting up a rehabilitation group. Age, sex, and the individual resources of each child are factors generally important to the formation of a treatment group.

The different physical and psychological backgrounds and capabilities of various patients with bronchial asthma often place greater demands upon the group leader in determining the type and intensity of activities than would a more homogeneous group. One child, who may take part to improve his general physical fitness, may already function at adequate social and psychological levels. Another group member may be extremely inhibited and exploit his asthma, retreating to a safe corner at the slightest provocation.

Ideally, the group should remain as stable as possible in order for the individual to achieve a sense of security and a sense of belonging. However, each individual member may be concerned only with himself and his own problems, and may not consider himself able both to give and to receive support and encouragement. He does not realize that group interaction can result in all achieving *together* what each member is unable to achieve alone. It takes time to feel secure within the group and to trust one another. Continual changes in group membership create a big handicap for both leader and child alike.

The group leader is often faced with the problem of follow-up when the child returns home. It is important for these children to continue with physical activity in their home environment. It is often suggested that they join some sort of club, for example, an athletics, jazz ballet, or swimming club. It is therefore necessary to inform the club leader/physical education teacher about how the child can be helped to function to the best of his ability.

In order to do this, the therapist must involve the parents as early as possible. Both individual and group meetings with parents allow the therapist to give the parents the information they need and have the right to know. These meetings provide the opportunity to learn of the experiences and the problems involved in having a severe asthmatic in the family. It is important for the parents to put their expectations into words, and, at the same time, for the therapist to explain to them what the child is taking part in and why. Parental cooperation is an essential factor in the follow-up of these patients.

The leader's attitude toward the group is a deciding factor in achieving an efficient yet lighthearted working atmosphere. It is important to be able to enter the group at its members' level, and to speak the same language. It is essential to be well prepared because a leader's uncertainty is quickly registered and reflected in the group. It may be necessary to alter the activities originally planned, often in the middle of a session. There are many reasons for this: the combination of children in the group may be unsuitable; the therapist may be uninspiring as group leader; or one of the children may suddenly become very wheezy.

With experience one learns how to remain in control of the situation: the therapist can often "save" the session by replacing a hard circuit training with an enjoyable ball game, for example. The choice of activities often seems limited because of the great need for variation. Groups at the Institute have certainly been outspoken when they were bored by scheduled activities. Therapists have often wished for an abundance of exciting, effective, and amusing exercises. The variety possible in group treatment offers an enormous advantage over individual treatment. Choice of activities is much easier when there are several children together.

Group treatment places great demands upon the leader. In addition to involvement in the various activities, the therapist must be constantly aware of what is happening within the group in case anyone becomes obstructive. It is therefore a great asset to have other adults taking part who can help in difficult situations. It should be unnecessary to be authoritative, but certain limits must be set so that each individual may function within the group. This delicate balance can be difficult. For instance, when one child climbs to the top of the rib bars, when another throws the contents of the ball basket around the room, and when a third sets off at full speed on the stationary bicycle, one feels like stamping one's foot and shouting "Attention!"

Reactions to group treatment vary. Some children react with tears or tantrums, while some may resort to violent protest. Group treatment can be frightening and self-revealing and can result in an asthmatic reaction, either consciously or unconsciously incurred. These reactions are often expressions of inadequacy caused by a lack of body awareness and a lack of self-confidence in the face of demands put upon the child. The attitudes people have toward their own bodies are part of how they look upon themselves generally. Improving a person's bodily awareness will result in his being more confident in himself, as a person, and will make him more positive and secure in other situations.

Most of these children react positively to group treatment, having often wanted to be a member of a group in which they can function despite their asthma. The togetherness they experience within the group is often new and exciting for them, because they have often been mere onlookers in their home environment.

The final aim of therapists must be to make themselves superfluous to the individual asthmatic, but only when the patient is ready for it. The supportive function should not be necessary for more than a limited period: therapy must work toward making the patient independent both in dealing with his asthma and in relating to the community. He belongs, after all, at home and at school. It is there that he must fit in and function. It is essential that the child be capable of taking part in a group with other asthmatic children, but this is just part of a process that extends beyond the boundaries of the asthmatic group. This demands reciprocal understanding and insight among patient, family, friends, and school.

In this regard, the therapist's role is a rewarding one. Whatever is given in knowledge and experience is returned tenfold—by the patient.

# Effects of Home Care and Prone Immersion Physical Exercise (PIPE) or Bicycle Ergometer Training on Patients with Chronic Obstructive Pulmonary Disease (COPD)

**L. W. Jankowski and L. E. Roy**

Chronic obstructive pulmonary disease (COPD) has been called the major public health problem in the western world (Lertzman and Cherniack, 1976). COPD is a degenerative disease of the small airways that is prevalent among working class adults characterized as long-time heavy cigarette smokers. The initial diagnosis is usually made when the patient is about 50 years of age and at the peak earning period of his career. Because roughly 80% of the patients are male "breadwinners," the disease has severe socioeconomic consequences, particularly in societies practicing socialized medicine.

The disease usually begins insidiously and progresses slowly but relentlessly until the patient is a dyspneic cripple, physically dependent on his family and friends and financially dependent on social welfare or disability payments. The patient's progressive deterioration proceeds imperceptively; thus the disease is usually well advanced before the patient realizes his abnormality and seeks medical treatment.

Current medical treatment is symptomatic and palliative (Macklem, 1974), emphasizing energy conservation, diaphragmatic breathing, and postural drainage, and relying heavily on bronchodilators and inhalation therapy. Such treatment has minimal effects

This study was supported in part by National Health and Welfare of Canada Grant 605-1013-30 and by the Quebec Christmas Seal Society, Inc.

and consequently the prognosis for COPD patients is poor. Patients suffering from exertional dyspnea avoid physical activity. This then predisposes to physiological deterioration that provokes even greater dyspnea upon exertion. As this vicious cycle continues, arterial hypoxia and pulmonary hypertension develop and in turn cause cor-pulmonale, pulmonary edema, and death. Epidemiological studies (Damsgaard and Kok-Jensen, 1974) have found that death occurs in most cases approximately 12 years after the initial diagnosis.

Since 1952 reports of the beneficial effects of physical exercise therapy programs have been presented by many investigators. Many researchers (Barach, Bickerman, and Beck, 1952; Miller, Taylor, and Jasper, 1962; Pierce et al., 1964; Pierce, Paez, and Miller, 1965; Haas and Cardon, 1969; Petty et al., 1969; Vyas et al., 1971; and Brundin, 1975) had their patients exercise in the vertical position, walking, cycling, or climbing stairs while breathing air or oxygen-enriched air mixtures. The general conclusion from these investigations was that regular and frequent participation in a progressive physical exercise rehabilitation program can improve the exercise tolerance and the physical working capacity of patients with COPD. These ameliorations apparently result from increased maximal oxygen consumption ($\dot{V}_{O_2}$ max) and an improved efficiency of motion. Patients in these studies almost always reported a greater sense of well being, better sleep, improved appetite, and a decreased dependence on oral bronchodilators. Most investigators agree that therapeutic exercise can improve the quality of life of the COPD patient. Curiously, these objective and subjective improvements are not generally associated with improved pulmonary function.

The COPD patient's maximal oxygen consumption is limited by a low ventilatory capacity, complicated by a poor ventilation-perfusion ratio ($\dot{V}A/\dot{Q}$). In the vertical position, the regional $\dot{V}A/\dot{Q}$ of healthy normals is high in the apices and low in the bases of the lungs (Anthonisen and Milic-Emili, 1966). This condition improves in the horizontal position, largely because of greater perfusion of the apices. A pilot study has been done to determine the feasibility and utility of using the horizontal position for exercise therapy in patients with COPD (Jankowski et al., 1976; Jankowski et al., 1977). The technique of "prone immersion physical exercise" (PIPE therapy) is illustrated in Figure 1. Four months of PIPE therapy produced all previously reported benefits and significantly increased the mean vital capacity (VC) of seven patients with moderate to severe COPD (Figure 2).

The purpose of this study was to compare the effects of PIPE therapy with those of traditional exercise training programs for COPD patients.

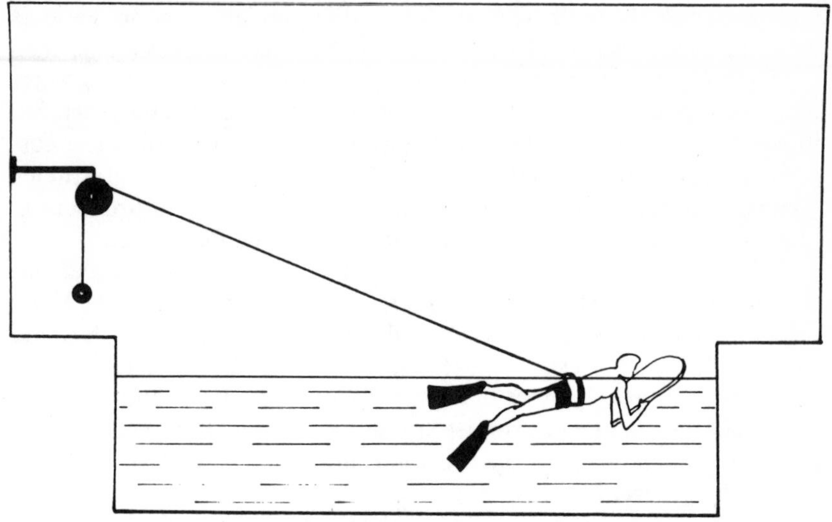

Figure 1. Prone immersion physical exercise (PIPE) is illustrated here.

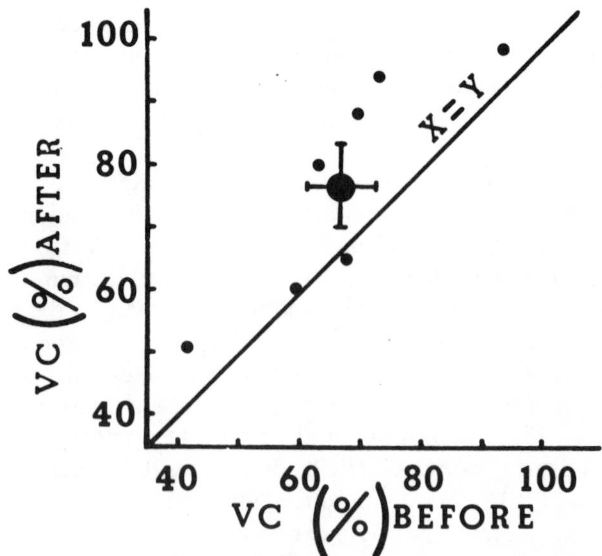


Figure 2. This graph shows individual and mean ± standard error for observed/predicted forced vital capacity (VC) (%) before and after PIPE therapy (Jankowski et al., 1976).

## METHODS

Eighteen patients (7 men and 11 women) ranging from 46 to 64 years of age ($\bar{X}$ = 55.8 years), diagnosed as having moderate to severe COPD but showing no clinical signs of serious cardiovascular or metabolic diseases, completed the 6-month study. Patients participated voluntarily and without pay, but free door-to-door transportation was provided.

The patient volunteers were randomly divided into three groups as follows: Group I served as controls and received routine home care including symptomatic medical treatment and physical therapy. In addition to receiving home care, Groups II and III exercised three times per week, on alternate days, at approximately 75% of their $\dot{V}_{O_2}$ max. Group II exercised on stationary bicycles, while Group III exercised by the experimental PIPE technique. The duration of exercise for both Groups II and III was increased progressively and identically from 15 to 60 min, and the work-to-rest ratio increased from 1:1 to 10:1. In other words, patients began with five 3-min bouts of exercise, each followed by 3 min rest, and progressed to four 15-min bouts of exercise, each followed by 2 min rest.

Before, during, and after training, each patient's submaximal and maximal oxygen consumption was measured during a progressive, intermittent bicycle ergometer test using an open circuit system. Minute ventilation was measured with a Parkinson Cowan dry gas meter, and expired $O_2$-$CO_2$ concentrations were measured with Beckman OM11 and LB2 gas analyzers. Exercise heart rates were calculated from precordial lead (C5-C5R) ECG tracings made during the final 15 sec of exercise at each level. Simple spirometric measurements, VC, forced expiratory volume ($FEV_1$), and mean forced expiratory flow ($FEF_{25\text{-}75}$) were measured before and after training with a Jones waterless spirometer.

## RESULTS

The results are summarized in Table 1. The physical work capacity, maximum oxygen consumption, and pulmonary function of those patients receiving symptomatic home care and routine physical therapy decreased dramatically during the 6-month observation period. Both exercise therapy groups demonstrated increased physical work capacity and increased $\dot{V}_{O_2}$ max.

While the respiratory function of patients in Group II apparently stabilized, the forced VC and the FEV of those patients performing PIPE exercise seem to have improved.

Table 1. Summary of changes in work capacity, oxygen consumption, and pulmonary function

| Variable | | Group I (control) (N = 6) Before | After | Δ%[a] | Group II (bicycle) (N = 6) Before | After | Δ%[a] | Group III (PIPE) (N = 6) Before | After | Δ%[a] |
|---|---|---|---|---|---|---|---|---|---|---|
| Maximum load | $\bar{X}$ | 35.4 | 32.0 | −9.6 | 22.2 | 37.5 | +68.9 | 33.3 | 54.2 | +62.8 |
| (Watts) | SE | 6.8 | 6.4 | | 7.7 | 10.2 | | 5.3 | 5.3 | |
| $\dot{V}_{O_2}$ max | $\bar{X}$ | 743 | 686 | −7.7 | 574 | 693 | +20.7 | 742 | 917 | +23.6 |
| (ml/min) | SE | 120 | 64 | | 92 | 119 | | 103 | 93 | |
| $\dot{V}_E$ max | $\bar{X}$ | 26.6 | 24.3 | −8.6 | 25.5 | 26.8 | +5.1 | 26.2 | 30.2 | +15.2 |
| (liters/min) | SE | 3.3 | 1.9 | | 5.3 | 4.6 | | 2.1 | 1.8 | |
| $f$ | $\bar{X}$ | 28.7 | 29.3 | +2.1 | 29.7 | 28.7 | −3.4 | 31.2 | 28.8 | −7.7 |
| (resp/min) | SE | 1.2 | 1.4 | | 4.0 | 6.0 | | 2.4 | 2.0 | |
| $\dot{V}_T$ | $\bar{X}$ | 944 | 838 | −11.2 | 856 | 934 | +9.1 | 756 | 1066 | +41.0 |
| (ml) | SE | 130 | 67 | | 124 | 139 | | 173 | 90 | |
| FVC | $\bar{X}$ | 1638 | 1489 | −9.0 | 1697 | 1763 | +3.9 | 1483 | 1901 | +28.2 |
| (ml) | SE | 184 | 148 | | 169 | 191 | | 107 | 167 | |
| $FEV_1$ | $\bar{X}$ | 606 | 547 | −9.7 | 611 | 584 | −4.4 | 551 | 667 | +21.0 |
| (ml) | SE | 132 | 92 | | 133 | 111 | | 60 | 106 | |
| $FEF_{25\text{-}75}$ | $\bar{X}$ | 307 | 238 | −22.5 | 376 | 329 | −12.5 | 259 | 255 | −1.5 |
| (ml/sec) | SE | 98 | 63 | | 147 | 135 | | 32 | 51 | |

[a] Δ% is percent change calculated as: (final − initial) value/initial value × 100.

## DISCUSSION

The observed similarity in increased physical work capacity and increased $\dot{V}_{O_2}$ max in Groups II and III was anticipated, because they followed identical training programs. The slightly greater percent increase in the bicycle ergometer training group was probably attributable to the fact that their initial values were lower; it may also reflect training specificity.

Improved pulmonary function in the PIPE group compared with that of the controls was evidenced by an average 41%, or 418 ml, increase in forced VC and by a 21% increase in $FEV_1$. The improved pulmonary function of those patients performing PIPE exercise seems to explain their ability to increase exercise tidal volume and, hopefully, to improve alveolar gas exchange.

Prone immersion physical exercise therapy is evidently the preferred rehabilitative exercise for patients with COPD.

## ACKNOWLEDGMENTS

The authors thank Miss Lina Gagné for typing the manuscript, and Mrs. Jeanette Labelle and Mr. Normand Montagne for their technical assistance.

## REFERENCES

Anthonisen, N. R. and Milic-Emili, J. 1966. Distribution of pulmonary perfusion in erect man. J. Appl. Physiol. 21:760.

Barach, A. L., Bickerman, H. A., and Beck, G. J., 1952. Advances in treatment of non-tuberculous pulmonary disease. Bull. NY Acad. Med. 28:353.

Brundin, A. 1975. Physical training in severe chronic obstructive lung disease. Scand. J. Resp. Dis. 55:25.

Damsgaard, T. and Kok-Jensen, A. 1974. Prognosis in severe chronic obstructive pulmonary disease. Acta Med. Scand. 196:103.

Hass, A. and Cardon, H. 1969. Rehabilitation in chronic obstructive pulmonary disease. Med. Clin. of North Am. 53:593.

Jankowski, L. W., Portman, M., Martin, P., Roy, L. E., and Vall'ee, J. 1977. Controlled leg exercise in water. Can. J. Appl. Sport Sci. 1:277.

Jankowski, L. W., Roy, L. E., Vallée, J., and Boucher, R., 1976. Effect of prone immersion physical exercise (PIPE) therapy in patients with chronic obstructive pulmonary disease (COPD). Scand. J. Rehab. Med. 8:135.

Lertzman, M. M. and Cherniack, R. M. 1976. Rehabilitation of patients with chronic obstructive pulmonary disease. Am. Rev. Resp. Dis. 114:1145.

Macklem, P. T. 1974. Workshop on screening programs for early diagnosis of airway obstruction. Am. Rev. Resp. Dis. 109:567.

Miller, W. F., Taylor, H. F., and Jasper, L. 1962. Exercise training in the rehabilitation of patients with severe respiratory insufficiency due to pulmonary emphysema. Southern Med. J. 55:1216.

Petty, T. L., Nett, L. M., Finigan, M. M., Brink, G. A., and Corsello, P. R. 1969. A comprehensive care program for chronic airway obstruction. Ann. Int. Med. 70:1109.

Paez, P. N., Phillipson, E. A., Masangkay, M. and Sproule, B. J. 1967. The physiological basis of training patients with emphysema. Am. Rev. Resp. Dis. 95:944.

Pierce, A. K., Taylor, H. F., Archer, R. K., and Miller, W. F. 1964. Responses to exercise training in patients with emphysema. Arch. Int. Med. 113:28.

Pierce, A. K., Paez, P. N., and Miller, W. F. 1965. Exercise training with the aid of a portable oxygen supply in patients with emphysema. Am. Rev. Resp. Dis. 91:653.

Vyas, M. N., Banister, E. W., Morton, J. W., and Gryzbowski, S. 1971. Response to exercise in patients with chronic airway obstruction: I—Effects of exercise training. Am. Rev. Resp. Dis. 103:390.

# The Use of the Pool in Rehabilitation

**M. Foyer, I. Sjöberg, and U. Ersson**

Akademiska sjukhuset in Uppsala, Sweden, is a University hospital for acute and outpatient care. The Physiotherapy Department, which comes under supervision of the rehabilitation unit, treats patients from all departments within the hospital and provides for outpatient care.

Patients with all kinds of diseases and handicaps are treated within the rehabilitation unit. This chapter describes the training and rehabilitation of patients with myocardial infarction, with special emphasis on the use of the pool as a supplement to the rehabilitation treatment. In statistics assembled by the National Board of Health and Welfare, the Uppsala region (total population, 1.25 million) had about 20,000 hospital stays with a diagnosis of myocardial infarction between 1964 and 1970. This indicates that heart infarction is one of the most common illnesses in Sweden.

Patients with myocardial infarction were chosen as a study for this Congress report because of radical changes in treatment during the past 10 years. The former treatment of infarct patients was very conservative. The patient had to stay in bed for seven weeks, compared with today's ten days at the ward department and only 2-3 days in bed. The patient was overprotected, forbidden to participate in his regular daily activities while the long period of bedrest increased the risks of thrombosis, contractions and bedsores. Today, training starts at the ward department only 2 days after the attack; six weeks after the heart infarct occurred, the patient starts rehabilitation and physical training at the Physiotherapy Department as an outpatient.

Myocardial infarction and the following period of convalescense make many patients anxious and desperate. They often lose their self-confidence and have difficulty in evaluating their own physical capacity. Favorable psychological effects have resulted from regular physical training conducted by a physiotherapist. Such training has been a contributing factor in faster return to work and in reducing sick leave expenses.

Many individuals from this group of 15 patients chose swimming as a sport activity. In this Chapter, one patient's training is followed from its start under strict supervision to the day he was able to manage his sport activity without being supervised by the doctor and the physiotherapist. In this study we call him "Mr. Heart."

Mr. Heart, who was born in 1916, was taken ill with a myocardial infarction January 16, 1976, and was treated at the cardiology ward in the hospital. Rehabilitation and training started at the Physiotherapy Department with a workload test on an electrically braked ergometer monitored by a continuous ECG at the clinical physiological laboratory. The workload test provided a picture of Mr. Heart's condition; preliminary training was individually structured accordingly. After a few workload tests, Mr. Heart joined the other group members, and the training intensity was increased in a varied program. Swimming was one of the activities. It was essential to be certain that Mr. Heart was not afraid of swimming so that his fitness could be improved.

When patients with myocardial infarction are trained in the hydrotherapy pool, the water temperature is lowered from 35°C to 28°C (95°F to 82°F). The higher temperature would increase the heart rate. Telemetric equipment can be used to make sure that the maximum permissible heart rate is not exceeded and that arythmia does not occur. As further security, a doctor is accessible and an oxygen tank and other emergency equipment are immediately available.

In the training period of 30–45 min, interval training system is used. Hydrotherapy exercises are performed first, followed by some sort of water polo, and swimming. During swimming, the patient wears a belt attached to a rope that is tied to the ceiling. Two springs that increase the workload are fastened in the end of the rope. This arrangement is used near the end of the training period, when the physical capacity of the patient has improved.

Mr. Heart and the other members of his group trained twice a week for three months. Workload test on the electrically braked ergometer was administered at the end of the training period; thus the results of the training could be evaluated.

None of the patients suffered any complications caused by the training. All achieved better physical and psychological fitness. After the training period, their self-confidence improved and they were able to continue their training on their own, outside the hospital. The patients in this group who finished their training at the hospital wanted to continue their physical training with swimming, although many of them never participated in any sport activities before they were taken ill.

Today, they swim twice a week outside the hospital program. One of them is Mr. Heart, who is now training in one of the public pools in Uppsala. Many of them are back at work, some fulltime, others part-time.

During regular information meetings with the patients and their relatives, questions arise as to any danger that may be involved in physical training. They are informed that, if they carry on their training as instructed, the risk is minimal. During the 10 years these myocardial infarction patients have been in training, no mortalities have been caused by the training. The feeling of security is the most positive experience the patients have obtained from the training period, and, in addition, they also improve their physical capacities for work and daily living. It must be concluded that swimming and physical training in general are very useful in complementing the rehabilitation of patients with myocardial infarction.

## REFERENCES

Cullhed, I., Smedby, B., and Waern, U. 1975. Inpatients statistics from the Uppsala region. National Board of Health and Welfare.

# Sinoatrial Blockade Development During Underwater Swimming

**J. Rouš and K. Kočnar**

Drinker (1949) and Irving, Scholander, and Grinnell (1941a) were interested in the details of physiology in breathing as related to diving. In studying this phenomenon they also found interesting circulatory changes. In the 19th century, Bert (1870) and Richet (1898) observed an expressive bradycardia during diving as a part of the adaptation mechanisms in water mammals. Particularly conspicuous was the seal (Figure 1), in whom occurred a sudden deceleration of heart rate to values below 10 beats/min and lasting throughout the stay under water. On emerging, the seal's heart returned to its normal rate of about 110 beats/min.

According to Irving, Sholander, and Grinnell (1941a), the stoppage of breath in the whale induces a reflex that stops the blood flow to the muscles, which have a great capacity for work without a continuous oxygen supply. From anaerobic sources, the muscles accumulate an oxygen debt that is repaid after emerging. By the vasodilatation of the cerebral and heart vessels, together with vasoconstrictions in the muscles, blood redistribution occurs and the circulation is limited to the two vitally important organs—the brain and the heart. A sufficient concentration of oxygen remains in the blood and the lungs at the disposal of the brain and the heart for the whole stay under water. The whale's heart rate drops 30 beats/min to values of about 5 beats/min after submerging. This phenomenon has been named "diving reflex."

Several investigations indicate that man has also retained this reflex partially in the course of phylogenesis; with a deep breath and in diving, the vagal heart rate deceleration occurs. (Gross et al., 1976; Williams and Bernauer, 1976). Mocellin (1974) referred to the heart rate deceleration in small children during diving within a discussion of swimming training.

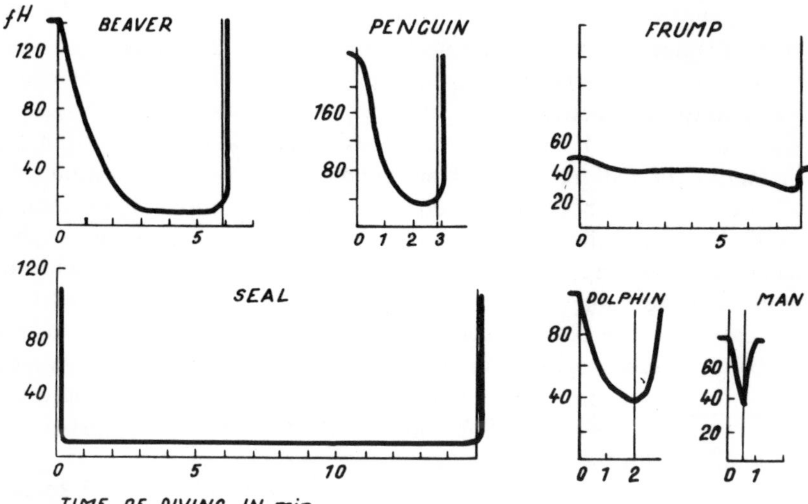


Figure 1. Diving reflexes of various water mammals.

## METHODS

The telemetry of sportsmen in training is a method in general use in research today. We have successfully used telemetry in rowing, cycling, ski running, mountaineering, track and field events, orienteering, canoeing, and in a series of games (Rouš and Kočnar, 1972; Kočnar, 1973).

Swimming belongs to the sport activities in which the researcher experiences many difficulties in utilizing telemetry in relation to the movement of a swimmer in an aquatic medium. An attempt has been made, however, to adapt the telemetric method to the conditions of the sport of swimming.

There is relatively little experience with radio wave propagation from the environment of water to that of air. Ultra-short waves of 56 and 57 MHz were utilized and it was found that the range of the transmitter encased in the caisson at a depth of 2 m during swimming has not been limiting in any way. Antennas that are commonly used over short distances are employed. There is a car antenna on the receiving side, and a soft wire antenna is used on the transmitting side. To achieve a good output from the transmitting antenna, it is necessary that the antenna float on the surface of the pool and that it not come into contact with the swimmer's body. This is achieved by using a polystyrene plate at the end of the antenna during swimming. The location of the transmitter must be such that it does not interfere with the swimmer's motions. Of the generally used locations for the transmitter telemetry, the position at the low part of the back has proven to be the best. It is necessary to secure perfect packing for the transmitter. It is placed in a small and light caisson from which the antenna and conductors rise to the electrodes.

Sintered $AgCl_2$ electrodes are used with adhesive rings from the Siemens firm. Differences have not been found between the swimmers' telemetry and the normal telemetry under dry conditions. In swimming itself, however, the turbulence of the water has been so great that mechanical tearing of the cables from the electrodes has occurred. Attaching the cables to the swimmer's body has failed, but affixing the cables to the bathing suit has provided a better solution to this problem. Therefore, in telemetry, girls' suits are worn by both women and men. The swimmers start in the water, without the racing dive. No swimming style, including somersaults and turns, has caused any difficulties with the telemetry.

Following swimmers telemetrically has worked with the Czechoslovak equipment, Teltest, placed in a small ambulance car that brings the receiver into close proximity with the pool. The equipment has a maximal range of 2.5 km and the transmitter a weight of 250 g. On the receiving side there are: a running signal check on the oscilloscope; an instantaneous automatic evaluation of the actual integrated heart rate; a simultaneous line record of the curve of the heart rate: a counter executing the summation of the pulse over each minute; an ECG recorder with the ability to provide an instantaneous record on paper of the trace on the oscilloscope; and a recording of the ECG curve. Simultaneously , a voice commentary on the training events may be recorded on the Tesla double-sound-track tape recorder, which provides for a permanent record that can be played back later and analyzed at the laboratory. The entire system allows for automatic storage for subsequent evaluation. The heart rate is secured by the electronic logic, thus removing possible artifacts.

## RESULTS

After seven repetitions of the 100 m freestyle with a pause of three expirations, the swimmer's heart rate was about 195–200 beats/min. After finishing the whole series, during a 30-sec pause the heart rate returns quickly to 150 beats/min. The next occasion of 100 m slow swimming resulted in a heart rate of about 150 beats/min.

When swimming under the water while holding one's breath, the situation is different. The so-called "diving-reflex" is usually encountered in this situation. In submerging and swimming under water, after having taken a deep breath, a sudden decrease in the heart rate to 90–110 beats/min occurs; after emerging from the water, the heart rate rapidly increases to 135–147 beats/min. During the course of a calm rest period at the edge of the swimming pool, the heart rate decreases in 30 sec to 140 beats/min (Figure 2). This phenomenon was very consistent and was repeated with only slight variations in values during each submergence. Therefore, the "diving reflex" is a physiological phenomenon in man.

A dangerous situation could occur in cases of extreme vagal reaction to the diving reflex. Such an extreme excitability of the vagus nerve may provoke an extreme deceleration of the heart rate and may even induce short-term asystole leading to short-term faintness. The hazard of drowning because of such vagal reaction is evident. It is a matter of a similar situation occurring in an atrioventricular block in which, after transition to the third degree, the Adams-Stokes syndrome develops. The high excitability of the vagus nerve can lead to a large deceleration in the automatism of the sinoatrial knot, a condition commonly in evidence during the rest period after extreme physical exertion.

Following are two examples of such a vagal expressive excitation in which the diving reflex could be associated with the development of

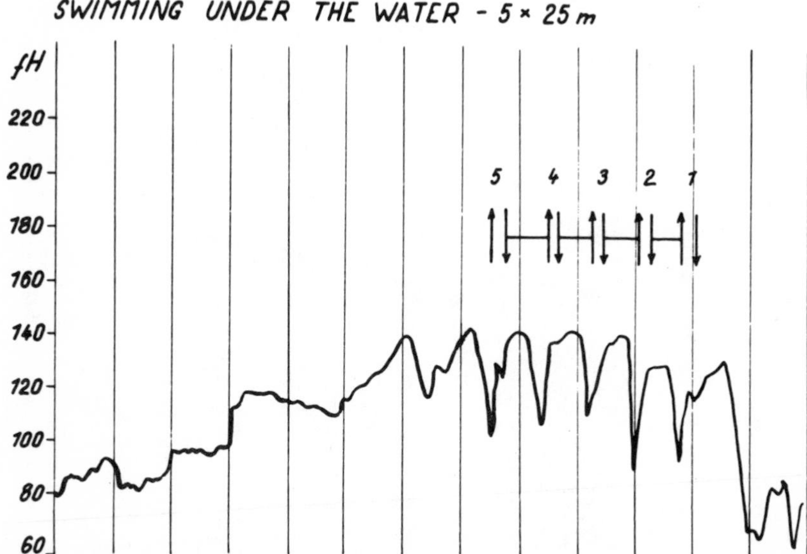


Figure 2. Diving reflex in man during underwater swimming shows the sudden decrease of the heart rate during the diving.

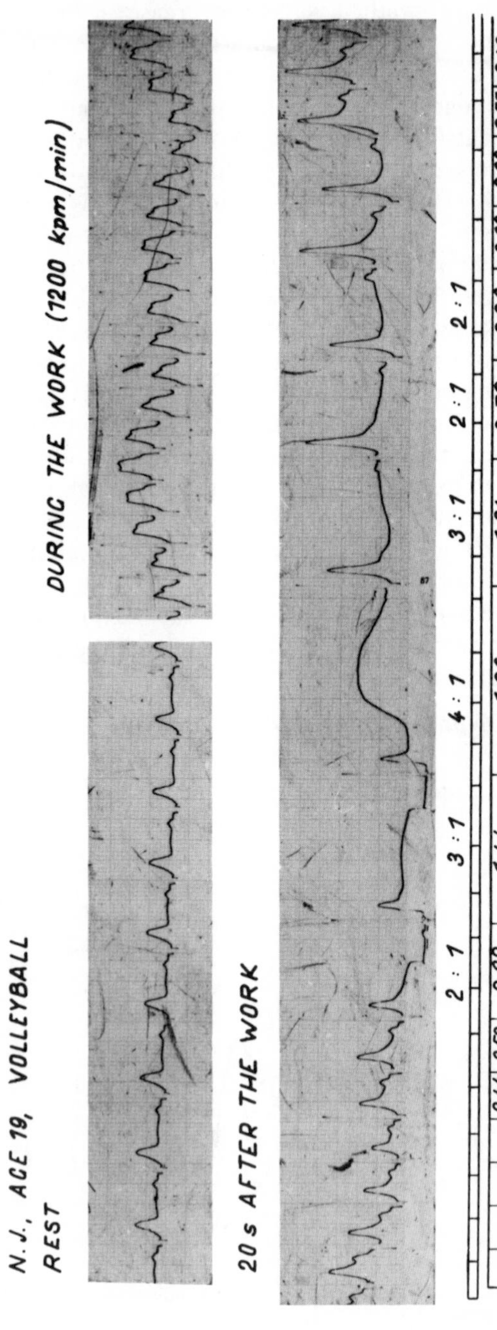


Figure 3. Occurrence of sinoatrial blockade in a volleyball player during 20 sec rest after a workout.

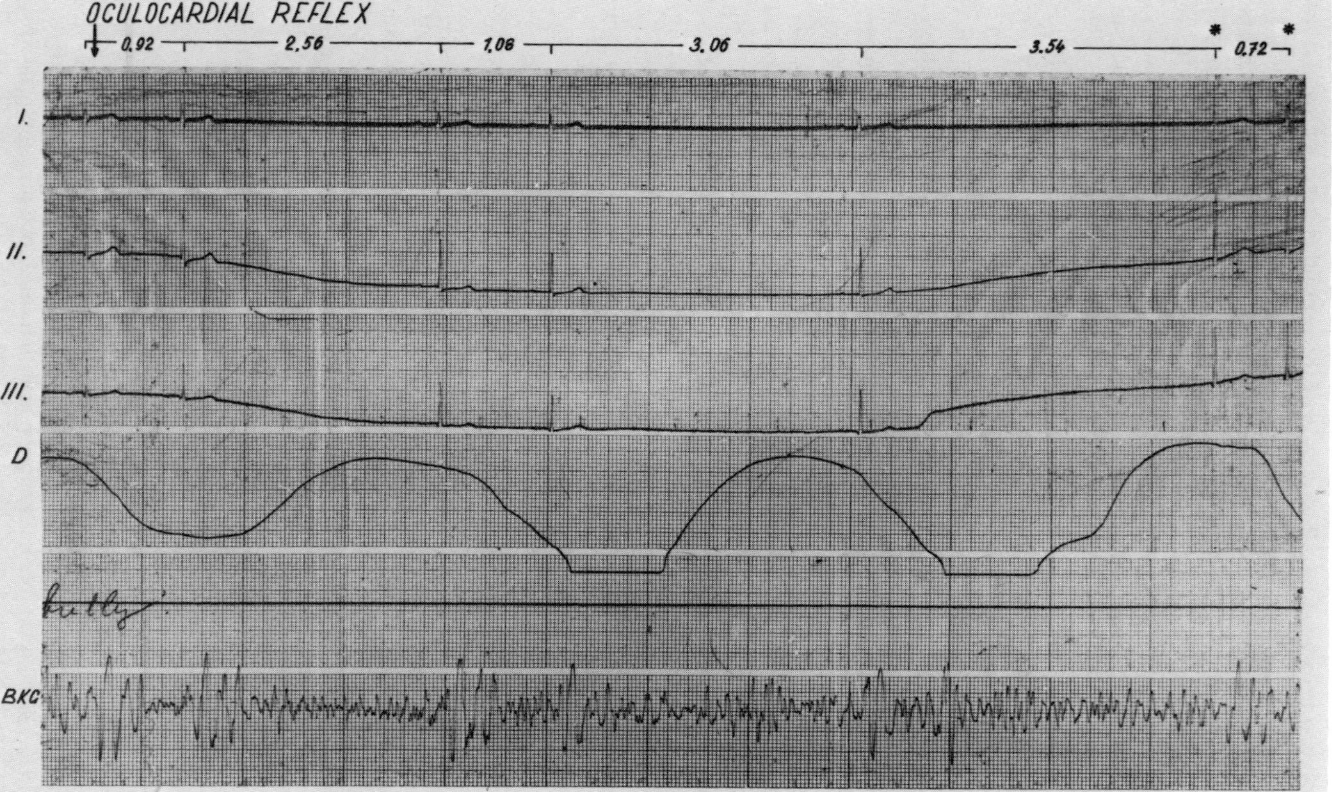


Figure 4. This figure shows a sinoatrial blockade of the third degree during the oculocardial reflex of an oarsman.

a short-term syncope and the danger of drowning. In a volleyball player, a heavy sinoatrial blockade of the second degree occurred during the rest period following a workout. Because of a sudden vagal intervention after a 2:1 blockade, a further failure of the heartbeats occurred, from 3:1 to 4:1, with a successive, gradual return to normal rhythm (Figure 3). It was analogous to the Wenckebach's periods in the atrioventricular blockade. With respect to rheumatic fever in history, a possible sinoatrial knot lesion should be considered. The sinoatrial blockade is perhaps a symptom of the "sick" sinal syndrome.

The SA blockades of the third degree are disproportionately infrequent and are usually pathological. They can develop for a short time, even with uneffected SA knots because of vagal maneuvers. In a 23 year old oarsman with a normal ECG at rest even after exertion, SA blockade of the third degree occurred because of a vagal maneuver, with a transition to a compensatory slow junctial rhythm (Figure 4). With the Valsava's maneuver and a simultaneous pressure on the eyeballs, a 3–4 sec asystole appears.

These examples are evidence of the fact that individuals with extreme vagal excitability exist. This is a cause of SA blockades of all degrees with expressively decelerated heart rate after a deep breath and with an accompanying increase in the intrathoracic pressure (Valsava's maneuver). With the third degree blockade resulting in a delayed start of compensatory rhythm, a short-term faintness may occur that could result in drowning if the swimmer were underwater at the time.

## CONCLUSION

For those individuals interested in scuba diving, a test of their vegetative, and especially, their vagal excitability is recommended. It is advantageous to follow the ECG curve in deep inspiration with the Valsava's maneuver, with a massage of the glomus caroticum and with the oculocardial reflex. Individuals with extremely high excitability of the vagus nerve should abandon scuba diving activity because of the potential risk involved.

## REFERENCES

Bert, P. 1870. In: V. Kruta (ed.), 1958. Some Aspects of Comparative Physiology of the Heart and Circulation. St. Zdrav. Nakl., Praha.

Drinker, C. K. 1949. The physiology of whales. Sci. Am. 7:52–55.

Gross, P. M., Whipp, B. J., Davidson, I. T., Koyal, S. N., and Wasserman, K. 1976. Chemoreceptors' influence on heart rate and blood pressure responses to breath holding in man. Med. Sci. Sports 8(1):63.

Irving, L., Scholander, P. F., and Grinnell, S. W. 1941a. Significance of heart rate to diving ability of seals. J. Cell. Comp. Physiol. 18:283–297.

Irving, L., Scholander, P. F., and Grinnell, S. W. 1941b. The respiration of the porpoise, tursiops truncatus. J. Cell. Comp. Physiol. 18:145–168.

Kočnar, K. 1973. Radiotelemetry in cycling. Cycling and Health, pp. 70–75. °Sport, Bratislava.

Kruta, V. (ed.) 1958. Some Aspects of Comparative Physiology of the Heart and Circulation. St. Zdrav. Nakl., Praha.

Mocellin, R. 1974. Swimming and diving in 3–10 year old boys and girls. Paper presented at the 6th International Symposium on Pediatric Work Physiology, June 13, Seč, Czechoslovakia.

Richet, C. 1898. In: V. Kruta (ed.), 1958. Some Aspects of Comparative Physiology of the Heart and Circulation. St. Zdrav. Nakl., Praha.

Rouš, J., and Kočnar, K. 1972. Telemetric measurements during sports performances of sportsmen with cardiac arrhythmias. In: Biotelemetry, pp. 256–263. Meander, Leiden.

Williams, C. I., and Bernauer, E. M. 1976. Diving reflex during exercise in man. Med. Sci. Sports 8(1):63–64.

# Comparison of LH and FSH Concentrations in Age Group Swimmers, Moderately Active Girls, and Adult Women

**A. Bonen, A. N. Belcastro, A. A. Simpson, and W. Ling**

The effect of athletic training on the human menstrual cycle has been of interest to both researcher and clinician, particularly during the past decade when training programs have become extremely rigorous. Unfortunately, little quantitative data are available; most of the information is anecdotal or was obtained via recall questionnaires (Zaharieva, 1965) in which the perceived incidences of menstrual cycle irregularities and/or disorders were recorded. Thus, while some clinicians have speculated that sports have a favorable effect on dysmenorrhea (Åstrand et al., 1963; Erdelyi, 1976), others suggested that athletes in endurance sports experience more menstrual disorders such as amenorrhea, oligomenorrhea, scanty menstrual flow, or completely irregular periods. It is also thought that swimmers may experience a greater incidence of dysmenorrhea than sedentary women (Erdelyi, 1976). It was reported that the menstrual cycles of female rowers were irregular or completely absent during training, but that they reverted to normal patterns during the off-season (Erdelyi, 1976).

Irregularities in menstrual cycles should be reflected in alterations of circulating hormonal concentrations because the menstrual cycle is regulated by the complex interaction of luteinizing hormone (LH), follicle-stimulating hormone (FSH), progesterone, and 17$\beta$-estradiol, and their releasing factors. In adult women, the patterns of change of these circulating hormones are well documented (Page, Villee, and Villee, 1972; Miyake, 1974). Thus, it is known that normal menstrual bleeding occurs when the progesterone support of the endometrium is withdrawn, but dysfunctional bleeding occurs in response to disturbances in the normal hormonal secretions (Vorys, Neri, and Boutselis,

1975). In addition, a chronically short luteal phase (< 10 days) is associated with a deficiency in the circulating level of FSH and a reduced FSH/LH ratio throughout the menstrual cycle (Strott et al., 1970; Sherman and Korenman, 1974; Dodson, MacNaughton, and Coutts, 1975).

There is some evidence to suggest that strenuous exercise may increase the circulating menstrual cycle hormones. Bonen et al. (in preparation) and Hall et al. (1975) showed that strenuous exercise can increase the concentrations of progesterone and estradiol in untrained women. However, in one study these increases were not observed after an 8–11 week training program (Bonen et al., in preparation). On the other hand, Sutton et al. (1973) found a 19% increase in the 17β-hydroxysteroid concentrations after 2-hr swimming workouts in 13–15 year old girl swimmers.

To determine whether strenuous swimming training programs have a persistent effect on some of the circulating menstrual cycle hormones, the resting concentrations of LH and FSH were measured daily during one complete menstrual cycle in young swimmers. In addition, these results were compared with those of an age-matched control group and those of a group of fertile, adult women.

## METHOD

Four teenage swimmers (age: 15–19 years; height: 161–168 cm; weight: 56.6–66.3 kg) participated in this study. These girls had been training for 3–6 years, 2–3 hrs per day, 6 days per week.

Prior to this study, each girl was examined by a gynecologist and was identified as having normal menstrual function for her age group, with freedom from complications and medical treatment. Menarche had occurred two to four years earlier in all subjects. Two subjects had occasionally been amenorrheaic.

From the day of onset of menses, blood samples (15 ml) were obtained daily at rest, from a forearm vein, for one complete menstrual cycle. The samples were allowed to clot for 1 hr; the serum was then divided into appropriate aliquots for the various assays and these aliquots were stored at −20°C.

For purposes of comparison, blood specimens were also collected from sedentary, healthy adult women. They had had regular menstrual cycles 26–34 days in length during the preceding year, were taking no medication, and were within the normal weight range.

Data were also obtained from four moderately active young students (age: 16–18 years; height: 156.5–172.5 cm; weight: 43.8–61.0 kg) who were selected to match, approximately, the gynecological age of the swimmers. Menarche had occurred 1–5 years previously in this control group. Blood samples were again obtained daily for one complete menstrual cycle and were treated and stored as described above.

For the radioimmunoassay of FSH and LH in serum of the swimmers and adult women, the standards, antibodies, and purified hormones for iodination were obtained as assay kits (Calbiochem, La Jolla, California). LER-907 (20 mIU FSH/ml; 48 mIU LH/ml) as granted by the National Institute of Arthritis, Metabolism and Digestive Diseases (NIAMDD) was used as a reference preparation (Albert et al., 1968). For samples from the teenage control group, the FSH and LH assays were based on a modified procedure described by Midgley (1966). Antisera for LH and FSH were obtained from Calbiochem and the standards were provided by WHO.

All data were expressed in terms relative to the day of the LH peak (Day 0): the days prior to the LH peak (follicular phase) were labelled negatively, and the days after the LH peak (luteal phase) were labelled positively. Data from Days −12 to +12 were used in this study. Hormone concentrations were compared against those of the adult women with the Mann-Whitney $U$ test (Siegel, 1956).

## RESULTS

Data were initially obtained only from the swimmers and the adult women, but because there were considerable differences in the durations of the menstrual cycles and the gonadotropin patterns of these two groups, further data were obtained from four other teenage subjects who were moderately active. In the swimmers, menarche had occurred 2, 2.5, 3 and 4 years earlier, and 1, 2.5, 4 and 5 years earlier, in the control group.

The menstrual cycle of the swimmers, 20.0 ± 1.8 days, was significantly shorter than that in the adults, 28.5 ± 3.4 days, ($P \leq 0.05$). This difference was attributable to the short luteal phase of 4.5 ± 0.3 days in the swimmers as compared with that in the adults of 13.5 ± 1.7 days, ($P \leq 0.05$). In the teenage control group, the duration of the menstrual cycle, 29.7 ± 4.4 days ($P > 0.05$), was similar to that of the adults, but three control subjects had a short luteal phase, 7.0 ± 0.6 days. This was slightly longer than the luteal phase duration in the swimmers ($P \leq 0.05$).

Gonadotropin comparisons were made among the adults, and the swimmers and control subjects ($N = 3$) with a short luteal phase. The concentrations ($\bar{X}$ ± 1SD) of LH and FSH during the normal adult menstrual cycle are illustrated in Figure 1. In Figure 2 the LH and FSH profiles of the swimmers are compared with those of the adults, and

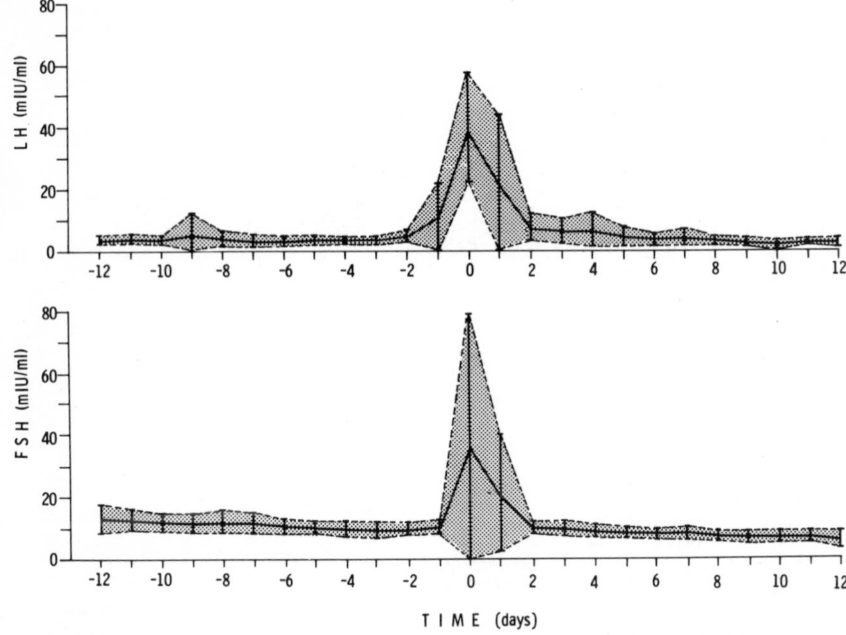


Figure 1. Serum concentrations ($\bar{X} \pm 1SD$) of LH and FSH during the menstrual cycle of normal adult women are illustrated. The cycle is centered on the day of the LH peak.

the FSH/LH ratios are compared in Figure 3. The LH pattern of the swimmers during the follicular phase prior to the LH peak was normal, but the average concentrations were higher than in the control group and the adult women ($P < 0.05$, Figure 4). Peak LH concentrations and early luteal phase LH concentrations were slightly lower in the swimmers and the control group than in the adults, but these differences were not significant ($P > 0.05$, Figure 4).

Surprisingly, the characteristic midcycle FSH peak was not observed in any of the swimmers; their FSH concentrations remained at basal levels throughout the cycle (Figure 2). In contrast, the FSH peak did occur in the control and adult groups. The concentrations of FSH peaks in these two groups were not significantly different from each other ($P > 0.05$), but they were significantly greater than the FSH concentrations of the swimmers ($P \leqslant 0.05$) on the same day (Figure 4). During the midfollicular and early luteal phases, FSH levels were greater in the control group and in the adults than in the swimmers ($P \leqslant 0.05$, Figure 4).

During the follicular phase, the FSH/LH ratio in the swimmers was significantly lower (Figure 3) than in the adult women and in the control group ($P \leqslant 0.05$, Figure 4). This also occurred on Day 0,

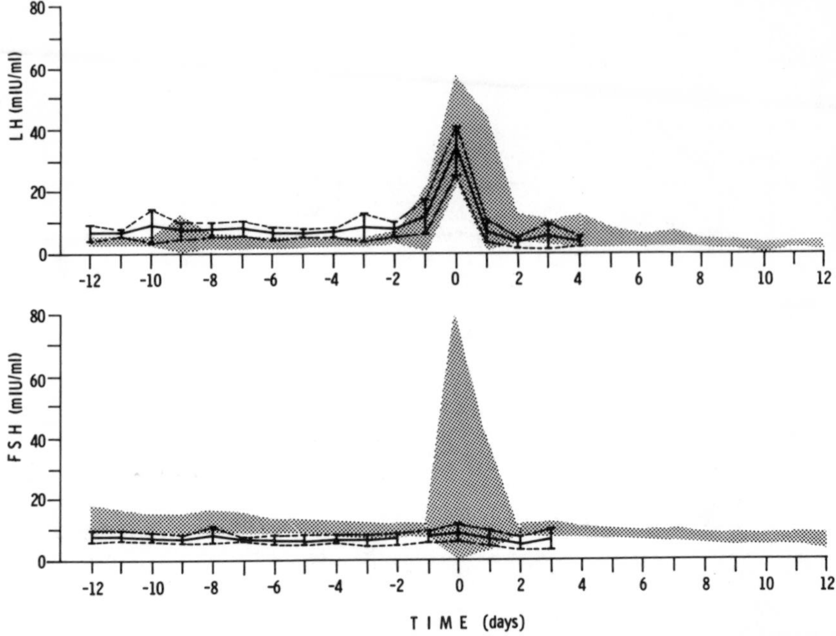


Figure 2. This shows comparison of serum concentrations ($\bar{X}$ ±1SD) of LH and FSH in four swimmers with those of adult women. The cycle is centered on the day of the LH peak. Gray area represents ±1SD of the normal adult.

but thereafter, during the early luteal phase, the FSH/LH ratios for the three groups were not different ($P > 0.05$, Figure 4).

## DISCUSSION

The elevated LH and depressed FSH concentrations in the four swimmers were very similar to those reported by Strott et al. (1970) for sedentary young women with short luteal phases. In this study, however, only the swimmers, and not the age-matched control group, had these FSH and LH imbalances. The absence of the characteristic FSH peak in swimmers was observed in mature rhesus monkeys with short luteal phases (Wilks, Hodgen, and Ross, 1976), but was not found in other studies with human subjects (Strott et al., 1970; Sherman and Korenman, 1974; Dodson, MacNaughton, and Coutts, 1975). Because a menstrual cycle with a short luteal phase is also characterized by low levels of estradiol during the follicular and the luteal phases (Sherman and Korenman, 1974; Dodson, MacNaughton, and Coutts, 1975; Wilks, Hodgen, and Ross, 1976), this strongly suggests that the corpus luteum is not functioning optimally.

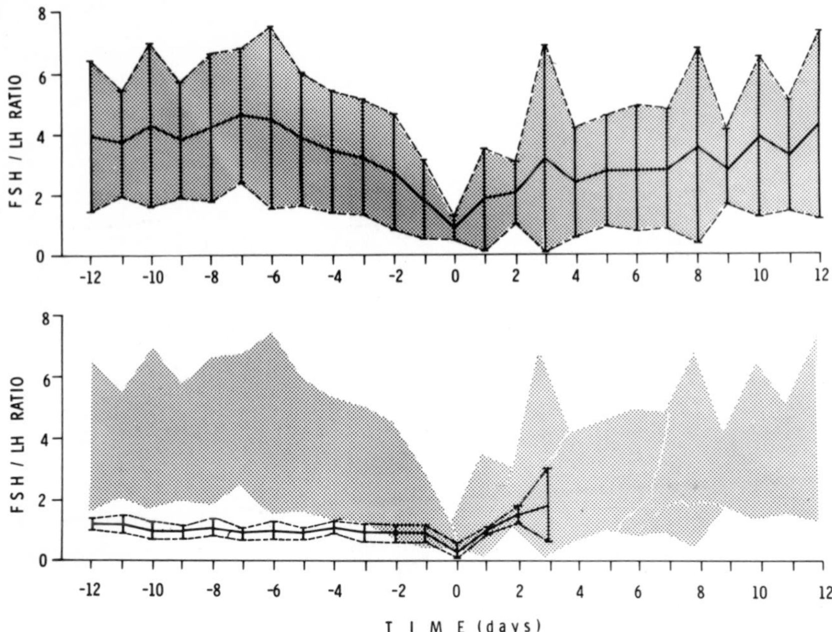


Figure 3. A comparison of the FSH/LH ratio in the adult group (upper panel) and four swimmers ($\bar{X}$ ±1SD) (lower panel) is given. Gray area represents ±1SD of the normal cycle.

Strott et al. (1970) have proposed that the origin of the short luteal phase should be sought in the hormonal events before ovulation. Because the gonadotropin levels in these cycles are abnormal, it has been suggested that the deficiency in FSH and its imbalance with LH during the follicular phase may be responsible for the improper follicular growth and maturation as reflected by the reduced luteal phase progesterone and 17 $\alpha$ hydroxyprogesterone concentrations (Sherman and Korenman, 1974; Dodson, MacNaughton, and Coutts, 1975; Wilks, Hodgen, and Ross, 1976). This hypothesis is well founded because luteal gonadotropin stimulation will not yield a normal luteal function if the FSH stimulation of the corresponding follicle has been suboptimal (Jones et al., 1969); and human granulosa cells achieve maximal progesterone production, in vitro, only after prolonged exposure to estradiol and FSH and after a simulated LH surge (McNalty and Sawers, 1975). Therefore, it is possible that the premature onset of menses in the swimmers may be precipitated by low levels of progesterone secreted from the corpus luteum. The origin of this problem occurs during the follicular phase, when the FSH levels and/or the FSH/LH ratios are insufficient to stimulate the development of a normal follicle to maturity.

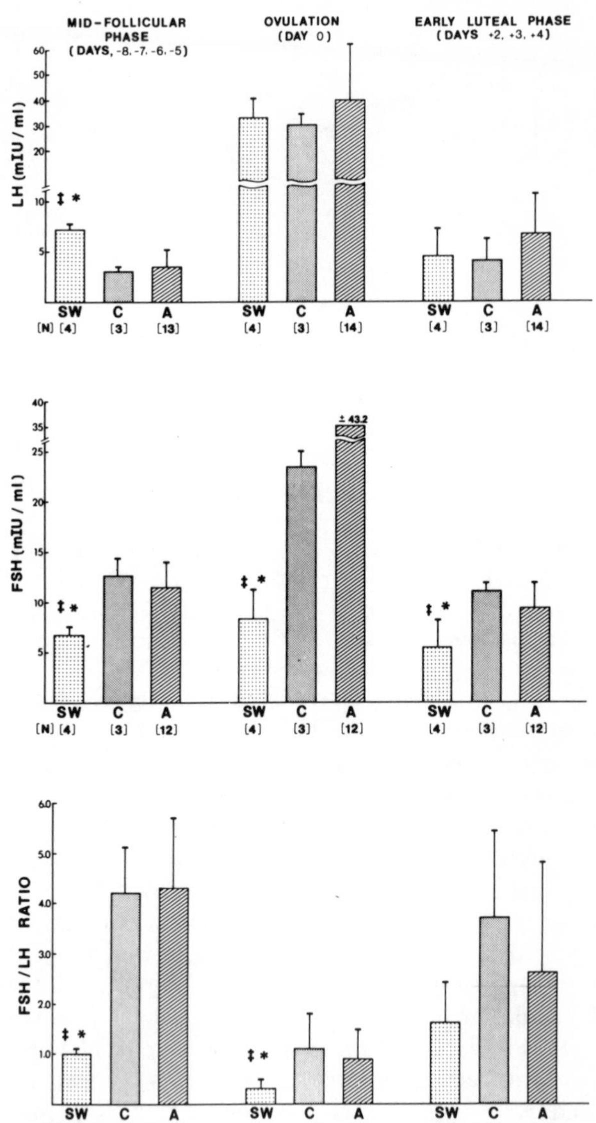


Figure 4. This figure compares the LH and FSH concentrations and the FSH/LH ratio during the midfollicular phase (Days −8 to −5), the day of the LH peak, and the early luteal phase (Days +2 to +4) in swimmers (SW), the control group (C), and adult women (A), Symbols: ‡, significantly different from adult data, $P \leq 0.05$; *, significantly different from teenage control group, $P \leq 0.05$).

The incidence of a short luteal phase seems to be age-related: this occurred in all of our young swimmers and in three of four teenage girls in the control group. In addition, there were two short luteal phases in the sample of 28 sedentary women (18–30 years). These occurred in the two youngest subjects (Bonen et al., in preparation). Similarly, Strott et al. (1970) found that the short luteal phases occurred in their youngest subjects. Among 155 fertile women investigated by Marshall (1963), a short luteal phase, determined from basal body temperatures, occurred in 9% of 1,088 menstrual cycles. With similar procedures, Collett, Wertenberger, and Fiske (1954) found that a short luteal phase (< 10 days) occurred in 17.8% of the menstrual cycles of 46 subjects 17–19 years of age. This incidence declined to 4.5% in 25–34 year old subjects, and increased again in older age groups. In two young girls (1 month and 1 year postmenarchial), Hayes and Johanson (1972) observed five short luteal phases in six menstrual cycles. Because the swimmers in this chapter's study were quite young (15, 15, 16, 19 yrs.), it may be quite normal for these girls to experience abbreviated luteal phases. Certainly, at their ages, these phenomena should probably not be considered abnormal. The differences in FSH concentrations in the swimmers and the control group remain interesting because depressed FSH levels in trained subjects have been observed after 30 min. of bicycle ergometer exercise (Bonen et al., in preparation). Thus, whether regular intense training programs could lead to depressed FSH levels remains to be investigated.

## ACKNOWLEDGMENTS

We thank Mr. Nigel Kemp, Coach of the Halifax Trojan Aquatic Club, for his cooperation in this study, and the swimmers and other subjects who participated willingly in this investigation.

## REFERENCES

Albert, A., Rosemberg, E., Ross, G. T., Paulsen, C. A., and Ryan, R. J. 1968. Report of the National Pituitary Agency collaborative study on the radioimmunoassay of FSH and LH. J. Clin. Endocrinol. Metab. 28:1214–1219.

Åstrand, P. -O., Engström, L., Eriksson, B., Karlberg, P., Nylander, I., Saltin, B., and Thorén, C. 1963. Girl swimmers: With special reference to respiratory and circulatory adaptation and gynecological and psychiatric aspects. Acta Paediatr. Scand. (suppl. 147):43–63.

Bonen, A., Ling, W., MacIntyre, K., Neil, R., and McGrail, J. C. 1977. Menstrual cycle hormone responses to exercise. In preparation.

Collett, M. E., Wertenberger, G. E., and Fiske, V. M. 1954. The effect of age upon the pattern of the menstrual cycle. Fertil. Steril. 5:437–448.

Dodson, K. S., MacNaughton, M. C., and Coutts, J. R. T. 1975. Infertility in women with apparently ovulatory cycles. I. Comparison of their plasma sex steroid and gonadotropin profiles with those in the normal cycle. Br. J. Obstet. Gynaecol. 83:615–624.

Erdelyi, G. J. 1976. Effects of exercise on the menstrual cycle. Phys. Sportsmed. 4:79–81.

Hall, J. E., Younglai, E. V., Walker, C., Jones, N. L., and Sutton, J. R. 1975. Ovarian hormonal response to exercise (Abstr.) Med. Sci. Sports 7:65.

Hayes, A., and Johanson, A. 1972. Excretion of follicle-stimulating hormone (FSH) and luteinizing hormone (LH) in urine by pubertal girls. Pediatr. Res. 6:18–25.

Jones, G. S., de Mordea-Ruehsen, M., Johanson, A. J., Salvatori, R., and Blizzard, R. M. 1969. Elucidation of normal ovarian physiology by exogenous gonadotropin stimulation following steroid pituitary suppression. Fertil. Steril. 20:14–34.

Marshall, J. 1963. Thermal changes in the normal menstrual cycle. Br. Med. J. 1:102–104.

McNalty, K. P., and Sawers, R. S. 1975. Relationship between the endocrine environment within the Graafian follicle and the subsequent rate of progesterone secretion by human granulosa cells in vitro. J. Endocrinol. 66:391–400.

Midgley, A. R. 1966. Radioimmunoassay: A method for human chorionic gonadotropin and luteinizing hormone. Endocrinol. 79:10–18.

Miyake, T. 1974. Blood concentration and interplay of pituitary and gonadal hormones governing the reproductive cycle in female mammals. In: R. O. Greep (ed.), Reproductive Physiology. MTP International Review of Science, Series 1, Vol. 8, p. 155. University Park Press, Baltimore.

Page, E. W., Villee, C. A., and Villee, D. B. 1972. Human Reproduction, p. 44. W. B. Saunders Co., Toronto.

Sherman, B. M., and Korenman, S. G. 1974. Measurement of plasma LH, FSH, estradiol and progesterone in disorders of the human menstrual cycle: The short luteal phase. J. Clin. Endocrinol. Metab. 38:88–94.

Siegel, S. 1956. Nonparametric Statistics for the Behavioral Sciences, pp. 116–127. McGraw-Hill Book Company, Toronto.

Strott, C. A., Cargille, C. M., Ross, G. T., and Lipsett, M. B. 1970. The short luteal phase. J. Clin. Endocrinol. Metab. 30:246–251.

Sutton, J. R., Coleman, M. J., Casey, J. and Lazarus, L. 1973. Androgen responses during physical exercise. Br. Med. J. 1:520–522.

Vorys, N., Neri, S., and Boutselis, J. G. 1975. Menstrual dysfunction. In: J. J. Gold (ed.), Gynecologic Endocrinology, pp. 213–244. Harper and Row, Hagerstown, Md.

Wilks, J. W., Hodgen, G. D. and Ross, G. T. 1976. Luteal phase defects in the rhesus monkey: The significance of serum FSH:LH ratios. J. Clin. Endocrinol. Metab. 43:1261–1267.

Zaharieva, E. 1965. Survey of sports women at the Tokyo Olympics. J. Sports Med. Phys. Fit. 5:215–219.

# Earaches and Adolescent Swimmers

**N. Roydhouse**

Earache is a common complaint among children; in a controlled study of adenotonsillectomy, earache occurred in 36% of the normal children, aged 2–12 years (Roydhouse, 1969). The most common causes of earache in such children are infections and disorders of the middle ear. After this age, there are other causes of earache, but these are often not recognized. Because many swimmers belong to this 2–12 year old group, the general practitioner tends to consider earache in the adolescent as he would consider earache in the child. Whether or not these doctors realize the exact mechanism with which water sports affect the protected middle ear, their general attitude in dealing with adolescents is to tell them to stay out of the water and even to give up swimming altogether. It is possible to make anyone's ears suitable for swimming and, with few exceptions, for scuba diving as well (Roydhouse, 1970a).

## HISTORIES

The case histories of 12 adolescent swimmers whose complaints were earaches were taken from the records and analyzed. Table 1 shows age and sex distribution of these subjects. The details of some cases are quoted and the overall symptoms and signs are tabulated.

### Case History 10: Female, 12 years

A 12 year old girl who liked competitive swimming because she said "I am good at it," had been seen by an ear surgeon because of recurrent earaches; he had said that he could find no abnormality but that she should give up swimming. No audiometry was performed. A second opinion and clinical examination showed small adenoids, retracted eardrums because of spasm of the tensor tympani, and a clicking right

Table 1. Age/sex distribution of 12 adolescent swimmers seen because of earache

| Age (years) | Female | Male | Total |
|---|---|---|---|
| 10–12 | 2 | 1 | 3 |
| 13–14 | 5 | 1 | 6 |
| 16–18 | 2 | 1 | 3 |

tempromandibular joint. Her earaches began within a few minutes of her entering unheated pools, but not in heated pools, although they also occurred at other times. The earaches were clearly related to exposure to cold and not to any form of infection; therefore, the opinion was that, because the earaches would have no effect on her hearing, she should continue to swim, and, if she kept herself protected from the cold, the earaches would occur less frequently.

The follow-up came 18 months later in a letter from her family doctor. It said:

> The lassie you saw with earache no longer comes to me as a patient. After consultation with you she continued to have earaches. She changed doctors and was given ear drops which cured her. It is significant that the child, although she has continued to swim in competition no longer has a coach, swims more or less at will. I have always been of the opinion that the child had a large psychosomatic element to her earaches. I think the child was being pushed beyond her desire. Brian Corrigan (a Sydney Sports Medicine Specialist) has found children who do a lot of training usually get abdominal pain, this one got earache.

### Case History 12: Female, 16 years

This is an example of the more acute earache. The participant arrived three days early at the New Zealand National Swimming Championships for intensive practice, but she developed an earache after an hour and a half air flight to the venue. She had a history of intermittent left earaches for the previous several months; this bout was slightly worse than she had had previously. She was taken by the team manager to a general practitioner who diagnosed an abscess in the middle ear although she did not complain of deafness nor was her hearing tested. Antibiotics were prescribed and she was told not to swim. There was no change in her condition, so although she missed practices, she ignored medical advice and swam in her three events, not winning but performing up to her standard.

Three days later her ears were examined intensively with an operating microscope. A full range of hearing tests was done, including measurements of the middle ear pressures and reflex contractions of the middle ear muscles. All tests showed normal results although she still had some earache. These tests were sufficient to exclude any infectious condition within the last 9 days, including the time she was under treatment for the abscess in the middle ear. Dentally she had some gaps because of removal of milk dentition, and there was undue wear showing on her incisor teeth, indicating excessive grinding of teeth. Within 10 days and with no treatment other than reassurance, and with continuing competitive swimming, her earache gradually subsided.

### Case History 11: Female, 13 years

Case 11, a competitive swimmer since September 1971, developed an earache in March 1972 at the age of 13. In April 1972, her tonsils and adenoids were removed, her nose cauterized, and her eardrums opened. Because the earache continued, she was told to give up swimming. When she was seen for the first time in November 1972, her second molars were erupting and she often complained of sore ears that became painful at times after swimming. She also had orthodontic problems. In August 1975, at 16, she was still getting sore ears at times, relieved by reducing training and also by taking 5 mg of Librium at bedtime.

Psychological problems probably existed in Case 10 (already described) and in Case 14, patient who had headaches and a history of grinding her teeth and of biting her nails.

External otitis is common in competitive swimmers and occurred in at least five of the swimmers, but it did not cause earache in any of the five. There was minor discharge from the ears and itchiness. Many of the swimmers used eardrops regularly to prevent this disorder from occurring. Table 2 shows the main symptoms of complaint other than earache. In a search for an obvious cause for the earache, the conditions listed in Table 3 were found.

## DISCUSSION

All these cases of referred sensations belong to the Mandibular Dysfunction Syndrome. Disorders of the molar teeth or excessive use of the jaw muscles as in grinding and clenching the teeth can result in all the complaints listed in Table 2.

Table 2. Symptoms other than earache

| Symptom | Number |
|---|---|
| Itching ears | 4 |
| Noises in ear | 3 |
| Ear discharge | 4 |
| Headaches | 1 |
| Deafness | 0 |

Table 3. Primary disorders discovered

| | |
|---|---|
| History of grinding teeth | 4 |
| Erupting molar teeth | 4 |
| Impacted molar teeth | 2 |
| Psychological background | 2 |
| No obvious cause | 2 |

It is clear that the earaches described were referred pains in view of the lack of signs of any middle ear disorder, as verified by operation microscope study, normal pure tone audiograms, and normal impedance audiometry. It is commonly known that impacted molar teeth and erupting molar teeth can cause earache, but in the cases cited the original examiner usually failed to discern these conditions. There is no excuse for failing to see partly erupted teeth, especially as the second molars erupt normally at about 12 years of age. Impacted and unerupted molar teeth are not visible, but the panoramic x-ray shows them clearly. If there are no ear signs and especially if there are other ear symptoms (see Table 2), such an x-ray is justified.

One of the features of this type of earache is its onset on exposure to cold water. This occurred as a complaint in five cases, one of whom volunteered the information that no earache occurred after swimming in a heated pool. Once out of the cold, the earaches subsided. It is well known that muscle pains occur with or are aggravated by exposure to cold. In these cases, spasm or overuse of the temporalis muscle produced the pain on exposure to cold.

Nocturnal earache can arise from grinding and clenching of the teeth. With infections it is unusual for the earache to come and go under such conditions. Table 2 shows that no patient complained of deafness as a recent accompaniment of the earache, although Case 12 had had deafness and earache in a bout of what was likely to have been an abscess in the ear 4 months prior to her examination. The prime sign of disease is loss of function, and there can be no middle ear disease of any significance without some measureable degree of hearing loss.

Some subjects complain of a blockage felt in the ear; this must be distinguished from deafness. In fact, in the Mandibular Dysfunction Syndrome, some patients strongly complain of deafness although pure tone audiometry shows normal acute hearing for the speech frequencies. In this disorder, spasm of the muscle tensing the eardrum from inside, the tensor tympani muscle, causes this symptom. This spasm gives a visible alteration of the shape of the eardrum, causes a tone deafness in notes below the speech frequencies, and can also be responsible for buzzing and ringing in the ears (Roydhouse, 1970b). The other hearing disorders that occur are an undue sensitivity to noise and the feeling of "tunnel hearing."

The itch in the ear or the blocked feeling from the dental disorder results in the swimmer rubbing in or around the ear or even poking objects into the ear. Once the skin is breached, organisms may gain entry and a state of infection or external otitis may occur. This infection in itself causes itching, and further poking can aggravate the condition or prevent recovery.

## PREVENTION

The most important advice that can be given is an explanation of the cause of the earache. Often the reassurance that no damage is occurring to the hearing apparatus disperses anxiety, especially of the patient's parents. The swimmer is then prepared to put up with what is mostly an intermittent discomfort.

Prevention of exposure to the cold can be helpful, either by using a heated pool or by wearing a thick rubber swimming cap. Reduction in or cessation of grinding and clenching of the teeth reduces the subthreshold pain stimulus to the ear so that earache occurs less frequently and is less marked. Once these habits have been shown harmful, some swimmers can give them up. A short course of a sedative such as Librium (5 mg) or Vallergan forte at bedtime with its specific effect on the chewing center can also break the nocturnal habit.

If there is any marked dental disorder, a dental specialist should be consulted. The average dental practitioner is not well versed in this disorder and is most likely to declare that there is nothing wrong with the teeth, so be prepared for his initial rebuff, but persist and request the opinion of a specialist. The panoramic x-ray view of the teeth is used especially in patients over 16 years of age to provide evidence of impacted wisdom teeth.

For the itchy ear, if there is external otitis present, the usual treatment of cleaning and steroid/antibiotic drops can be used. For prevention, 5% Glacial Acetic Acid in SVR or similar preparations should be used. For the persistent itch, whether caused by a dental disorder or a local skin condition, the anti-itch lotion Eurax (Geigy) is very effective.

## CONCLUSION

Earache is erroneously perceived by many doctors as a reason for the adolescent to give up swimming. In the adolescent, middle ear infection is uncommon, especially among trained swimmers, who are taught to breathe out through the nose whenever the head enters the water (Roydhouse, 1970a). Beware of the doctor who wants to operate and seek out the doctor with a sports medicine background or affiliation. The most common causes of earache in adolescents are erupting molar teeth, impacted wisdom teeth, and referred pain from excessive use of the jaw muscles, all aggravated by exposure to cold and by anxiety states.

## REFERENCES

Roydhouse, N. 1969. The effects of tonsils and adenoids on children, ch. 6, p. 106. University Publications, Auckland.

Roydhouse, N. 1970a. The ear and water sports. Aust. J. of Sports Med. 3(4):11–27.

Roydhouse, N. 1970b. In defense of Costen's Syndrome. J. Otolaryngol. Soc. Aust. 3(1):106–114.

# Iron in Young Sportsmen

**L. Ehn, B. Carlmark, and S. Höglund**

To improve performance, top sportsmen of today often consult so-called experts to find support for using drugs, nutritional items, hormones, etc. Medical experts also often act as advisers to the trainers in the planning of the season for the sportsmen.

Iron deficiency has sometimes been reported among athletes, especially in long distance runners and in young female swimmers. In those groups and in cross-country skiers, this deficiency has been looked upon as a possible cause of poor performances. In an attempt to standardize training methods and diets and to support them with possible scientific information, a group of researchers in the Hematological Department at Karolinska Hospital were contacted by Riksidrottsförbundet. This research group had previously performed pilot studies on young military men and on a group of long distance runners.

The purpose of this study was to compare a group of rigorously training young swimmers with a group of long distance runners and a control group of military men of the same age. Initial hematological status was examined in each of the three groups and changes in peripheral blood values were followed continuously.

Thus far, eight runners, whose weight, weekly training, energy, and iron intake have been controlled have been studied. The investigation has progressed over 2 years with a break planned after a total of 5 years (Table 1).

The group of swimmers consists of 11 young boys without prophylactic iron. These studies have so far progressed for 2–4 months and this group is just in its starting period (Table 2).

The control group is a group of military men of the same age as the runners but 2–3 years older than the swimmers.

All these groups at the time of this investigation were undergoing hard physical training programs. For the control group, only a short, concentrated program was involved, but the other two groups had trained for years.

Table 1. Description of runners and their training

| Number | Weight | Training km/week (km) | Energy intake (kcal) | Iron supplement (mg/daily) |
|---|---|---|---|---|
| 8 | 54–66 kg | 120–200 | 3–3,500 | 20–100 |

Table 2. Description of swimmers and their training

| Number | Weight (kg) | Training (hr/week) | Energy intake (kcal) | Iron supplement |
|---|---|---|---|---|
| 11 | 61–85 | 14–20 | 2–3,700 | None |

At the time of investigation, there were no signs of subnormal hemoglobin, hematocrit or serum iron values in any of the groups. De Wijn (1971) reported latent iron deficiency in hard training athletes and swimmers before the Olympic Games in Mexico City on the basis of low serum iron values. In the present group of subjects, however, all serum iron values were well above the lower normal level (Table 3).

To obtain more detailed information about the iron situation, storage iron was estimated from bone marrow sections and iron kinetics from iron absorption. The bone marrow was poor in stainable iron (Table 4). Thus, although peripheral blood showed no signs of iron deficiency, the bone marrow showed complete lack of iron in five of the eight subjects and only traces of iron in the remainder of the runners' group. In the group of swimmers, eight had stainable iron and three showed a complete lack of iron. Of 76 controls, however, none had a complete lack of bone marrow iron.

Cellularity was estimated in the two groups of sportsmen. In the swimmers, it was normal in all cases, but three of the runners were classified as hypocellular by the pathologist. The smears were examined by three independent investigators.

The iron absorption of $^{59}Fe$ measured with a whole body counter was shown earlier to be high in latent iron deficiency (Höglund, Ehn,

Table 3. Peripheral blood concentrations

| Group | Hb | Hct vol% | SeFe | Saturation |
|---|---|---|---|---|
| Swimmers | 14.7 ± 0.6 | 42.8 ± 1.6 | 20.1 ± 5.8 | 38.8 ± 9.5 |
| Runners | 14.9 ± 0.2 | 42.5 ± 0.8 | 25.9 ± 2.6 | |
| Controls | 14.4 ± 0.4 | 42.7 ± 1.1 | 17.3 – 0.8 | |

Table 4. Bone marrow biopsies

| Group | Hemosiderin iron | | Cellularity | |
|---|---|---|---|---|
| | + | 0 | Normal | Reduced |
| Swimmers | 8 | 3 | 11 | 0 |
| Runners | 3 | 5 | 5 | 3 |
| Controls | 76 | 0 | | |

Table 5. Absorption of 3.5 mg $^{59}Fe$

| Group | Number | Absorption percent Mean ± SE |
|---|---|---|
| Swimmers | 5 | 8.7 ± 3.1 |
| Runners | 8 | 16.4 ± 4.7 |
| Blood donors | 8 | 30.0 ± 11.7 |

and Lieden, 1970). However, the mean values for the two groups of active sportsmen were lower than a group of blood donors with the same amount of bone marrow iron (Table 5).

Increased loss of iron from the body usually indicates bleeding, whereas losses via sweat and urine are usually considered negligible.

With the whole body counting technique the elimination of $^{59}Fe$ has been studied over a period of 6–8 months in the runners but for not more than two months in the swimmers. Therefore, it is not possible to comment upon this last group.

The findings are corrected for cobalt contamination and show an increased loss of iron for runners even when compared with blood donors and menstruating women (Figure 1). An attempt has been made to continue measurements of the group of swimmers, and it is anticipated that the results will be presented when it is possible to calculate a daily iron loss.

Table 6. Increased iron requirement in runners

| | Difference from normal | Iron requirement |
|---|---|---|
| Muscle mass | +10% | 170 mg |
| Blood volume | +9% | 200 mg |
| Physiological loss | | 350 mg/year |

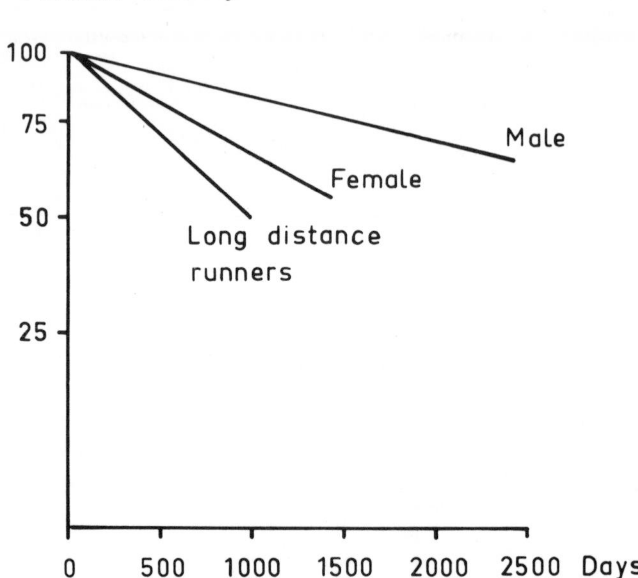


Figure 1. Total body elimination of iron is shown as measured by $^{59}Fe$ in the group of long distance runners in comparison with one group of female and one of male blood donors.

In summary, earlier studies have shown an increased loss of iron measured with the whole body counting technique. Active sportsmen have been shown to have reduced iron stores with peripheral blood values. This has been regarded as normal in previous studies. The studies have also shown 10% increase of muscle mass, measured through the 40 K technique and an increase in blood volume of 9% (Table 6). With this in mind, the hemoglobin values can be regarded as suboptimal. To test this hypothesis, iron supplements are given to the group of swimmers in the form of hemoglobin capsules (HemoJärn) to permit a controlled regular iron absorption and to avoid side effects.

Although these studies are preliminary, the iron status in the swimmers does not indicate an iron deficiency. Because of the increased need for iron in young people undergoing hard physical training for growing bodies, iron supplements are recommended, preferably as hemoglobin iron and/or a low dose of iron salts.

## REFERENCE

de Wijn, J. E. 1971. Hemoglobin pack cell volume, serum iron, and iron binding capacity of selected athletes during training. J. Sports Med. Phys. Fitness 11:42.

Höglund, S., Ehn, L., and Lieden, G. 1970. Studies in iron absorption. VII. Iron deficiency in young men. Acta Haemt. 44:193.

# Orthopaedics

# Orthopaedic Manifestations

**J. C. Kennedy**

Swimming is a recreational and competitive sport that, like tennis and jogging, is rapidly increasing in popularity. It is one of the few athletic endeavors where proficiency may save a life.

Remarks on swimmer's shoulder need not be limited to that sport and may be applied equally to other activities such as gymnastics and weight lifting, where repetitive movements over years of training and competition may eventually result in irreversible pathology in the tendons.

## THE PROBLEM

While attending the 1972 Olympic Games in Munich as orthopaedic consultant for the Canadian team, the author noticed a high incidence of orthopaedic complaints among swimmers, and on returning to Canada, immediately began a survey of orthopaedic visits to the Medical Clinic at Munich. These were tabulated as follows:

| | |
|---|---|
| Size of overall team | 296 |
| Size of swimming team | 35 |
| Total orthopaedic consultations | 127 |
| Total orthopaedic swimming consultations | 43 |

The survey of the Canadian Swimming Team at the Munich Olympics was as follows:

| | |
|---|---|
| Orthopaedic consultations | 43 |
| Specific areas | |
| shoulder | 16 |
| knee | 12 |
| calf and foot | 8 |
| miscellaneous | 7 |

To pursue this problem further, an all-Canada survey was made involving competitive swimmers. This survey included the most prominent swimming clubs in the nation and attempted to gain information on the size of the club, the average yardage swum per day, specific orthopaedic complaints, and the eventual fates of such swimmers.

It became obvious that only major problems found their way to either the family doctor or the orthopaedic consultant. In many instances, therapists, trainers, and coaches were quite familiar with the common ailments of swimmers and changed their training programs and techniques with beneficial results.

## ANATOMICAL AREAS

In the all-Canada swimming analysis, the original premise was readily substantiated. The primary anatomical areas involved in 90% of competitive swimmers were the shoulder, the knee, and the calf and foot.

Included in the analysis were 2,496 swimmers. The average club consisted of 90 competitors and the average distance swum per day was 5,000 yards. It must be emphasized that this is considered short yardage; many clubs are now swimming 20,000 yards per day.

With reference to the shoulder, there were 81 specific complaints, with freestyle and butterfly strokes being the most common offenders and the backstroke occasionally producing symptomatology. The reason for this is evident as the pathogenesis develops.

A personal review of the Canadian Olympic Swimming Team in Montreal (1976) revealed far fewer orthopaedic complications. There were 38 athletes, 14 of whom won medals. Only three were repeaters from the 1972 team. Of the 38, four had shoulder problems that required concentrated treatment during the Olympic Games; two of these four were repeaters from the 1972 Munich Olympics.

### The Shoulder

In analyzing both freestyle and butterfly strokes, it is obvious that the supraspinatus tendon is called upon to do far more than nature originally intended. This observation may also be applied to the biceps tendon. Because the supraspinatus tendon is the most superior component of the rotator cuff, it passes over the humeral head directly beneath the coracoacromial arch to insert on the superior facet of the greater tuberosity.

The biceps tendon arises from the supraglenoid tubercle, immediately runs intra-articularly in close proximity to the head of the humerus, and exits from the joint in its bicipital groove. These two structures have a very intimate intra-articular relationship. The work of MacNab and Rathbon (1970) in Toronto using micropaque injections in the subclavian artery supplying the rotary cuff produced a large series of microangiograms which aided greatly in the understanding of supraspinatus pathology.

Microangiograms reveal a distinct and characteristic vascular pattern with particular relationship to the functioning position of the arm. With the shoulder abducted, there is almost complete filling of all vessels of the tendon to its point of insertion. However, with infusion of micropaque carried out with the arm by the side, there is a constant area of avascularity extending from 1 cm proximal to the point of insertion directly to the areas of insertion. Such a zone of avascularity is present in specimens of all ages, even cadavera under the age of 20 years.

These experiments suggest that the supraspinatus tendon is subjected to constant pressure from the head of the humerus that tends to wring out its blood supply when the arm is held in a resting position of adduction and neutral rotation. With a maximum abduction, as in the recovery phase of the freestyle stroke, this area of avascularity in the supraspinatus tendon may impinge on the coracoacromial arch or, indeed, on the acromion itself.

If such observations are transferred to the freestyle or butterfly stroke, it is readily seen that the underwater pull and early arm recovery in repetitive fashion over months or even years of training invites early degenerative changes in a critical area of the supraspinatus tendon. Such changes will be reflected in symptoms of pressure impingement on the rotator cuff as the swimmer approaches the phase of maximal abduction.

At present, there are two theories in vogue in reference to the pathogenesis. The MacNab theory recognizes a constant avascular pattern as these tendons are employed in a dependent position. The Neer theory concerns itself with cuff impingement on anatomical structures as repetitive abduction of the extremity is carried out. It is unfortunate that these diverse theories cannot be resolved because their differences could readily lead to changes in training programs.

To summarize the pathology, chronic irritation in the avascular area of either biceps or supraspinatus leads to focal cell death. This leads in turn to inflammatory response, reflected in tendonitis of both supraspinatus and biceps tendons, eventually complicated by subacromial bursitis, calcific tendonitis, and actual rotator cuff tear.

Diagnosis is usually not difficult. Discomfort is first noticed only after swimming activities, progresses to pain during training and, in the ensuing hours, finally increases to the extent that performance of the stroke becomes difficult. This may be reflected in a painful arc of movement between 60° and 120° of abduction, tenderness over the supraspinatus and biceps tendon, a positive straight arm raising test, and, the final and distressing stage, eventual restriction of movement at the glenohumeral joint.

It may be helpful to divide swimmer's shoulder into three phases: Phase 1 includes pain only after activity; Phase 2 includes pain after and during activity, but not disabling pain; and Phase 3 occurs when disabling pain is in evidence during and after activity, eventually affecting the swimmer's performance. This classification has been employed by Blazina (1973) for "Jumper's Knee."

Coaches and therapists can be of great help with this problem. If a swimmer is developing shoulder symptomatology at a reasonably early competitive age and has reached only Phase 1 or 2, it may be necessary to make major decisions as to the swimmer's future training program. *The impression is that the vascular and anatomical pattern of the rotator cuff dictates in many ways the future yardage to which a coach may submit his swimmer.* For this reason, the coach may have to decide that a young swimmer should be a sprinter rather than a distance swimmer; consequently, the average training yardage would be reduced considerably. It is important that the swimmer not train continuously in the stroke that hurts him. It is a well known peculiarity that many swimmers experience pain with the freestyle stroke but not with the butterfly, or vice versa.

It is most important to be absolutely certain that the range of motion in the swimmer's shoulder is not restricted. Swimmers must be supple and flexible. It is amazing how the limitation of range of motion may slowly creep in if a swimmer actually substitutes by dipping the opposite shoulder to a minor degree for accommodation.

Experience with a Nautilus pullover apparatus has been encouraging, improving the swimmer's performance while reducing shoulder complaints. Using two different sets of exercises, the Nautilus equipment was utilized for both strength and endurance. In a specific review of 10 swimmers, all but one performed lifetime bests, the improvement being most noticeable in the shorter events (i.e., 100 and 200 m). This accomplishment took place with only moderate daily yardage in training. Strength gains were not great but initial strength, of course, was relatively high in these athletes.

Studies that emphasize specificity of muscle fiber recruitment also have important implications for both dry land and water training.

In summary, a swimmer should ice his shoulder after workouts and maintain his range of shoulder motion. Affected swimmers should change their training pattern by reducing yardage, training in another stroke, and perhaps concentrating on a sprinter's workout rather than a long distance swimmer's average yardage.

### The Coracoacromial Ligament

Occasionally, athletes who engage in repetitive shoulder activity may not be relieved of disabling pain by any or all forms of conservative management. There are scattered and very isolated reports of relief of swimmer's shoulder by division of the coracoacromial ligament. Dissections of both cadaver and fresh autopsy material have aided the writer's understanding of the role of this ligament in pathological conditions of the shoulder area.

The coracoacromial ligament is a very strong, flat, triangular band extending between the coracoid process and the acromion. It arises from a wide base at the outer edge of the coracoid and tapers to a narrow band, inserting into the anteromedial border of the acromion just anterior to the acromioclavicular joint. It frequently is composed of two dense, isolated bands with a thinner intervening portion. The outermost border of the ligament tapers to form a sharp, firm leading edge.

From anatomical studies, the biceps and supraspinatus tendons do not impinge against the coracoacromial ligament when the arm is at rest or in a purely abducted position. In abduction, the biceps and supraspinatus are at some distance from the coracoacromial ligament. However, when the shoulder is partially abducted, brought into forward flexion and extreme internal rotation, these structures are forcibly impaled against the sharp edge of the coracoacromial ligament, producing extreme discomfort and a positive impingement test.

Rehabilitation of swimmers who have exhausted conservative treatment may be successfully achieved by dividing the coracoacromial ligament.

### Transcutaneous Stimulation

For a group of swimmers who were resistant to other forms of conservative therapy and who did not fit a pattern of surgical impingement, transcutaneous nerve stimulation has produced surprising success. The discovery that peripheral stimulation can alleviate chronic pain if applied to the site of pain has resulted in its use in at least a dozen of the swimmers under study. The reader is certainly familiar with the type of needle electrodes and percutaneous stimulation. Most of the study group employed the technique for one-half hour prior to workouts. Statistics are not available at this time but initial impressions are very encouraging.

### Tibial Collateral Ligament

In the Canadian survey, there were 70 swimmers affected by "Breast Stroker's Knee."

The tibial collateral ligament is one of the two main components of the medial collateral ligament arising from the adductor tubercle and extending downward and forward to insert approximately 4–5 cm distal to the knee joint on the anteromedial surface of the tibia. The tibial collateral ligament is probably and by far the main offender in "Breast Stroker's Knee."

For this reason, the concentration is on the tibial collateral ligament, although it is recognized that other etiologic factors must be ruled out. These include the hypermobile or torn medial meniscus, the mobile patella with early chondromalacia, repetitive stretching of the capsular ligament that may progress to rotatory instability, and finally the well known and well documented swimmer suffering from osteochondritis dissecans.

In studying the pathomechanics of the whip kick in the breast stroke, it is noted that the tibial collateral ligament increases in tension as the knee moves from flexion to extension. Tension is increased by a valgus strain and, most importantly, by external rotation of the tibia, ankle, and foot. An analysis of the whip kick reveals the dramatic valgus and final external rotation force superimposed on a knee moving from flexion into full extension.

While investigating the tension developing in various ligaments about the knee joint using miniature instrumentation, it was found that the strain gauges could be readily adapted to the pathomechanics of the whip kick in the breast stroke. A mercury filled strain gauge was sutured directly onto the tibial collateral ligament in a series of fresh autopsy specimens. With concentration of the tibial collateral ligament and its attached strain gauge, the whip kick was simulated in its entirety.

The strain gauge readings indicated a constant buildup in tension in the tibial collateral ligament as three forces were applied in sequence. The cadaver knee was extended to 20° short of full extension, a valgus force was superimposed, and an external rotation force was applied. Marked tension developed in the ligament.

***Diagnosis*** Point tenderness is usually located at the origin of the tibial collateral ligament at the adductor tubercle, although naturally this tenderness may be found at other areas along the distribution of the tibial collateral ligament. Other specific tests include pain on forced abduction and external rotation of the tibia with the knee in 20–30° of flexion. It is also important to rule out other pathology in the knee joint.

***Treatment*** It must be recognized that what is involved is chronic ligamentous irritation. The kick may have to be modified so there is less external rotation of the tibia; the training program should be altered so that the important breast stroke swimmer trains infrequently with the whip kick and swims other strokes during his workout. Ice is a simple and useful modality following workouts if pain has been experienced during or after exertion. Ultrasound may be of help over a short period of time.

Steroid or cortisone injections should play only a minor role here, but they have been used occasionally. Results are not spectacular and certainly are most unrewarding when compared with treatments for complaints in and about the shoulder. This may be because an isolated ligament is involved rather than specific tendonitis in an intra-articular region.

Unfortunately, total rest may be necessary from time to time. Of all the competitive strokes, only the breast stroke requires at least 2 months of total rest per year when the knee joints are not subjected to this most abnormal stress. Occasionally, the Breast Stroker's Knee has become so chronic that in spite of all forms of treatment the competitor must quit. This naturally applies only to the mature swimmer. It is hoped that, in the adolescent age group, early diagnosis and intelligent management would preclude this fate.

### The Ankle and Foot

There seems to be no pattern of complaints here concerning a particular stroke. The extensor tendons of the ankle and foot are firmly bound over the dorsum of the ankle by the extensor retinaculum. In this area, the tendons enclosed in their sheaths are particularly liable to irritation.

***Pathomechanics*** The foot position has been studied with particular reference to the backstroke and flutter kick. The ankle and foot are carried in an extreme and abnormal plantar flexion, stretching the extensor tendons in their narrow compartment. Chronic overuse in this peculiar position creates friction between the tendons and their surrounding sheaths with resultant edema, inflammation, and adhesions. The diagnosis is obvious and crepitations are often noted as the foot is passively brought from plantar flexion into dorsiflexion.

***Treatment*** The condition is not common and its chronicity is not worrisome. However, if it does arise and if it recurs in unpredictable fashion, it may be necessary to change the type of leg kick. The Australians are known to be emphasizing the arm stroke more and more, far more than the leg kick, and training on a two-beat crossover leg kick instead of the six-beat kick of the American sprinter. It may well be that the sprinter with this recurring problem may have to change his leg kick pattern.

Local modalities are of great help. Particularly useful are icing after workouts and occasional wrapping of the foot at night at a 90° angle. Injection of steroids into the tendon sheaths at the foot and ankle may be very helpful, particularly if gross crepitations arise and, most importantly, if there is a serious competition in the near future.

Competitive athletes require help from everyone to reach their full potential. Swimming requires hard work; of countless age group swimmers, few become national champions. The swimmer's anatomy is subjected to repetitive strains in most unusual positions. Coaches, trainers, and physicians must be alert for early manifestations of difficulties.

## REFERENCES

Blazina, M. E. 1973. Jumper's Knee. Ortho. Clin. No. Am. 4(3):655.

Macnab, I., and Rathbon, J. B. 1970. The microvascular pattern of the rotator cuff. Br. J. Surg. (Bristol) 52-B:540–553.

# Insertion Tendonitis Among Swimmers

J. A. Merino and M. Llobet

Swimming as a sport produces relatively few lesions. If ophthalmologic and otorhinolaryngological conditions are excluded, the number is very small indeed.

Insertion tendonitis is a common lesion among swimmers and water polo players. It is a mild but annoying condition because of pain that, though slight, influences the swimmer's output. Coaches are usually concerned that a period of rest during the training season will keep swimmers from reaching top form in time for important meets. Only rarely does tendonitis require stopping practice altogether.

Muscular hypertrophy occurs in the swimmer just as in other athletes, increasing tractions on the tenomuscular system. Sudden, violent, and repeated muscular contractions cause tiny fibrillar ruptures leading to "insertion tendonitis." The individual experiences pain that is hard to localize and that intensifies when the corresponding muscle or muscle group contracts. A painful swelling also characterizes superficial tendonitis. In the deeper lesions, mobility is not affected and pain is felt only when the muscle contracts. X-rays and laboratory studies are negative.

Sixty-nine cases of insertion tendonitis have been observed over the past 13 years. Most of them occurred during the second half of June, shortly after the beginning of the summer training period. The condition was localized in the shoulder, elbow, knee, or groin (Table 1).

The type of tendonitis suffered usually depends on the particular stroke the swimmer practices. Shoulder tendonitis is especially frequent among water polo players and backstroke and crawl swimmers, probably because these athletes exercise rotation muscles such as the supraspinatus, infraspinatus, teres major, and subscapularis. Tendonitis of the long head of the biceps brachii is not uncommon, sometimes leading to the rupture of the tendon.

Table 1. Relationship between localization of insertion tendonitis and strokes of swimmers in 69 cases

| Stroke | Shoulder | Elbow | Groin | Knee | Total Cases |
|---|---|---|---|---|---|
| Crawl | 17 | | | | 17 (25%) |
| Water polo | 11 | 12 | | | 23 (33%) |
| Breast | | | 1 | 4 | 5 (7%) |
| Back | 14 | | 1 | | 15 (22%) |
| Butterfly | 2 | | 4 | 2 | 8 (12%) |
| Dive | | 1 | | | 1 (1%) |
| Total | 44 (64%) | 13 (19%) | 6 (9%) | 6 (9%) | 69 (100%) |

The differential diagnosis of shoulder tendonitis includes:

Periarthritis: All movement, even passive, is painful, although pain is dull. Pain in tendonitis is felt only when the muscle contracts.

Arthritis: There is swelling and heat within the affected part. The general condition is impaired and the slightest movement is accompanied by pain.

Bursitis: The differential diagnosis may be very difficult to establish in cases of deep bursitis. Sometimes crepitation can be detected.

Neuritis: It is characterized by irradiated pain and a selective painful point.

## THERAPEUTIC PROTOCOL

In treating tendonitis, the prescription included 3 g of buffered aspirin per day combined with physical therapy consisting of extra-short wave radiation, mobilizations, and massage. Trainers were also advised to apply a light schedule during the period of treatment. If this was not successful, local infiltrations with corticosteroids (1 cc of betamethasone per week for 2 or 3 weeks, at the longest) and novocaine were given.

Tendonitis of the groin and knee have been treated successfully with local infiltrations. All patients responded satisfactorily except one swimmer with tendonitis of the groin that lasted several months and forced the athlete to desist from competition. Most lesions in the groin occur in swimmers performing the butterfly stroke, and pain appears when adductors are contracted. Tendonitis of the knee is more frequent among swimmers practicing the breast stroke. It affects the insertion of the patellar ligament either at the borders or at its lower end.

Pain in the elbow occurs in water polo players and has been noted in one diver. It is interesting to notice that the majority of cases are not classic epicondylitis but epitrochleitis. It is thought they are produced by twisting the forearm (forced supination) at the same time the hand is flexed when the player catches and holds the ball before shooting at the goal. Epicondylitis would occur at the moment of thrust. Excellent results were obtained in all cases treated without exceeding three infiltrations.

Lastly, in only two cases, satisfactory results were not obtained. One was the swimmer mentioned above with tendonitis of the groin that forced him to give up the sport. The other case was a tendonitis of the shoulder that was treated in various ways, including absolute rest, over a 2-year period without achieving total healing.

## RESULTS

In view of the results, it is obvious that these lesions very seldom have an important influence on the swimmer's life. This is especially true if they are treated quickly and properly with the coach's cooperation.

In evaluating the results, the complete disappearance of the symptoms and a return to full performance in a period of 1 month or less is considered to be good (N=58). Results are considered average when mild malaise lasts for more than 1 month but does not interfere with the swimmer's output. (N=9). Results are considered unsatisfactory when the athlete cannot return to training or when his performance is definitely impaired (N=2).

## CONCLUSIONS

Although 69 cases are not enough to establish definite conclusions, certain considerations may be justified if it is remembered that the majority of these individuals swam competitively.

The low percentage of women—five cases—was of no consequence because they do not play water polo, their training programs do not usually include exercises with weights, and they have a lower muscular potential.

The largest group to present tendonitis was the water polo players. The violent and rapid contractions involved in shots and long passes and the difficulty in holding onto the ball explain the higher incidence of tendonitis, despite the greater number of competitive swimmers. Good results were obtained, although there were a few cases of recurrence.

Tendonitis of the shoulder was most common in swimmers practicing the crawl and backstroke. The complete rotation of the arm in this specific stroke makes the supraspinatus muscle more vulnerable. In some cases it was noted that the lesion coincided with the use of weights in training.

Water polo players typically develop tendonitis of the elbow at the insertion of the epitrochlea. This is believed to be caused by the motion of catching and holding the ball, while epicondylitis is produced by shooting and long passes. In divers, the condition appears during training exercises outside the pool.

Tendonitis of the lower extremities was found almost exclusively among breast stroke and butterfly swimmers. These strokes require a more forceful use of the legs than do other styles.

Recommended therapeutic protocol includes a combination of drugs, physical therapy, and the cooperation of the trainer in adapting the workout program to the patient's condition.

# Shoulder Pain in Age Group Swimmers

**R. H. Dominguez**

Organized swimming for children under the age of 3 years is a subject of some controversy. However, once past the age of 3, swimming is generally recommended from a safety standpoint (Diamond, 1975). In the United States, competitive swim meets are organized by the Amateur Athletic Union (AAU), YMCA, and other public and private organizations. These meets are usually organized using age group classifications. The usual categories are 8 and under, 9 and 10, 11 and 12, and 13 and over; occasionally, 6 and under is included as an additional category. No deleterious effects of competitive swimming have been documented. An increase in nail biting (Hendry and Whiting, 1968) and possibly a slight increase in skeletal maturity in age group champion swimmers have been noted (Bugyi and Kausz, 1970).

Most swimming coaches agree that the main power in swimming comes from the shoulder girdle and that the lower extremities function only as assistors in the stroke (Counsilman, 1968). Coaches and most competitive swimmers agree that shoulder pain is the swimmer's single most common orthopaedic complaint. However, "swimmer's shoulder" is not listed in the AMA Standard Nomenclature of Athletic Injuries (1966), O'Donohue's textbook on athletic injuries (1967), Bateman's text *The Shoulder and Neck* (1972) or DePalma's textbook *Surgery of the Shoulder* (1973). Kennedy and Hawkins (1974) first called attention to swimmer's shoulder when they stated it was the single most common complaint of swimmers on the Canadian Olympic Team. They claimed it occurred in approximately 3% of 2,496 Canadian swimmers. However, informal conversations with coaches and swimmers in the United States seem to indicate that shoulder pain occurs in more than 3% of the competitive swimmers in the United States. This study sought to determine the incidence of shoulder pain in age group swimmers in the United States.

## METHOD

The first year, 144 swimmers from a championship YMCA age group swimming team and a private boys' high school team were examined. All swimmers were examined during or immediately after the close of a practice session at poolside. Swimmers were classified by the standard age groupings of 8 and under, 9 and 10, 11 and 12, and 13–18. Blazina's (1973) classification for jumper's knee was used:

1. pain only after activity
2. pain, not disabling, during and after activities
3. disabling pain during and after activity that eventually affects the swimmer's performance

## RESULTS

### Eight and Under

Fifty-seven swimmers were examined, 25 females and 32 males. During the first year, 23 swimmers were examined and 11 of them had definite tenderness along the course of the coracoacromial arch. During the second year, no objective abnormalities or tenderness could be found. For the first year of the study in this age group, a physical therapist volunteered to aid in screening the children and recording their range of motion. While the writer examined all of the children in both years, no therapist was used the second year. Dr. Peter J. Fowler, in his critique of the preliminary report of the first year, felt that the findings for this age group were suspect (Dominguez, 1976). For this reason, great care was taken the second year to examine the children gently; the second year's results are considered accurate. Because it was felt that no reliable history could be obtained from this group, only objective findings were considered. These children practiced 4 days a week and each swam approximately 650 m per day. The coaches stated that none of this group ever complained of shoulder pain.

### Nine and Ten Year Olds

There were 55 swimmers examined in this age group, 32 females and 23 males. One female and two males complained of pain. All three complained of pain in the region of the trapezius muscle, but only when swimming. None of the three had objective findings at the time of examination. Three females and three males all had objective tenderness along the coracoacromial arch; all six denied a history of pain. This age group practiced 4 days a week and each swam approximately 1,400 m per day.

### Eleven and Twelve Year Olds

In this age group, 67 swimmers were examined, 38 females and 29 males. Six females complained of pain, one of the Class 3 variety. Nine males complained of pain. All six females and six of the nine males had tenderness along the coracoacromial arch. The swimmers with objective findings averaged 4 years' experience in competitive swimming. All of these swimmers practiced 4 days a week and each swam approximately 1,800 m per day.

In addition, one case of a true apprehension shoulder (Kennedy and Hawkins, 1974) was diagnosed on the basis of physical examination and history. Close questioning revealed the swimmer was troubled with inferior subluxation of the shoulder whenever she touched the wall during her backstroke. She denied pain, however, and it was apparent that she was afraid that she would be taken out of swimming if she revealed this information.

### Thirteen to Eighteen Year Olds

There were 84 swimmers who were examined in this group, 38 females and 46 males. There were 28 females who complained of pain, and four of these claimed to have Class 3 pain; of 27 males who complained of pain, five were of the Class 3 type. A total of 19 females and 14 males had objective findings of tenderness along the course of the coracoacromial ligament. The swimmers with Class 3 pain had averaged 8.5 years of competitive swimming. This group was usually divided into two separate groups that practiced 6 or 7 days a week. Distance varied from 3,000–9,000 m per day.

In this age group, there seemed to be an inverse correlation between distance swum at practice and shoulder pain; that is, the group swimming shorter distances seemed to have a higher incidence than those swimming longer distances. As a general rule, however, the group swimming the shorter distances did not do weight training, while the group swimming the longer distances did. No breast strokers had shoulder pain in this study.

While no limitation of motion was found in any swimmer examined, it was clear that some swimmers were more flexible than others. No significant increased flexibility could be found.

Paddles on the upper extremities seemed to have no significant effect on causing or relieving shoulder pain.

Six male swimmers noted a significant decrease in pain after they had been on a weight lifting program. In the preliminary report on the first year, however, several female swimmers complained of increasing pain after being placed on an isometric weight lifting program. This problem seemed to have been solved in the second year by conversion to an isotonic weight lifting program.

Most of the swimmers that lacked objective tenderness but complained of shoulder pain reported pain in the region of the trapezius muscle that usually ceased after the practice session had begun or started at the close of the practice session. Further clarification revealed that most of the swimmers either failed to warm up properly or were experiencing muscle fatigue at the close of a vigorous training session.

## DISCUSSION

It rapidly became apparent that a significant proportion of swimmers complaining of shoulder pain had tenderness along the course of the coracoacromial ligament and/or the supraspinatous tendon and bicipital tendon. Kennedy and Hawkins (1974) believed that devascularization of the supraspinatous tendon and bicipital tendon leads to a significant tendonitis. Once this tendonitis occurs, mechanical impingement of the supraspinatous tendon against the coracoacromial ligament can also become a significant factor and can cause pain.

Another group of swimmers who complained of shoulder pain had diffuse shoulder pain with no objective findings or pain in the trapezius region. The pain in most of these swimmers occurred while swimming if they failed to warm up properly or were fatigued. Most of these swimmers were aware of this finding.

The term "swimmer's shoulder" should be used to refer only to pain along the course of the coracoacromial arch, supraspinatous tendon, or bicipital tendon. Apprehension shoulder and trapezius pain appeared to be separate entities with apparently different etiologies. It also appears that lack of weight lifting training may be a significant factor in the development of shoulder pain in competitive swimmers. Most of the swimmers with significant coracoacromial ligament impingement either did not lift weights, did not swim during both winter and summer seasons, or had swum a significantly increased distance at practice. None of the swimmers with Class 3 pain discontinued their competitive swimming; they persisted in swimming with the pain after varying modes of treatment including modifications of training schedules and rest.

## CONCLUSIONS

In the 8 and under age group, no significant shoulder problems could be found from competitive swimming.

In the 112 swimmers aged 9–12 examined, one case of mild apprehension shoulder and one case of Class 3 pain were noted. This is an incidence of less than 1% of significant shoulder problems in this age category, and this pain did not preclude continuation of swimming.

About 65% of the 13–18 year old swimmers examined complained of some type of shoulder pain. Objective evidence of coracoacromial ligament tenderness at the conclusion of a practice session was found in 39%. Another 10.9% of the swimmers in this age group had Class 3 symptoms. However, all nine Class 3 pain sufferers planned to continue competitive swimming.

Weight lifting training seems to be of some benefit in decreasing the incidence of shoulder pain.

Shoulder pain appears to be a significant orthopaedic problem for the competitive swimmer. This 2-year study of competitive age group swimmers indicates that, in the 13–18 age group, over 50% of swimmers will have some complaints of shoulder pain. Slightly more than 10% will have shoulder pain significant to the degree that it will cause them to miss practice or swimming meets.

## REFERENCES

American Medical Association. 1966. Standard Nomenclature of Athletic Injuries. American Medical Association, Chicago.

Bateman, J. F. 1972. The Shoulder and Neck. W. B. Saunders Co., Philadelphia.

Blazina, N. E. 1973. Jumper's knee. Orthop. Clin. North Am. 4(3):665.

Bugyi, B., and Kausz, I. 1970. Radiographic determination of the skeletal age of the young swimmers. J. Sports Med. Phys. Fit. 10:269–270.

Counsilman, J. E. 1968. The Science of Swimming. Prentice-Hall, Inc., Englewood Cliffs, N.J.

DePalma, A. F. 1973. Surgery of the Shoulder. 2nd Ed. J. P. Lippincott Co., Philadelphia.

Diamond, E. F. 1975. Swimming instruction for preschool children. J. Sports Med. 3(2):58–60.

Dominguez, R. H. 1976. Swimmer's shoulder: A preliminary report and report of a case. Presented to the American Orthopaedic Academy of Sports Medicine, New Orleans.

Hendry, L. B., and Whiting, H. T. A. 1968. Social and psychological trends in national calibre junior swimmers. J. Sports Med. Phys. Fit. 8(4):198–203.

Kennedy, J. C. and Hawkins, R. J. 1974. Swimmer's shoulder. Phys. Sports Med. 2(4):34–38.

O'Donohue, D. H. 1967. Treatment of Injuries to Athletes. W. B. Saunders Co., Philadelphia.

# Coracoacromial Ligament Resection for Severe Swimmer's Shoulder

**R. H. Dominguez**

Shoulder pain is the most common orthopaedic complaint of competitive swimmers. Kennedy and Hawkins (1974) first coined the term "swimmer's shoulder" when they stated it was the single most common complaint of swimmers on the 1972 Canadian Olympic Team. They claimed that shoulder pain occurred in approximately 3% of the 2,496 Canadian swimmers. Dominguez, in a less extensive study in the United States, suggested that the incidence of significant shoulder pain is slightly greater than 10% in competitive swimmers over the age of 13 years (see pp. 109).

Most swimmers with shoulder pain are treated by their coaches with minor alterations in the angle of hand entry, height of arm recovery, or distance swum at practice. Alternate breathing in swimmers with pain who only breathe on one side frequently gives significant relief. Few competitive swimmers in the United States present themselves to physicians because of universal frustration in seeking medical attention. The frequent experience is that the physician will diagnose tendonitis and prescribe an anti-inflammatory agent or administer a local steroid injection into the tender shoulder region. If these treatment modalities fail, the swimmer is told to stop swimming. At this point the athlete will often cease seeking medical attention.

Isotonic exercises with weights seem to be of some benefit in decreasing pain, but isometric exercises may be of no value and may be harmful. For those few swimmers who have severe disabling shoulder pain that has failed to respond to prolonged conservative measures, resection of the coracoacromial ligament is a possible solution. However, no report of this procedure being performed on competitive swimmers is available in the literature. Excision of the coracoacromial ligament is an accepted procedure in other degenerative lesions of the rotator cuff (Neer, 1972). This chapter presents case histories of three competitive swimmers treated with coracoacromial ligament resection for severe disabling swimmer's shoulder.

## CASE 1

The patient is a 17 year old white female who began competitive swimming at the age of 5. At age 12, she began to complain of right shoulder pain and occasional mild left shoulder pain. At age 15, at a swimming camp in Canada, a physician injected her right shoulder with steroids, but this had no effect whatsoever on her shoulder pain. The pain continued to increase in severity. At age 16, she sought an orthopaedic surgeon's consultation. She was told her shoulder was "normal." Chiropractic consultation was also sought to no avail. She retired from swimming at the completion of the winter season at age 16 because of severe shoulder pain.

At age 15, she had been a 182-m (200-yard) freestyle and 91-m (100-yard) butterfly YMCA state champion. She was ninth in the 450-m (500-yard) freestyle at the YMCA national meet.

At age 16, she did not win the YMCA state meet and could not swim at the YMCA national meet because of pain. She continued to have pain for a year after her retirement. She had severe disabling shoulder pain whenever she put on a coat or attempted to demonstrate swimming strokes when she worked as a swimming instructor and coach. She was unable to play sports such as volleyball. She was pain free as long as she avoided an arc of abduction or flexion of the right shoulder between 60° and 90°.

Physical examination demonstrated an exquisite tenderness along the course of the coracoacromial arch with the extremely painful arc of motion between 60° and 90°. There was an unusually full range of motion of the shoulder; in fact, her flexibility was quite remarkable with full circumduction of the shoulder without difficulty. X-rays of the right shoulder were within normal limits despite careful inspection for the osteophytes described by Neer (1972).

A frank discussion with the patient and her mother about the paucity of medical literature on this subject was held. Excision of the coracoacromial ligament was offered as a possible solution to her symptoms because it is an accepted procedure in other degenerative lesions of the rotator cuff. Excision of this ligament is said not to weaken the shoulder (DePalma, 1973). Phenylbutazone failed to affect her symptoms in any way.

After thorough contemplation, excision of the coracoacromial ligament was performed under general anesthesia. The midportion of the standard deltopectoral incision was made. Great care was taken to use muscle splitting just lateral to the deltopectoral groove and to disturb the deltoid as little as possible. The muscle was not detached from the clavicle. The coracoacromial ligament was exposed and completely excised from both of its attachments on the coracoid and acromion. An attempt was made to keep this operation as pure as possible, and no further procedures were performed. However, it was evident at surgery that there was virtually no clearance; this extremely sharp ligament abutted against the rotator cuff, expecially through her symptomatic arc of motion. The patient had an uneventful postoperative course, was immobilized in a sling for comfort for approximately 5 days, and then began a gentle active range of motion.

Three weeks postoperatively, she was able to swim without pain and claimed full relief of preoperative symptoms. She had full painless shoulder motion. She has remained pain-free now for 2½ years.

## CASE 2

The second patient was an 18 year old white male with a 1 year history of disabling left shoulder pain. In 1975 he was the state champion in the 450-m (500-yards) freestyle. In 1976 he was unable to swim this event because of disabling pain. The pain began when he was doing "pulls with paddles" of 14,000 m per day during workouts. He had had bilateral shoulder pain, but the left remained disabling. Six months after the onset of pain, he had to stop swimming altogether for 5 months. When he returned to swimming, the pain recurred and became acute and disabling. He had had two steroid injections that had failed to relieve his symptoms. After discussion of the alternatives with the family and the patient, they requested that excision of the coracoacromial ligament be done. This was performed without incident.

The patient made an uneventful postoperative recovery and in one month was able to return to a full, heavy schedule of collegiate swimming training and over the course of the next swimming season reduced his times in all events by 1–2 sec. One year after surgery he remains completely asymptomatic and has a complete range of motion.

## CASE 3

The third patient was a 16 year old male with a 3-year history of right shoulder pain and a history of left shoulder pain. He had had steroid injections into both shoulders; the pain was relieved in the left shoulder but not in the right. An anti-inflammatory agent was also tried for relief of pain, to no avail. At the time of examination, he had significantly decreased his level of training and was unable to work out to any significant degree. His best strokes were the freestyle and butterfly sprints.

Examination demonstrated a full range of motion of both shoulders. There was exquisite tenderness along the coracoacromial arch of the right shoulder, especially through an arc of 60–100° of flexion and abduction. X rays demonstrated several benign cystic lesions in the right humeral head; compared with results in previous films, these lesions had almost completely healed. One could also feel some crepitation through this arc of motion. Coracoacromial ligament resection was offered to this patient and his parents as a mode of treatment. Exploration of the right shoulder with excision of the coracoacromial ligament and partial anterior acromionectomy were performed, the latter procedure because there seemed to be some bony impingement upon the anterior acromion even after the coracoacromial ligament was excised. Once the inferior anterior acromionectomy had been performed, there seemed to be complete clearance of the humeral head under the shoulder.

The patient made an uneventful postoperative recovery and was able to return to full training and swimming 1 month after surgery, including sessions of 10,000–15,000 m per day without difficulty. Nine months after surgery, his 200-m freestyle time was reduced by 5 sec; his 100-m freestyle and 100-m butterfly times were each 2 sec less as well. He was totally asymptomatic and quite pleased.

## RESULTS

All three swimmers had complete relief of pain and were back to swimming, free of pain, one month postsurgery. The two males were able to swim faster and train harder than they had ever been able to do in the preoperative period. The female patient had retired from swimming a year prior to surgery and had not planned to return to swimming regardless of the result of the surgery.

The three have remained free from pain for 1–2½ years postoperatively. All three swimmers had full and complete arcs of motion and circumduction of both shoulders. No detectable disability or weakness was evident postoperatively. None complained of any loss of function; in fact, all three noted a definite improvement in their ability to function.

## CONCLUSION

Coracoacromial ligament resection in three competitive swimmers with severe chronic shoulder pain from impingement of the rotator cuff or bicipital tendon on the coracoacromial ligament seemed to be a safe, effective way to treat this type of "swimmer's shoulder."

## REFERENCES

DePalma, A. F. 1973. Surgery of the Shoulder, 2nd Ed. J. B. Lippincott Co., Philadelphia.

Kennedy, J. C. and Hawkins, R. J. 1974. Swimmer's shoulder. Phys. and Sports Med. 2(4):34–38.

Neer, C. S., III. 1972. Anterior acromioplasty for the chronic impingement syndrome in the shoulder. JBJS 54(A):41–50.

# Low Back Pain in Butterfliers

**Y. Mutoh**

Recently, sports records and techniques in various fields, especially in competitive swimming, have been greatly improved. As new records have been set, the number of cases and kinds of sports injuries have increased. In general, competitive swimmers are younger than competitors in other sports, and are more apt to be greatly affected by damage. In swimming, therefore, early diagnosis, correct treatment, and preventive steps have been strongly recommended. According to Mizumachi (1958), low back pain has been the most frequent sign of injury in competitive swimming.

## PURPOSE OF THE STUDY

The purpose of the study was to investigate the nature of low back pain in competitive swimmers, especially in butterfly strokers, who seemed to be most affected because of the mechanical stress on their lumbar spines.

## MATERIALS & METHOD

Investigation was carried out on 53 well trained Japanese competitive swimmers—5 females and 48 males, aged 13–21 years. These swimmers included 12 butterfliers, 22 crawl strokers, 5 backstrokers, 7 breast strokers, and 7 individual medley relay strokers. Nine of the swimmers were former butterfliers who had been switched over to other strokes.

The procedures included the taking of individual histories of low back pain, evaluation of the strength and flexibility of the muscles related to the low back, orthopaedic physical examination, and x-ray examination of the lumbar spine. As seen in Figure 1, for evaluation of the strength and flexibility of the muscles related to the low back, a

EVALUATION

Abdominal muscle strength

Back muscle strength

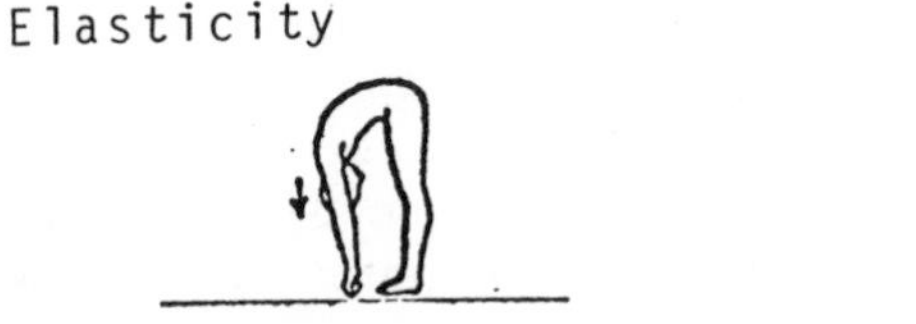


Figure 1. Tests for evaluation of muscle function.

modified Kraus-Weber test as described by Ichikawa (1976) was used. Swimmers who could maintain the respective positions for 20 sec were assumed to possess normal muscle strength. Stature, weight, and back muscle strength were also measured.

As shown in Table 1, physical examinations were performed in the orderly and systematic manner used in examinations done on patients complaining of low back pain. That is, limitation of mobility of the lumbar spine, tenderness, straight leg raising test, reflexes, sensory disturbance, and muscle weakness were investigated. Plain lumbar spine x-ray films were taken on 39 subjects, including all of the butterfliers and the swimmers in other styles who experienced low back pain.

Anteroposterior, lateral, and oblique roentogenograms were taken in the standing position. As seen in Table 2, radiographic abnormalities, especially spondylolysis, spondylolisthesis, intervertebral disc narrowing, and lumbosacral angle, were checked with great care on the lumbar spine x-ray films. The lumbosacral angle was studied by measuring the angle made by the upper margin of the third lumbar vertebral body and that of the sacrum (Williams, (1948).

Table 1. Abnormalities found in physical examinations of 53 subjects[a]

| Abnormality | Swimming style | | | | | Total |
|---|---|---|---|---|---|---|
| | Butterfly (N = 12) | Crawl (N = 22) | Back (N = 5) | Breast (N = 7) | Individual medley relay (N = 7) | |
| Limitation of mobility of the lumbar spine | 1 | 2 (0) | 1 (0) | 0 | 0 | 4 (0) |
| Tenderness | 4 | 5 (2) | 2 (0) | 3 (0) | 1 (1) | 15 (3) |
| Straight leg raising test | 0 | 0 | 0 | 1 (0) | 1 (1) | 2 (1) |
| Diminished or absent patellar jerk | 1 | 2 (1) | 0 | 2 (0) | 0 | 5 (1) |
| Diminished or absent ankle jerk | 1 | 1 (0) | 0 | 1 (0) | 0 | 3 (0) |
| Babinski reflex | 0 | 0 | 0 | 0 | 0 | 0 |
| Sensory disturbance | 2 | 2 (1) | 0 | 1 (0) | 1 (1) | 6 (2) |
| Muscle weakness | 2 | 1 (1) | 0 | 1 (0) | 1 (1) | 5 (2) |

[a] Figures in parentheses indicate the number of former butterfliers

Table 2. Roentogenographic abnormalities in 39 subjects[a]

| Abnormality | Swimming style | | | | | Total |
|---|---|---|---|---|---|---|
| | Butterfly (N = 10) | Crawl (N = 16) | Back (N = 1) | Breast (N = 7) | Individual medley relay (N = 5) | |
| Scoliosis | 2 | 2 (1) | 0 | 1 (0) | 1 (0) | 6 (1) |
| Kyphosis | 0 | 0 | 0 | 0 | 0 | 0 (0) |
| Spina bifida occulta | 0 | 3 (0) | 0 | 2 (0) | 0 | 5 (0) |
| Spondylolysis | 4 | 0 | 0 | 0 | 0 | 4 (0) |
| Spondylolisthesis | 1 | 0 | 0 | 0 | 0 | 1 (0) |
| Transitional vertebrae | 1 | 3 (1) | 0 | 1 (0) | 0 | 5 (1) |
| Intervertebral disc narrowing | 3 | 1 (1) | 0 | 0 | 0 | 4 (1) |
| Deformity or sclerosis of vertebrae | 1 | 1 (0) | 0 | 0 | 1 (0) | 3 (0) |
| Persistent apophysis | 1 | 1 (0) | 0 | 0 | 0 | 2 (0) |
| Osteophyte formation | 0 | 0 | 0 | 0 | 0 | 0 (0) |
| Schmorl nodule | 0 | 1 (1) | 0 | 0 | 0 | 1 (1) |
| Change of intervertebral joints | 0 | 0 | 0 | 0 | 0 | 0 (0) |
| Change of spinous processes | 0 | 1 (0) | 0 | 0 | 0 | 1 (0) |
| Change of lumbosacral joints | 0 | 0 | 0 | 0 | 0 | 0 (0) |

[a] Figures in parentheses indicate the number of former butterfliers.

## RESULTS AND DISCUSSION

Of 53 swimmers, 32 (60.4%) experienced low back pain; 22 of the 32 (68.8%) felt low back pain during or immediately after swimming or after completion of exercises done outside the pool. Only seven of the 22 (31.3%) asked for a coach's advice; coaches, however, must be careful not to force training upon swimmers who are suffering from low back pain and/or other illness in order to prevent injuries during competitive swimming, and swimmers must also be careful. It is therefore necessary that the doctor involved acquaint himself with each sports event.

Analyses of the data were carried out on 21 butterfliers (including former butterfliers) and on 32 swimmers in other styles. The percentage of swimmers experiencing low back pain and showing abnormalities in orthopaedic physical examinations tended to be higher in butterfliers than in nonbutterfliers. Butterfliers also tended to show greater back muscle strength than nonbutterfliers.

Next, x-ray films were taken of 18 butterfliers and 21 nonbutterfliers. Both spondylolysis and intervertebral disc narrowing were found in 22.0% of butterfliers; examples of these conditions are shown in Figure 2. The occurrences of spondylolysis and intervertebral disc narrowing were statistically more common to butterfliers than to nonbutterfliers. The lumbosacral angle also tended to be greater in butterfliers than in nonbutterfliers.

In the butterfly stroke, repeated stress is assumed to be directed to the lower lumbar spine of the swimmer by vigorous extension of the back and by the strong dolphin kick. In general, swimming training starts at an early age, when the spine is not yet completely developed and is therefore, susceptible to trauma caused by stress. Consequently, the repeated trauma and stress to the lumbar spine may cause spondylolysis or intervertebral disc degeneration. Kono et al. (1975) stated that spondylolysis resulted mostly from a stress fracture of the neural arch caused by repetitive athletic activities. They found patients with spondylolises in 11.8% of 55 swimmers. This writer also feels that most cases of spondylolyses are nothing more than stress fractures because they always appear as a result of repeated trauma and stress rather than of an acute traumatic episode.

Figure 3 shows spondylolisthesis with the defects of pars interarticulares of the fourth and fifth lumbar vertebrae, as indicated by arrows. The patient was a 20 year old swimmer who had been a butterflier for 8 years. The lumbosacral angle was 42°. He was suffering from low back pain.

Figure 4 shows the remarkably increased lumbar lordosis observed in a 21 year old female swimmer who had competed as a butterflier for 11 years. Her abdominal muscle strength was found to be

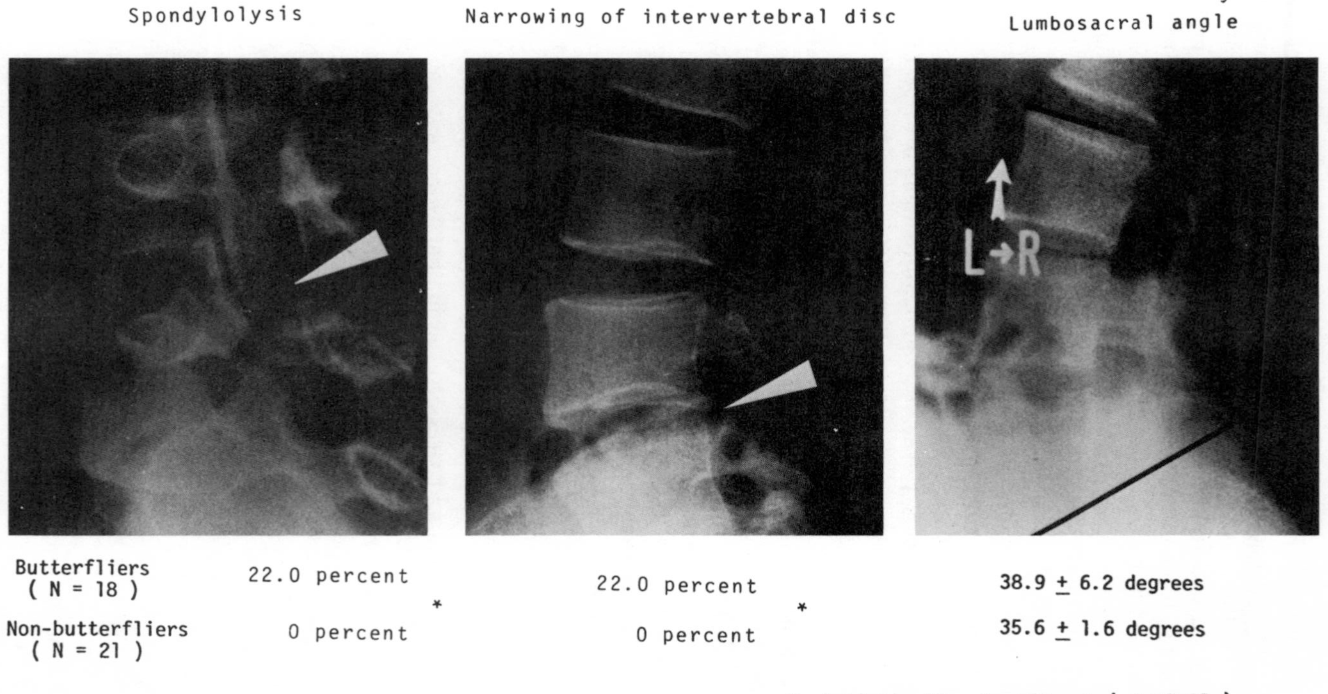


Figure 2. Results of the radiological survey are illustrated.

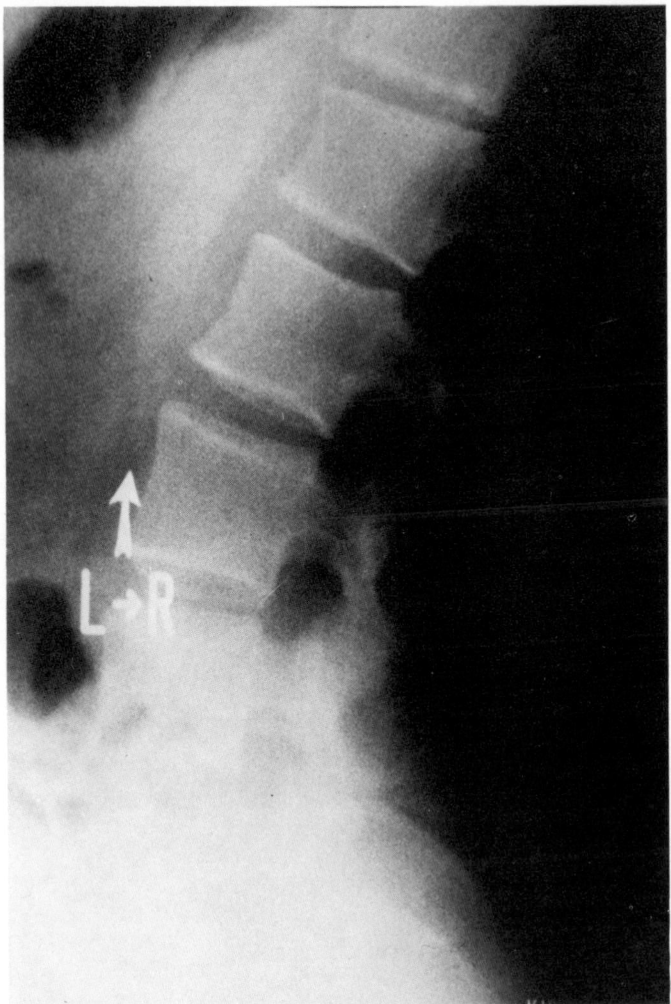


Figure 3. The x-rays show spondylolisthesis with defects of pars interarticulars of the third and fourth vertebrae, as observed in a 20 year old male butterflier.

weak in the test previously described. The lumbosacral angle was 47°. She was also suffering from low back pain.

Principally, the back muscles, the iliopsoas muscle, and the quadriceps extend the spine, while the abdominal, the gluteal, and the hamstring muscles flex the spine. Well trained butterfliers seem to have stronger spine extensors than spine flexors because of a special breathing action and the dolphin kick. Wide lumbosacral angles in butterfliers are indicative of the increased lumbar lordosis that is supposedly associated with low back pain; it is assumed that the butterfly

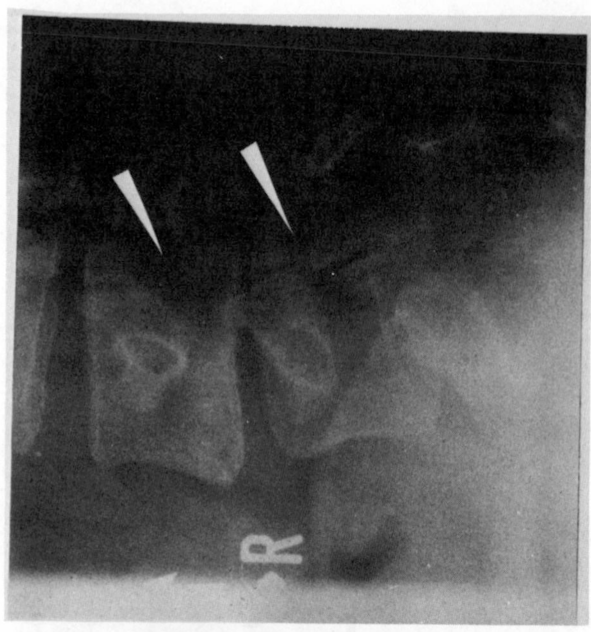


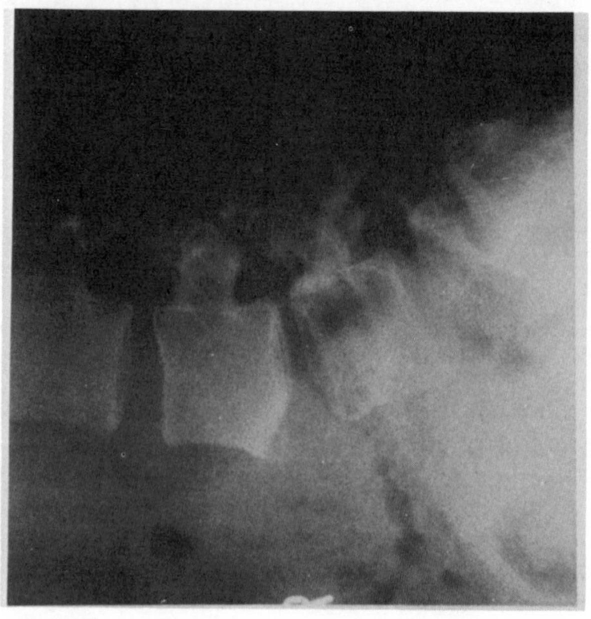

Figure 4. This remarkable lumbar lordosis was observed in a 21 year old female butterflier (Lumbosacral angle: 47°)

stroke requires vigorous spine extensors that would cause increased lumbar lordosis, thus giving rise to low back pain.

Therefore, it is necessary for a coach of the butterfly swimmers to be very careful about the following items:

1. Instruction should be avoided by beginning swimmers unless they have enough physical strength.
2. The training program for butterfliers should be composed of various swimming styles. Long-term training limited to the butterfly stroke should be avoided.
3. For the butterfliers, exercises to strengthen the muscles related to the low back are very important. The training, however, should be done with gradually increased workloads.

In summary, to study the nature of low back pain in competitive swimmers, especially in butterfliers, various investigations were performed. The investigations consisted of taking the histories, evaluation of muscle functions, various physical examinations, and x-ray examinations. In the radiological surveys, spondylolysis and intervertebral disc narrowing were statistically more common to butterfliers than to nonbutterfliers. It was made clear that the butterfly stroke occasionally caused increases in lumbar lordosis accompanied by spondylolysis and/or degeneration of intervertebral disc giving rise to low back pain.

## REFERENCES

Ichikawa, N. 1976. Low back pain in young athletes. Surg. Ther. 35(3):294–305.

Kono, S., Hayashi, N., Kasahara, T., Akimoto, T., Kaneko, F., Sugiura, Y., and Harada, A. 1975. A study on the etiology of spondylolysis with reference to athletic activities. J. Jap. Orthop. Assoc. 49:125–133.

Mizumachi, S. 1958. Sports medicine. Lecture of Modern Biology X (Jap.). Kyoritsu Shuppan, Tokyo.

Williams, P. C. 1948. Diagnosis and conservative management of lesions of the lumbosacral spine. In: Regional Orthopaedic Surgery and Fundamental Orthopaedic Problems, Vol. 2, pp. 103–116. American Academy of Orthopaedic Surgeons. Edwards Brothers, Ann Arbor, Mich.

# Physiology

# Aerobic Power

**P.-O. Åstrand**

This chapter is an attempt to present a survey of the physiology of the oxygen transport system, i.e., the discussion is limited primarily to the aerobic part of the energy yield during exercise. It should be pointed out that each exercise and work situation is unique because each has a specific pattern in its demands on the body—on energy yielding processes (aerobic and anaerobic), on neuromuscular function (strength and technique), and on psychological factors (motivation, tactics). Therefore, it becomes difficult or impossible to predict the performance in one activity from data obtained in studies from a different activity. However, there is one factor operative in all types of muscular movement, i.e., an increased energy demand, and (disregarding the anaerobic contribution) this is mirrored in an elevated oxygen uptake. Therefore, with a known potential for an individual's oxygen transporting system, one can actually predict his potential for vigorous muscular exercise. (One liter of oxygen when used yields about 20 kJ or 5 kcal.) There are studies indicating that the maximal oxygen uptake in exercises involving large muscle groups is not limited by the capacity of the muscle mitochondria to consume oxygen. Slight variations in the volume of oxygen offered to the tissue produce almost proportional variations in the volume of oxygen utilized (Åstrand and Rodahl, 1977).

Exercise with the arms (in swimming) as well as with one leg (bicycling) includes muscle groups that are also engaged in normal swimming and two-leg work, respectively. It is remarkable, however, that the combined exercise does not dramatically increase the maximal oxygen uptake (Davies and Sargeant, 1974; Holmér, 1974; Clausen, 1976).

It should be emphasized that a period of physical conditioning increases the volume of mitochondria in trained muscles, thus increasing their aerobic energy potential (Holloszy, 1973; Howald and Poortmans, 1975). However, Gollnick et al. (1972) concluded from their studies of enzyme systems in skeletal muscles of untrained and trained men that the metabolic capacities of both the conditioned and unconditioned muscles normally exceed the actual uptake of the muscles. The increase in enzymes noticed with conditioning also far exceeds the noticeable improvement in maximal oxygen uptake (Henriksson, 1977). The local adaptations in trained skeletal muscles, including an increase in capillary density and myoglobin content, modification of enzyme systems, and size of the muscle fibers, may be important factors behind the well known "specificity of training" (Åstrand and Rodahl, ch. 12).

The physiology of swimming is examined in the following paragraphs. (Part of this text has been published in Åstrand and Rodahl, 1977.) Swimming engages practically all muscle groups of the body. It is therefore not surprising that very high oxygen uptakes have been obtained on swimmers (Åstrand et al., 1963; Holmér, 1974). A maximal oxygen uptake of 3.75 liters $\times$ min$^{-1}$ was attained by the female silver medallist in the 400-m freestyle in the Olympic Games in Rome, 1960. In male swimmers of world caliber, a maximum of around 6 liters $\times$ min$^{-1}$ has been measured.

Because the specific gravity of the body is not much different from that of water, the weight of the body submerged in water is reduced to a few kilograms. The obese individual especially may stay afloat with very little energy expenditure. Swimming may therefore be an easy task when performed at a low level of intensity. For this reason, swimming and various exercises performed in water are common forms of training for physically handicapped individuals.

The functional demands of competitive swimming were evaluated in 22 female swimmers on the basis of the relationship between oxygen uptake during work on a bicycle ergometer and oxygen uptake during swimming at competitive speed (Åstrand et al., 1963). A very high correlation was observed, but the oxygen uptake during swimming averaged only 92.5% of the maximum reached during cycling. Five girls, however, attained higher values in swimming.

The high correlation is also evident from the fact that the blood lactate concentration after swimming was of the same order of magnitude as after maximal cycling (10.3 and 10.5 mM, respectively). Similar results were reported by Åstrand and Saltin (1961) and Holmér (1974): 12.8 mM after maximal swimming and 12.9 mM after running for male swimmers.

The quotient of pulmonary ventilation to oxygen uptake ($\dot{V}_E/\dot{V}_{O_2}$) was significantly lower during maximal swimming (27.7) than during cycling (35.5). The reason for this relative hypoventilation may be different mechanical conditions of breathing. The water pressure on the thorax makes respiration more difficult. Furthermore, the breathing is not as free during swimming as in most other types of work because respiration during competitive swimming is synchronized with the swimming strokes.

When the body was submerged, Holmér (1974) noted that the vital capacity was reduced by 10% and the expiratory reserve volume was less than 1 liter as compared with 2.5 liters in air. The increase in tidal volume in water was achieved exclusively by the use of the inspiratory reserve volume. Holmér et al. (1974) noted a similar difference in the ratio between maximal pulmonary ventilation and maximal oxygen uptake when comparing the data obtained during swimming and running (29.8 and 37.4, respectively, for five subjects). However, despite the relative hypoventilation in the subjects when swimming as compared with running, the arterial oxygen pressure and content were the same in the two types of exercise.

In recent years, world records have been attained by girls at increasingly younger ages. Girls 13–14 years of age not engaged in hard physical training have almost reached the maximal power of their aerobic processes. During puberty, the organism may respond more strongly to training. In the previously mentioned study of girl swimmers, it was found that the swimmers had significantly greater functional dimensions than girls who had not taken part in competitive sports or undergone any special physical training. Vital capacity and heart volume were highly correlated with maximal oxygen uptake.

Thus, young girls may exhibit very high motor power. It has been shown that women doing the breast stroke at a certain speed have a lower oxygen uptake (greater mechanical efficiency) than men. This may be explained by the fact that the lower specific gravity of women, attributable to their greater fat content, reduces the effort required to keep the body afloat. However, considerable individual variations in technique are characteristic of swimming (Holmér, 1974). The oxygen uptake during swimming at a given submaximal speed depends on the degree of swimming training, body dimensions, swimming technique, and swimming style. Thus, oxygen uptake at a given submaximal speed is higher for untrained swimmers than trained ones, and for tall subjects than for short ones. It is the arm stroke that has the higher efficiency, not the leg kick. In fact, the maximal speed in freestyle swimming that could be maintained for about 5 min with arm strokes was almost the same ($1.31 \text{ m} \times \text{s}^{-1}$) as for the whole stroke ($1.34 \text{ m} \times \text{s}^{-1}$) but at a significantly lower oxygen uptake. One might speculate that over long distances the leg kick should be deemphasized because it may waste oxygen and blood flow.

In the breast stroke, the leg kicks are probably as important as or more important than the arm strokes. The mechanical efficiency was 6–7% in freestyle and 4–6% in breast stroke in elite swimmers. Most costly from the standpoint of energy expenditure is the butterfly stroke (Holmér, 1974; di Prampero et al., 1974).

The increase in oxygen uptake with increased swimming speed is linear or slightly exponential. Maximal oxygen uptake during swimming for elite swimmers, was 6–7% lower than during running (on the average) and approximately the same as during cycling. For subjects untrained in swimming, maximal oxygen uptakes during swimming were, on the average, 80% of the running maximum. Heart rate, cardiac output, and stroke volume during submaximal swimming were of the same magnitude and increased with increasing speed in approximately the same way as during running.

Heart rate was significantly lower in maximal swimming than in maximal running. The mean intra-arterial blood pressure at submaximal as well as maximal rates of work was higher in swimming than in running. The significance of this finding when recommending exercises for cardiac patients is at the present time difficult to evaluate. (The circulatory data were obtained on five subjects who were studied when running and swimming.) (Holmér et al., 1974).

Holmér (1974) presented data on maximal oxygen uptake measured on a champion swimmer when swimming in a flume and also when running on a treadmill. For about 4 years his maximum was the same when running, but varying oxygen uptake values were measured during maximal swimming, because of variations in training intensities, illness, etc. The variation was most pronounced in freestyle swimming using only the arms. Peaks were noted when the swimmer was most successful (winning two Olympic gold medals in 200- and 400-m medleys, 1972).

Identical twin sisters reached similar maximal oxygen uptake values when running (3.6 liters $\times$ min$^{-1}$), but the sibling who had been training for competitive swimming attained a 30% higher oxygen uptake than her untrained sister. When swimming with arms only, the trained sister could reach a 50% higher maximum (Holmér and Åstrand, 1972; Magel et al., 1975).

The conclusion is that a treadmill test is not a good predictor of performance in other types of activities. Secondly, in order to utilize the aerobic potential in an optimal way in a given activity, one must train in that activity. This is a good illustration of the specificity of training.

The engagement of the different types of muscle fibers depends on the exercise and the rate of work. It is logical to assume that a training protocol should cover a large range of swimming speeds. (It should be emphasized that the motor units in the skeletal muscles recruited at a low intensity are most likely active at high intensities also.) Therefore, it is essential to devote time to interval training at competitive speed.

The writer is unconvinced that many hours of daily training at a submaximal speed are essential for achieving a good performance.

Running and cross-country skiing are very efficient types of exercises for improvement of the maximal oxygen uptake. It is an open question whether or not an increased potential of the central circulation thus obtained could be utilized in swimming, although the two types of training should run parallel. As previously mentioned, most well trained swimmers cannot reach the same maximum in swimming as in running. In a given swimmer, is the maximal oxygen uptake in swimming a given percentage of the running maximum? That is one question that needs an answer.

## REFERENCES


Åstrand, P.-O., Engström, L., Eriksson, B. O., Karlberg, P., Nylander, I., Saltin, B., and Thorén, C. 1963. Girl swimmers. Acta Paediat. (suppl. 147):43–63.

Åstrand, P.-O., and Rodahl, K. 1977. Textbook of Work Physiology, p. 185. 2nd Ed. McGraw-Hill Book Company, New York.

Åstrand, P.-O., and Saltin, B. 1961. Maximal oxygen uptake and heart rate in various types of muscular activity. J. Appl. Physiol. 16:977–981.

Clausen, J. P. 1976. Circulatory adjustments to dynamic exercise and effects of physical training in normal subjects and patients with coronary artery disease. Progress. Cardiovasc. Dis. 18:459–495.

Davies, C. T. M., and Sargeant, A. J. 1974. Physiological response to one- and two-leg exercise breathing air and 45% oxygen. J. Appl. Physiol. 36:142–148.

di Prampero, P. E., Pendergast, D. R., Wilson, D. W., and Rennie, D. W. 1974. Energetics of swimming in man. J. Appl. Physiol. 37:1–5.

Gollnick, P. D., Armstrong, R. B., Saubert, C. W., IV, Piehl, K., and Saltin, B. 1972. Enzymatic activity and fiber composition in skeletal muscle of untrained and trained man. J. Appl. Physiol. 33:312–319.

Henriksson, J. 1977. Training induced adaptation of skeletal muscle and metabolism during submaximal exercise. J. Physiol. 270:661–675.

Holloszy, J. O. 1973. Biochemical adaptations to exercise: Aerobic metabolism. In: J. H. Wilmore (ed.), Exercise and Sport Sciences Reviews, Vol. 1, pp. 46–71. Academic Press, New York.

Holmér, I. 1974. Physiology of swimming man. Acta Physiol. Scand. Suppl. 407.

Holmér, I., and Åstrand, P.-O. 1972. Swimming training and maximal oxygen uptake. J. Appl. Physiol. 33:510–513.

Holmér, I., Stein, E. M., Saltin, B., Ekblom, B., and Åstrand, P.-O. 1974. Hemodynamic and respiratory responses in swimming and running. J. Appl. Physiol. 37:49–54.

Howald, H. and Poortmans, J. R. (eds.). 1975. Metabolic Adaptation to Prolonged Exercise. Birkhäuser Verlag, Basel.

Magel, J. R., Guido, R., Foglia, F., McArdle, W. D., Gutin, B., Pechar, G. G., and Katch, F. J. 1975. Specificity of swim-training and maximum oxygen uptake. J. Appl. Physiol. 38:151–155.

# Use of Heart Rates in the Determination of Swimming Efficiency

**R. Treffene, J. Alloway, and J. Shaw**

Swimming efficiency has been investigated by many researchers, including di Prampero et al. (1974) and Holmér (1974). Di Prampero and colleagues deduced a relationship between swimming efficiency (e), body drag (Db), swimming speed (v), and net oxygen uptake ($\dot{V}_{O_2}$ net). He verified the relationship

$$\frac{e}{Db} = \frac{v}{\dot{V}_{O_2}net}$$

and his research at two submaximal speeds (0.55 and 0.9 m s$^{-1}$) showed that e/Db remained constant within this range. Furthermore, Treffene (1975) used the assumption of linearity of HR to $\dot{V}_{O_2}$ net to deduce that

$$\frac{e}{Db} \propto \frac{v}{HR}$$

Investigation of the velocity to heart rate relationship for swimmers by Treffene suggested that there exists a linear relationship between velocity and HR and, therefore, a constant value for e/Db. Therefore, if v(max) is the lowest steady speed at which the swimmer swims with his maximum heart rate, then

$$\frac{e}{Db} = \frac{v(max)}{0.93\ \dot{V}_{O_2}\ (bicycle\ max)}$$ (Treffene et al., 1976)

Holmér (1974) showed that for well trained swimmers the maximum oxygen uptake for a subject swimming is 93% of his oxygen uptake calculated on a bicycle ergometer. Therefore, the net oxygen uptake could be determined on a bicycle and the value, 0.93 $\dot{V}_{O_2}$ (bicycle), used for the swimming net oxygen uptake.

By measuring v(max) for a swimmer and a bicycle $V_{O_2}$ (max), the efficiency to drag ratio can also be calculated. This has been done for two swimmers and the results are shown in Table 1.

Table 1. Efficiency to drag ratio with the speed at which heart rate first reached a maximum value v(max) for two subjects

| Subject | e/Db ($kg^{-1} \times 10^{-2}$) | v(max) ($m\ s^{-1}$) |
|---|---|---|
| JC | 0.9 ± .05 | 1.13 |
| RW | 1.0 ± .05 | 1.26 |

## METHODS

Female (N = 15) and male (N = 15) swimmers participated in this study. The group was comprised of nationally ranked and club swimmers.

Heart rates were determined using stainless steel electrodes and a Telescan telemetry unit and transmitter. In addition, a permanent record of HR was made with a two-channel MK 2 recorder. In addition to this, velocity was calculated by timing each split 50 m with stopwatches. Later, values were recorded using a heart rate meter specifically designed for this purpose. This unit is now commercially available (from Heart Rate Industries, 48 Goldieslie Road, Indooroopilly. Queensland, 4068. Australia).

Using freestyle, backstroke, or breast stroke, all swimmers were required to swim four different but relatively constant speeds for a number of lengths of a 50-m pool. These speeds were predetermined and varied depending on the ability of various swimmers. In an attempt to ensure a steady state for the exercise HR (after 3 min or longer), six laps were chosen for the first two slower speeds and eight laps were chosen for the relatively faster two speeds. Furthermore, each swimmer was assigned an individual timekeeper whose task it was to indicate to the swimmer the consistency of each lap time.

Resting HR was calculated at the beginning of each test with the subject standing in the water with his/her hand placed on the stainless steel electrode. HR after each particular workload was determined by requesting the swimmer stand up and place his/her hand on the electrode immediately after finishing the set of laps. Maximum HR was determined by a maximal effort over a distance of 200 m.

Oxygen uptake ($\dot{V}_{O_2}$) was determined by analysis of the expired air using Douglas bag collection. Volume of expired gas was measured in a dry gas meter (Parkinson Cowan) and analyzed for oxygen content with a calibrated paramagnetic method (Servomex). Samples were analyzed for carbon dioxide concentration using a Godard capnograph. Maximum oxygen uptake ($\dot{V}_{O_2}$ max) was measured using the bicycle ergometer.

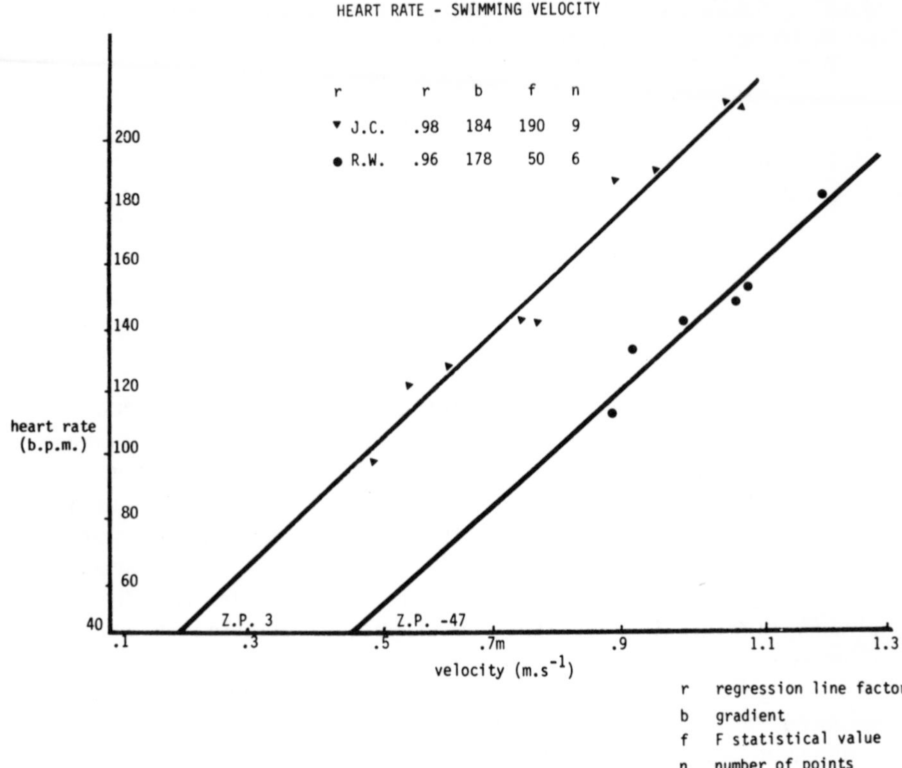


Figure 1. This graph shows heart rate versus velocity for two well trained swimmers.

## RESULTS

Table 1 shows the e/Db for two subjects taken over five separate days. The linear relationship between HR and velocity found in two swimmers is shown in Figure 1; the two lines illustrate how the curves differed for the two swimmers.

Other subjects displayed a significant change in the linear relationship with increasing velocity. This observed phenomenon is illustrated in Figure 2 (JH). Of the 30 subjects, each can be represented by a graph that reflects present swimming ability. The characteristic variation among individuals is also shown in Figure 2.

## DISCUSSION

The results provided HR-to-velocity curves for all subjects that were specific for each subject (Figure 2). The gradients of these curves were calculated to give an index of ability: the lower the gradient, the more efficient the swimmer.

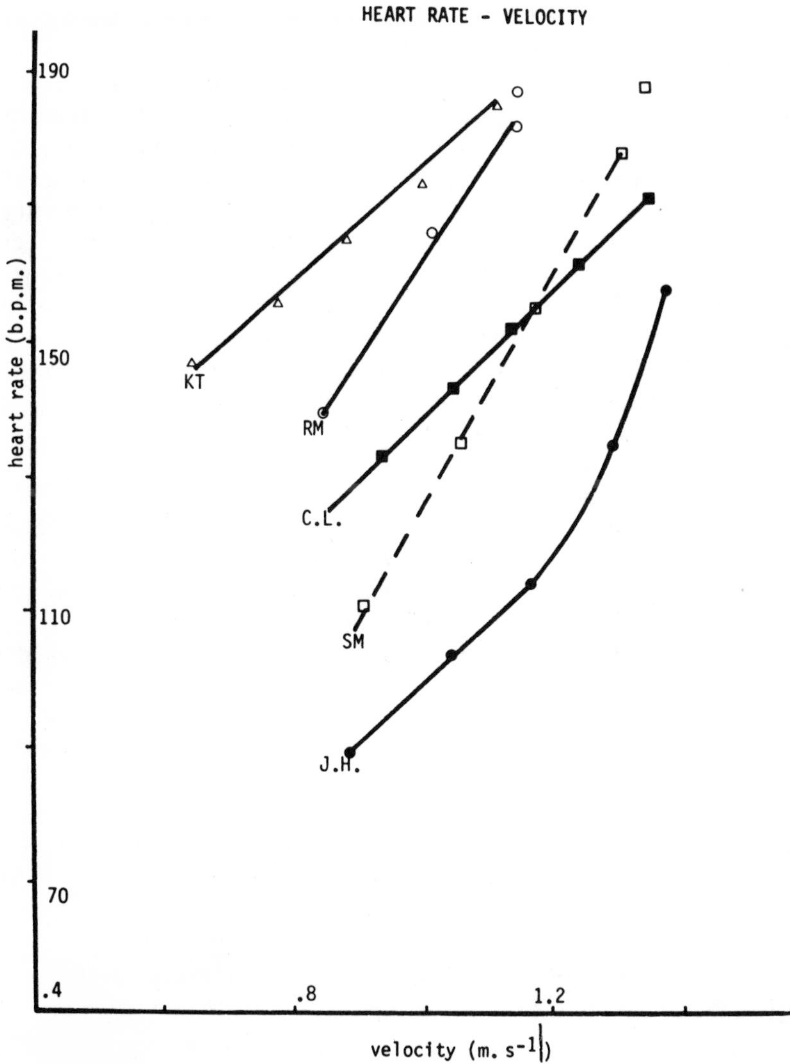


Figure 2. This graph represents heart rate versus velocity for five swimmers.

In the case of a swimmer who showed a change in gradient during a set of velocities (Figure 2., J.H.), it would be expected that at the point where the gradient increased, the stroke efficiency decreased because there was a great increase in HR relative to the increase in velocity. Such a gradient change would indicate that a swimmer's technique had deteriorated at the point (i.e., velocity) where the gradient increased.

Consequently, it is suggested that the coach pay particular attention to the swimmer's style at this critical speed to establish what variation in stroking has occurred in order to reduce the efficiency-to-drag ratio.

On repeated performances of the sets of velocities on different days, curves were calculated that were similar in gradient to previously calculated curves, but in a different position. This occurred because the resting HR was different from day to day (Åstrand and Rodahl, 1970) as a result of factors such as fatigue and drugs. With the increased resting HR, the work HRs that followed were higher than would have been recorded for the same velocities preceded by lower resting HRs. In recording HR in this study, the resulting data were used to obtain HRs by measuring the HR from the consecutive R-R waves; thus the HR was an instantaneous value. This procedure allowed the determination of maximal HR at the instant work ceased rather than as an average taken over the span of a minute.

Furthermore, the lowest velocity at maximum HR may be calculated by extrapolation of the linear relationship to the maximum heart rate. This may serve as a means of determining the training load for any particular swimmer. The coach may decide on a percentage value of the known maximum HR and therefore calculate the appropriate velocity at which the swimmer must train to elicit the desired HR.

At low submaximal speeds, all swimmers in this study displayed a definite linear velocity-to-HR relationship. This relationship continued through to maximum heart rate for some. For others, however, a radical change in gradient occurred, indicating a change in efficiency caused by a breakdown in swimming form.

For two swimmers an estimate of their e/Db ratio was also obtained. Unfortunately, no correlation could be drawn between the e/Db values obtained by this method and the e/Db ratio of the same subject obtained using a swimming flume. However, the e/Db ratios obtained are within the high values recorded by di Prampero et al. (1974). This would be expected for the two above average swimmers tested.

## REFERENCES

Åstrand, P.-O., and Rodahl, K. 1970. Textbook of Work Physiology. McGraw Hill Book Company, New York.

di Prampero, P. E., Pendergast, D. R., Wilson, D. W., and Rennie, D. W. 1974. Energetics of swimming in man. J. Appl. Physiol. 37:1–5.

Holmér, I. 1974. Physiology of swimming man. Acta Physiol. Scand. Suppl. 407.

Treffene, R. J. 1975. Investigation of the ECG in sports and sports medicine using radiotelemetry. Masters thesis. University of London.

Treffene, R. J., Frampton, C., Tunstall Pedoe, D., and Idle, M. 1976. Energetics of swimming using heart rate telemetry. Annual Proceedings of Australian Sports Medicine Conference, Brisbane.

# Dynamics of Oxygen Intake During Step-by-Step Loading in a Swimming Flume

**L. Kipke**

Many publications confirm the importance of determining the oxygen intake during sport-specific load conditions (Åstrand et al., 1963; Volkow, Gordon, and Sirkovec, 1968; Holmér, 1974). Oxygen intake measurements are being applied in sport medical performance diagnosis throughout the world because oxygen is a measure of energy metabolism that simultaneously provides an indirect assessment of physical fitness.

In 1974, oxygen intake values were found to be lower after swim loads than values determined under bicycle ergometer and free swimming loads using the same load periods and methods of analysis. In addition to reduced oxygen intake, other respiratory values, such as respiratory volume per minute and respiratory volume per breath, were also reduced. These findings were reported during the Third International Congress for Sport Medicine in Swimming held in Barcelona in 1974. Holmér (1974) described similar results.

The respiratory stereotype established within a highly trained swimmer led to the conclusion that other respiratory dynamics during swimming must differ from those during bicycle ergometer loads. Further investigations on the swimmer's respiration, repeatedly revealed significant relationships among respiration, swimming velocity, and specific strokes.

The members of the German Democratic Republic National Swimming Team, which included numerous World and Olympic champions, were the subjects in the investigation to determine how respiration changes during swimming. Testing was conducted in the flume of the Flygt Co., Stockholm, using step-by-step loads and water velocities of 1.20–1.50 m/sec for female swimmers and from 1.40–1.65

m/sec for male swimmers; their individual 200-m racing speeds were selected as the individual maximum loads. Exhaled air was fractionally collected in Douglas bags by means of a mask system (Nöding et al., 1975) that allowed the swimmers to breathe in an unrestricted manner by opening their mouths wide, and that also included their noses within the system. Respiratory volume was determined by using a gasometer, frequency by a thermistor as described by Schumann (1966), and oxygen differentiated from carbon dioxide by the performance-test-set "Spirolyt II" (Dessau Junkalor Co., GDR). Respiratory volume/minute, respiratory volume/breath, and respiratory rate were calculated from these data.

A linear increase of oxygen intake was found with the increasing load. (Michailow (1971) and Holmér reported the same results in similar investigations.) If, however, the velocity was increased to the level of the individual racing speed, a decrease of oxygen intake was observed.

Evaluation of the findings revealed that respiration is appreciably affected by swimming technique; because respiratory frequency, depth, and volume change from one technique to another, oxygen intake also changes. Three reasons were found for lower oxygen intake following changed respiration during swimming at high load levels:

1. At the maximum stroke frequency, the respiratory frequency of the swimmer increases, thus lowering the respiratory volume/minute and, consequently, oxygen intake as well (Figure 1).
2. The swimmer attempts to achieve greater velocity by increasing his effort. This leads to a decrease in stroke and breathing frequencies. The respiratory volume/breath remains constant; the respiratory volume/minute, however, decreases, and the oxygen intake is thus lowered (Figure 2).
3. Because of the heavier work at maximal loads, the swimmer must inhale more air to take in the same volume of oxygen and his/her work becomes less efficient. The small decrease in respiratory volume/breath is compensated for by increasing the breathing frequency. By doing so, respiratory volume/minute is kept constant; oxygen intake is, however, lowered by the increase in the breathing equivalent (Figure 3).

This decrease in oxygen intake during maximal swimming loads was mentioned earlier by Holmér, who described the establishment of a steady-state level of oxygen intake during step-by-step imposition of loads.

It must be concluded from the results of this investigation that a swimmer does not completely utilize his full oxygen intake capacity during competition. It is well known, on the other hand, that the maxi-

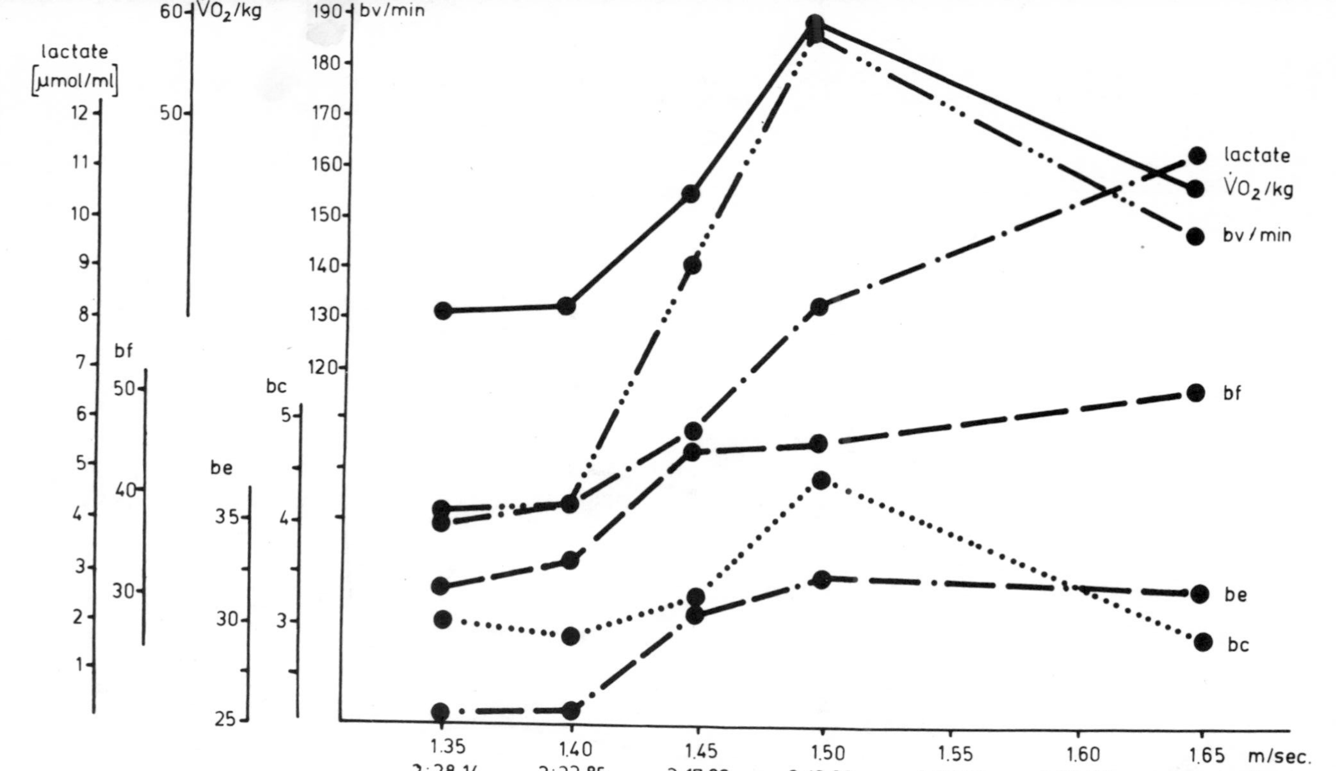


Figure 1. This graph illustrates oxygen intake, breathing volume/min, lactate, breathing frequency (bf), breathing equivalent (be), and breathing capacity (bc) in top swimmers with increasing swimming loads step-by-step in a flume at maximum stroke frequency.

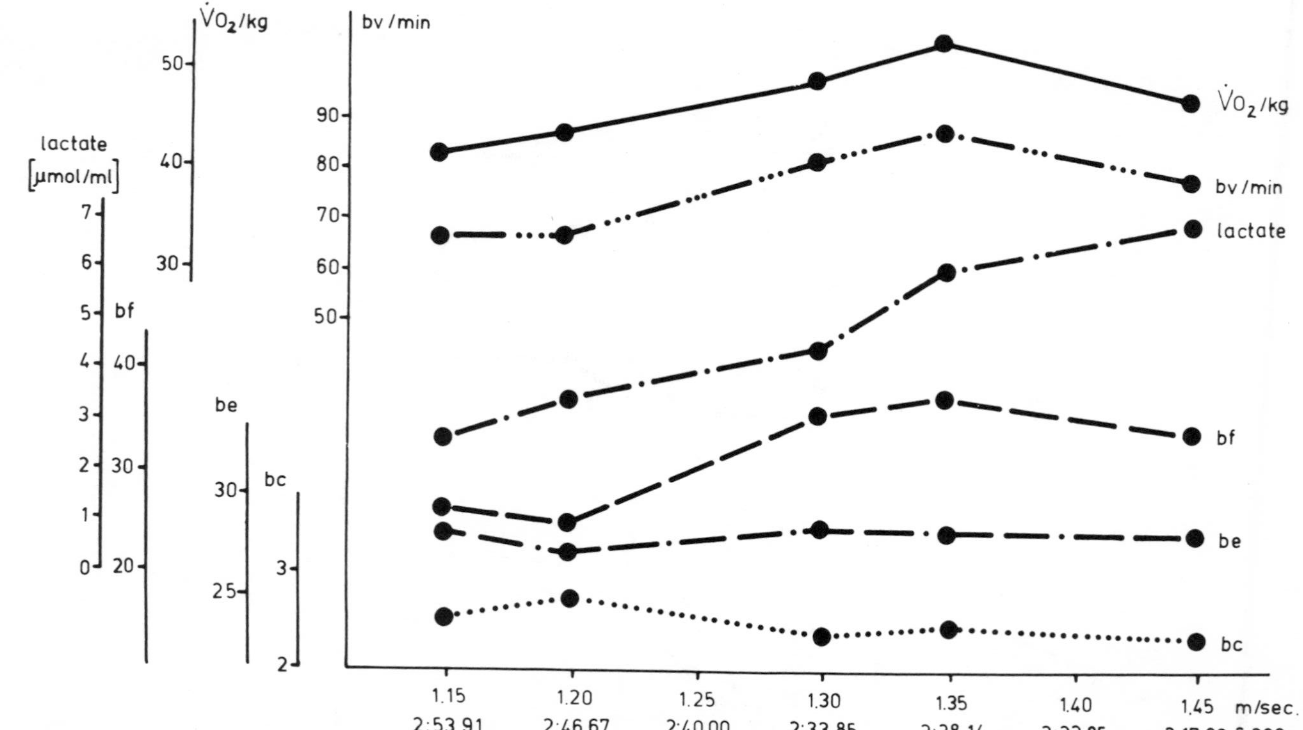


Figure 2. This graph depicts oxygen intake, breathing volume/min, lactate, breathing frequency, breathing equivalent, and breathing capacity in top swimmers with increasing swimming loads step-by-step in a flume with decreased stroke and breathing frequencies. Abbreviations as in Figure 1.

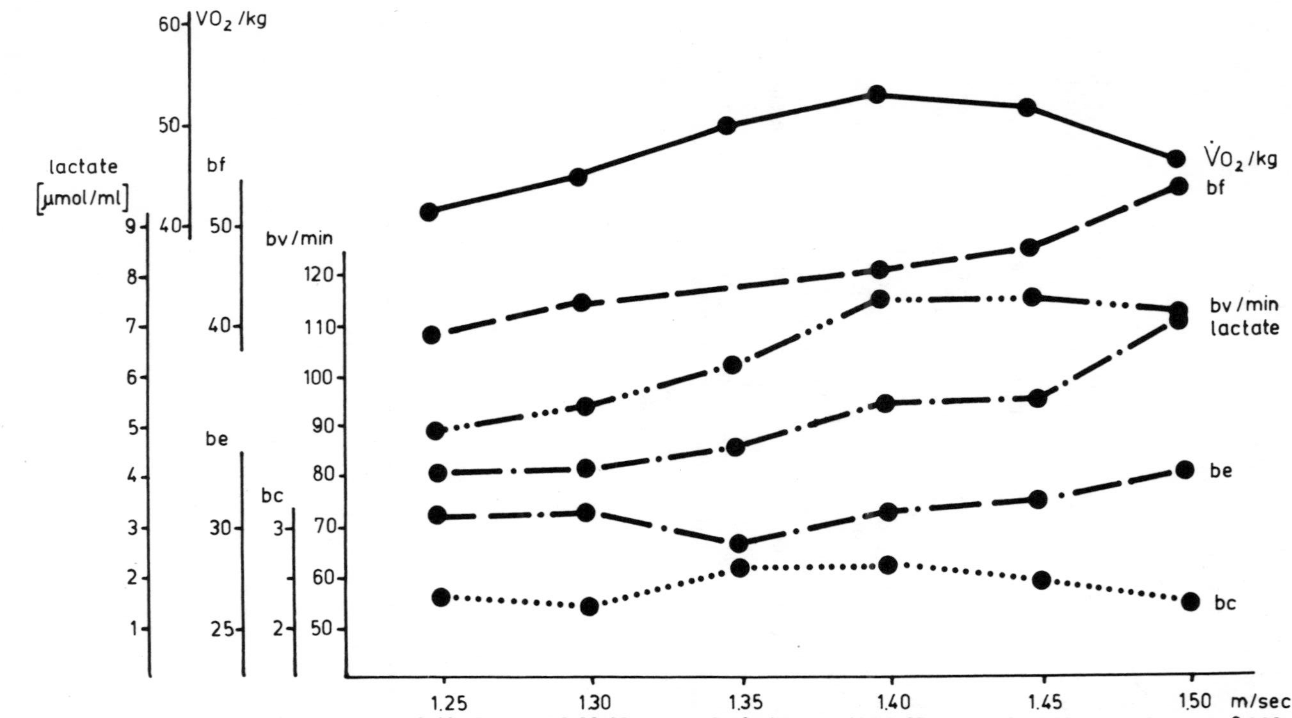


Figure 3. This graph shows oxygen intake, breathing volume/min, lactate, breathing frequency, breathing equivalent, and breathing capacity in top swimmers with increasing swimming loads step-by-step in a flume with increased breathing frequency. Abbreviations as in Figure 1.

mal oxygen intake of top athletes today is no higher than that of athletes of twenty years ago; nevertheless, there is an obvious difference in performances. We should, therefore, look for performance-limiting aspects in swimming which should be sought in factors other than oxygen intake.

## REFERENCES

Åstrand, P.-O., Engström, L., Erikson, B., Karlberg, P., Nylander, J., Saltin, B., and Thorén, C. 1963. Girl swimmers. Acta Paediat. Scand. (suppl. 147):43–63.

Holmér, I. 1974. Physiology of swimming man. Acta Physiol. Scand. (suppl. 407).

Kipke, L. 1974. Oxygen intake differences between bicycle ergometer and free swimming loads. 3rd International Congress for Sport Medicine in Swimming, Barcelona.

Michailow, W. W., Abrassimow, W. W., and Petrow, S. W. 1971. On problems of respiratory volume and the frequency regulation with athletes during high cyclic loads. Med. Sport 11:331–335.

Nöding, R., Gabler, U., Kipke, L., and Jankowski, R. 1975. The application of a modified Douglas bag method to examine respiration and gas metabolism in swimming. Med. Sport 15(8):238–241.

Schumann, H. 1966. A thermistor to measure the frequency and depth of respiration during athletic loads. Med. and Sport 6:122–124.

Volkow, N. J., Gordon, S. M., and Sirkovec, E. A. 1968. Investigations on the physiology of swimmers. Teor. Prakt. Fiz. Kult. 31:29–33.

# Maximal Oxygen Uptake in Older Male Swimmers During Free Swimming and Stationary Cycling

**F. W. Kasch**

Recent emphasis on cardiovascular fitness programs for adults has caused a need for evaluating various modes or types of exercise training. Although jogging has been one of the more popular training media, swimming has certain advantages, particularly for persons with musculoskeletal problems. The criteria measurement for various training modes usually involves maximal oxygen uptake ($\dot{V}_{O_2}$ max) on a treadmill or bicycle ergometer.

Åstrand et al. (1963) and Holmér (1974) found that stationary cycling and treadmill running gave a $\dot{V}_{O_2}$ max higher by about 6–8% than in swimming. Magel and Faulkner (1976) reported free swimming to give a $\dot{V}_{O_2}$ max 4–5% higher than in treadmill running. In each case, elite or highly skilled subjects were measured. The question then arises when evaluating swimmers as to which method truly measures the $\dot{V}_{O_2}$ max. It is the purpose of this chapter to investigate this problem as it relates to older swimmers.

## PROCEDURE

The subjects were nine men, aged 44–63 years ($\bar{x}$ = 47.9) participating for 1–4 years in an organized swimming fitness program (Table 1). All were essentially at a steady-state training level. Frequency of training was 3 days per week with an average of 87 days per year. Distances swam ranged from 900–1600 m per session. Intensity of training was regulated by heart rate (HR) with a mean rate of 155 beats/min (139–172), or about 85% of (PWC).

Table 1. Physical characteristics of subjects

| Age | N | Height cm | Weight kg | Resting HR | Resting Syst. BP | Resting Dias. BP |
|---|---|---|---|---|---|---|
| 47.9 | 9 | 174.6 | 85.2 | 68 | 135 | 86 |
| (44–63)[a] | | (166–181) | (72–115) | (45–90) | (108–164) | (70–100) |

[a] Denotes range of scores

$\dot{V}_{O_2}$ max was measured in the laboratory with a Monark bicycle ergometer and in free swimming in the pool with the Douglas Bag method as previously reported (Kasch et al., 1966; Kasch et al., 1973). $\dot{V}_{O_2}$ measurement in the pool was accomplished by suspending a meteorological collection bag from a pole manipulated by a technician. A snorkel arrangement permitted a one-way airflow. Heart rate (HR) was measured by telemetering in the water and by direct ECG in the laboratory. Each swimmer swam freestyle in a lane adjacent to the longitudinal edge of the 25-yd pool. Several bags were collected after four to five warm-up laps followed by three to four laps of greater intensity (85%) and then two to three all-out laps, during which time a $\dot{V}_{O_2}$ collection was made. The swimmers had been familiarized with the mouthpiece and entire pool procedure on a previous day. Ventilation ($\dot{V}_E$) collection per bag was minimally 1 min and maximally less than 1.5 min.

## RESULTS AND DISCUSSION

Maximal $\dot{V}_{O_2}$ results were 2.75 and 2.90 liters/min ($P < 0.01$) on bicycle ergometer and in free swimming, respectively. When compared with body weight, $\dot{V}_{O_2}$ results were 32.5 and 34.5 ml/min kg (6%) for cycling and swimming, respectively (See Table 2).

$\dot{V}_E$ collections were 123.4 and 96.1 liters/min BTPS ($P < 0.01$); HR max were 179 and 171 beats/min ($P < 0.01$); $0_2$ pulse and estimated stroke volume (SV) were 15.4 and 17.0 ml/beat and 106 and 114 ml on the ergometer and in swimming, respectively. The R (respiratory exchange ratio) was 1.10 and 0.94 by the two respective methods of cycling and swimming (see Table 3).

The difference in the $\dot{V}_{O_2}$ max measurements was probably a result of the specificity of training, indicating that the bicycle ergometer may not be a valid measurement of the PWC of swimmers. Running on a treadmill in the laboratory gives a $\dot{V}_{O_2}$ max about 9% greater (Davis and Kasch, 1975) than the finding on the bicycle ergometer. The results in this study give a difference of about 6% in favor of swimming over the bicycle ergometer, which was approximately the same $\dot{V}_{O_2}$ max

Table 2. Comparison of $V_{O2}$ max cycling and swimming

| Method | N | $\dot{V}_{O_2}$ max l/min | $\dot{V}_{O_2}$ max ml/min kg |
|---|---|---|---|
| Cycling | 9 | 2.75 (298) | 32.5 (4.7) |
| Swimming | 9 | 2.90 (310) | 34.5 (4.4) |

reported by other investigators using similar subjects (Robinson, 1938; Hartley et al., 1969; Åstrand and Rodahl, 1970; Kasch et al., 1973; Kasch, 1976).

Of great interest was the difference in the $\dot{V}_E$ apparently caused by the limited respiratory rate imposed by the swimming technique, yet the $\dot{V}_{O_2}$ was greater in the water. The difference was the result of a greater percent $O_2$ extraction (true $O_2$) from the pulmonary circuit during swimming (3.56% and 2.73%). Åstrand and Rodahl (1970) reported a $\dot{V}_E/\dot{V}_{O_2}$ ratio of 27.7 swimming and 35.5 cycling, whereas, with the older subjects in this study, the corresponding data were very similar—28.5 and 36.7, respectively.

The variation in max HR may be explained by the horizontal position used in swimming compared with the upright position employed in cycling. Åstrand and Rodahl (1970) reported a greater SV and lower HR in supine versus upright cycling. Using an indirect measure of Q from the formula of Åstrand et al. (1964) the SV can be estimated. A greater value (7%) was found during horizontal swimming than that in cycling.

From the foregoing it appears that swimming in older subjects gives a greater $\dot{V}_{O_2}$ max than does cycling. This may be because of the specificity of training and the lack of work by the lower extremities in free swimming. The $\dot{V}_{O_2}$ in the laboratory, lower on the bicycle ergometer than on the treadmill, may be similarly explained. It also seems logical to assume that swimming is an effective method of training the oxygen transport systems of middle-aged men.

Table 3. Comparison of $O_2$ pulse, Q, and stroke volume

| Method | N | $O_2$ pulse ml/beat | Estimated cardiac output liters per min | Estimated stroke volume ml |
|---|---|---|---|---|
| Cycling | 9 | 15.4 (3.4) | 18.86[a] (2.0) | 106 (14.3) |
| Swimming | 9 | 17.0 (2.5) | 19.35 (1.3) | 114 (9.9) |

[a] Estimated from Åstrand et al. (1964) formula ($\dot{Q} = \dot{V}_{O_2} \times 3.23 + 9.98$)

## REFERENCES

Åstrand, P.-O., Engström, L., Eriksson, B., Kurlberg, P., Nylander, I., Saltin, B., and Thorén, C. 1963. Girl swimmers. Acta Paediatr. (suppl. 147):43–63.

Åstrand, P.-O., Cuddy, T. E., Saltin, B., and Stenberg, J. 1964. Cardiac output during submaximal and maximal work. J. Appl. Physiol. 19:268.

Åstrand, P.-O., and Rodahl, K. 1970. Textbook of Work Physiology. McGraw-Hill Book Company, New York.

Davis, J. A., and Kasch, F. W. 1975. Aerobic and anaerobic differences between maximal running and cycling in middle-aged males. Aust. J. Sports Med. 7(4):81–84.

Hartley, L. H., Grimby, G., Kilbom, A., Nilsson, N. J., Åstrand, I., Bjure, J., Ekblom, B., and Saltin, B. 1969. Physical training in sedentary middle-aged and older men. Scand. J. Clin. Lab. Invest. 24:335–344.

Holmér, I. 1974. Physiology of swimming man. Acta Physiol. Scand. Suppl. 407.

Kasch, F. W., Phillips, W. H., Ross, W. D., Carter, J. E. L., and Boyer, J. L. 1966. A comparison of maximal oxygen uptake by treadmill and step test procedures. J. Appl. Physiol. 21:1387–1388.

Kasch, F. W., Phillips, W. H., Carter, J. E. L., and Boyer, J. L. 1973. Cardiovascular changes in middle-aged men during two years' training. J. Appl. Physiol. 34:53–57.

Kasch, F. W. 1976. The effects of exercise on the aging process. Phys. Sports Med. 4(6):64–68.

Magel, J. R., and Faulkner, J. A. 1976. Maximum oxygen uptakes of college swimmers. J. Appl. Physiol. 22(5):929–933.

Robinson, S. 1938. Experimental studies of physical fitness in relation to age. Arbeitsphysiologie 10:251–323.

# Physiological Analysis of Young Boys Starting Intensive Training in Swimming

**B. O. Eriksson, K. Berg, and J. Taranger**

Top athletes in endurance sports differ from ordinary people in many respects, e.g., in aerobic capacity and the dimensions of circulatory and respiratory organs (Saltin and Åstrand, 1962; Åstrand et al., 1963; Bevegård, Holmgren, and Jonsson, 1963; Hollman, 1963; Åstrand and Rodahl, 1970; Miyashita, Hayashi, and Furuhashi, 1970). It is not known whether these rather marked differences between athletes and nonathletes can be attributed mainly to constitutional factors or to the hard, protracted physical training these athletes have undergone (Åstrand et al., 1963). Only prospective, longitudinal studies starting before or at an early stage of long-term training could provide an answer. In many sports, however, this would entail following presumptive top athletes for a long period of time, making such studies both difficult to perform and extremely time-consuming.

Swimming is one of the best sports to study to obtain some answers within a reasonable period of time, because top performances are achieved early in life. This is especially true for girls. That was one reason for the study of girl swimmers (Åstrand et al., 1963) and for a recently completed prospective, longitudinal study of young girls followed from the age of 8–12 years to age 16 (Engström et al., 1971; Eriksson et al., in preparation). In recent years, there has been a tendency for top performances to be attained among males at increasingly early ages. Thus, the winner of the 1500-m event at the 1973 World Swimming Championships was only 15 years old. Therefore, a prospective, longitudinal study of young boys starting regular swim-

This report is the first on a prospective, longitudinal study supported by the Research Council of the Swedish Sports Federation.

ming training was felt to be of some value. Such a study would also make it possible to ascertain whether the constitution of these boys at the start of training differed from that of normal boys. This latter topic is the subject of this study.

## SUBJECTS

The subjects were 18 boys, aged 7.6–11.8 years (mean age: 10.1 years), from a larger group of boys selected for regular physical training by the coaches of the Swedish S02 and GKKN swimming clubs. These two Göteborg clubs have achieved total scores placing them first and third at the Swedish Swimming Championships during the last three years. The criteria for the coaches' selection were hard to ascertain. One criterion must have been results attained. However, many other reasons, such as the way the boys moved in water, the coordination of their arm and leg movements with breathing, etc., were of importance. The 18 boys were chosen for this study from the total group of boys selected for intensive swimming training because the subjects had not engaged in training for more than a few months and each was approximately 10 years of age.

## METHODS AND PROCEDURE

A carefully standardized anthropological program, including the following 17 measurements, was carried out: standing height, body weight, sitting height, head and chest circumferences, femur and humerus bicondylar widths, biacromial and biiliac widths, upper arm and calf circumferences, chest width and depth, and skinfold measurements—biceps, triceps, subscapular, and subiliac skinfolds (Karlberg et al., 1968). The progress of puberty was determined according to Tanner (1962). Eruption of permanent teeth was recorded. Estimates of the skeletal maturity of the hand and wrist were estimated according to Tanner and Whitehouse (1959). Cortical bone thickness was evaluated according to Garn (Frisancho, Garn, and Ascoli, 1970). All values used with the exception of those for cortical bone thickness, where the standard values published by Garn were used, were compared with Swedish standards (Taranger, 1976). In order to facilitate comparisons among the boys without regard to the age difference, standard deviation scores were calculated.

Total body potassium (K) was determined using the $K^{40}$ method and whole body gamma radiation counting within a lead shield, employing a plastic scintillator in a fixed position over the recumbent subject (McNeill and Grenn, 1959). Counting time was 100 sec. Total body water (TBW) was measured using the tritiated water dilution method (Berg and Isaksson, 1970). Heart volume (HV) was determined by means of biplanar radiograms with the subject in a prone position (Kjellberg, Rudhe, and Sjöstrand, 1949). Total hemoglobin (THb) and blood volume (BV) were measured employing the $J^{125}$ method (Williams and Fine, 1961). Pulmonary residual volume (RV), functional residual capacity (FRC) and total lung capacity (TLC) were measured using the closed circuit helium dilution method (Comroe et al., 1967); values for vital capacity (VC) and forced expiratory volume 1 sec ($FEV_1$) were established with a Bernstein spirometer.

Maximal oxygen uptake ($\dot{V}_{O_2}$ max) was measured at least twice on two separate days using an electrically braked bicycle ergometer (Elema) at a pedal rate of 60 rpm. Åstrand's (1952) levelling-off criterion was used in the determination of $\dot{V}_{O_2}$ max. Expired air was collected in Douglas bags and its volume measured in a balanced Tissot spirometer. At least two bags were collected on each occasion. A micro-Scholander technique was used for $O_2$ and $CO_2$ determinations (Scholander, 1947). Heart rate was obtained from ECG tracings. Blood lactate concentration was established in assays of blood drawn from a prewarmed fingertip and analyzed using an enzymatic method (Scholz et al., 1959).

All examinations were performed in March–April, 1974. The design of this longitudinal study entails the measurement of anthropological parameters, skeletal maturity, tooth eruption, total potassium, and total body water every 6 months; other examinations are performed once a year.

## RESULTS

Mean values with SD for the 18 boys are listed in Table 1. Body height exceeded a Swedish growth standard by 0.3 SD (Taranger, 1976), and body weight by 0.5 SD. Calf and upper arm circumference, triceps, and subscapular skinfold as well as bicondylar femur and humerus width were also above this growth standard (Figure 1). Body potassium (K) amounted to 76.83 g and total body water (TBW) to 24.02 liters. Vital capacity (Figure 2) and total lung capacity (Figure 3) were greater than expected on the basis of body size (Engström, Karlberg, and Schwartz, 1962). This was also the case for RV and FRC. Total hemoglobin (THb), blood volume (BV) and hemoglobin concentration were within the normal ranges for Swedish children (Karlberg and Lind, 1955). Individual values for heart volume (HV) displayed a more heterogenous picture (Figure 4). However, the mean values exceeded the anticipated values (Kjellberg et al., 1954).

Table 1. Mean values with SD for some physiological variables and body composition in boy swimmers

| Variable | Mean | SD |
|---|---|---|
| Age, years | 10.07 | 1.06 |
| Height, cm | 140.84 | 6.75 |
| Weight, kg | 33.82 | 5.49 |
| TLC, liters BTPS | 3.302 | 0.409 |
| VC, liters BTPS | 2.738 | 0.391 |
| FRC, liters BTPS | 1.438 | 0.249 |
| RV, liters BTPS | 0.562 | 0.150 |
| $FEV_1$ liters BTPS | 2.336 | 0.408 |
| THb, g | 309.4 | 62.8 |
| BV, liters | 2.42 | 0.42 |
| HV, ml | 420.7 | 79.5 |
| $\dot{V}_{O_2}$ max, liters/min STPD | 1.759 | 0.238 |
| $\dot{V}_E$ max, liters/min BTPS | 66.43 | 8.38 |
| $\dot{V}_E$ max/$\dot{V}_{O_2}$ max | 37.99 | 3.82 |
| HR max, beats/min | 198.6 | 6.2 |
| Lactate max, mmol/liter | 8.2 | 1.6 |
| K, g | 76.83 | 8.69 |
| TBW, liters | 24.02 | 3.18 |
| ICW, liters | 13.09 | 1.53 |
| ECW, liters | 11.39 | 2.33 |
| BCM, kg | 16.84 | 1.91 |
| BF, kg | 1.37 | 3.43 |

Mean maximal oxygen uptake ($\dot{V}_{O_2}$ max) amounted to 1.76 liters/min (range: 1.38–2.22 liters/min) (Figure 5) and maximal ventilation ($\dot{V}_E$ max) was 66.4 liters/min. The ventilatory coefficient in maximal exercise, $\dot{V}_E/\dot{V}_{O_2}$, was 38.0. Maximal blood lactate concentration amounted to 8.2 mmol/liter and maximal heart rate to 198.6 beats/min.

## DISCUSSION

The results obtained were in some instances quite striking, but the small size of the sample makes it impossible to draw too many conclusions. Moreover, there were differences in both body sizes and in ages. Thus, all values had to be corrected for these differences. The system described by Asmussen and Heeböll-Nielsen (1955) and by von Döbeln and Eriksson (1972) was used to adjust the differences in the dimensions and functions of the respiratory and circulatory system. Thus all volume values were divided by body height cubed and volume per time

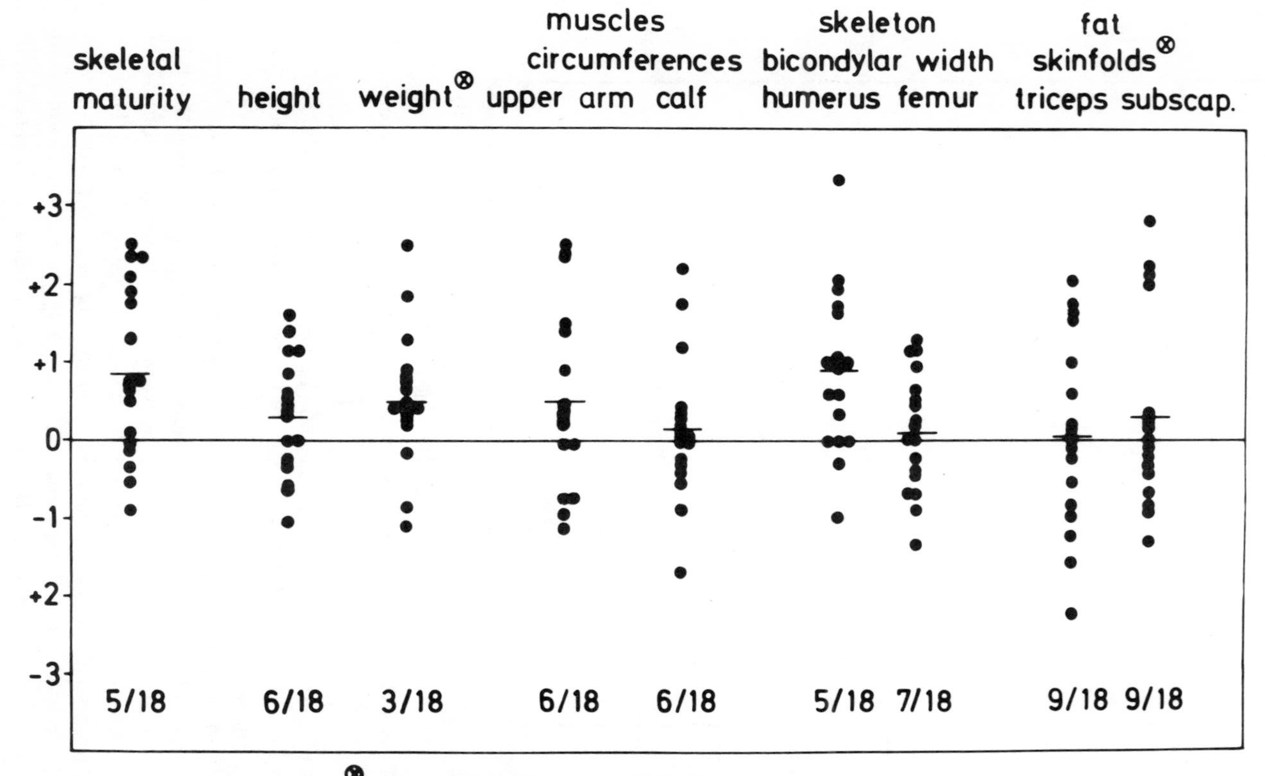


Figure 1. Individual and mean values for skeletal maturity, body weight, body height, muscle circumferences, skinfolds and skeleton bicondylar widths in relation to Swedish growth standards (Taranger, 1976). All values are expressed in standard deviation scores.

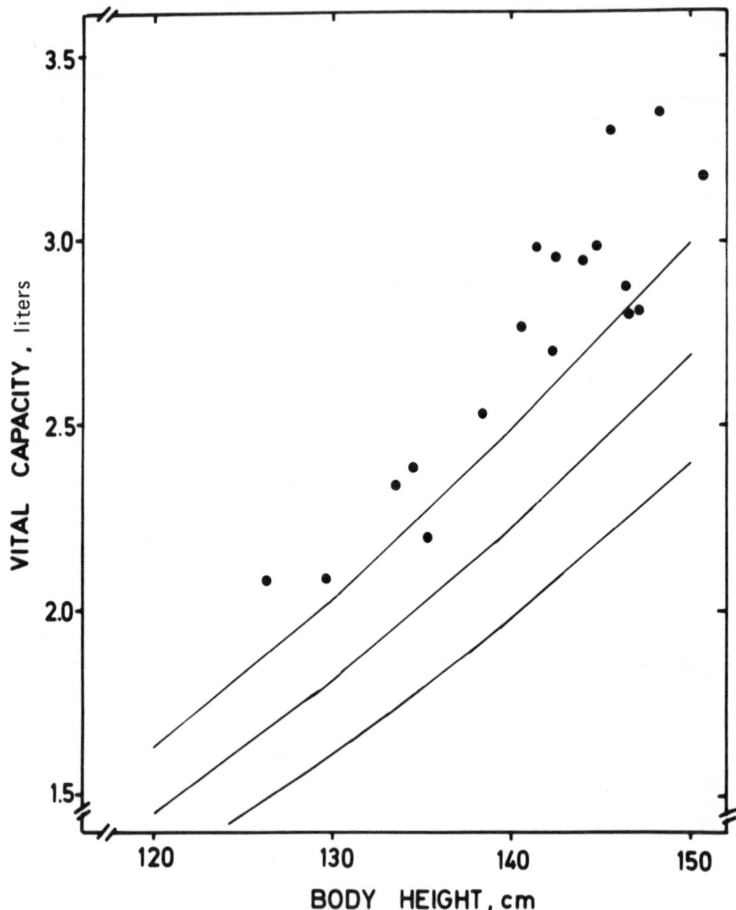


Figure 2. Individual values for vital capacity in young boy swimmers are compared with norms for Swedish boys (±2 SD) (Engström, Karlberg, and Schwartz, 1962).

values were divided by height squared (Table 2). Similar measurements for a group of Swedish boys 2 years older were also included for comparison purposes (Eriksson, 1972).

Standard deviation scores were used for anthropological measurements. The anthropological measurements indicate that the boy swimmers as a group appear to be somewhat taller and somewhat heavier without having more fat than normal boys (Figure 1), thus indicating increased muscle mass. This finding is in accordance with the total potassium values found. Since the boys had only trained at swimming for a few months, the increased muscular mass can scarcely be attributed to the training. Thus, one criterion for selection for training might be increased muscle mass.

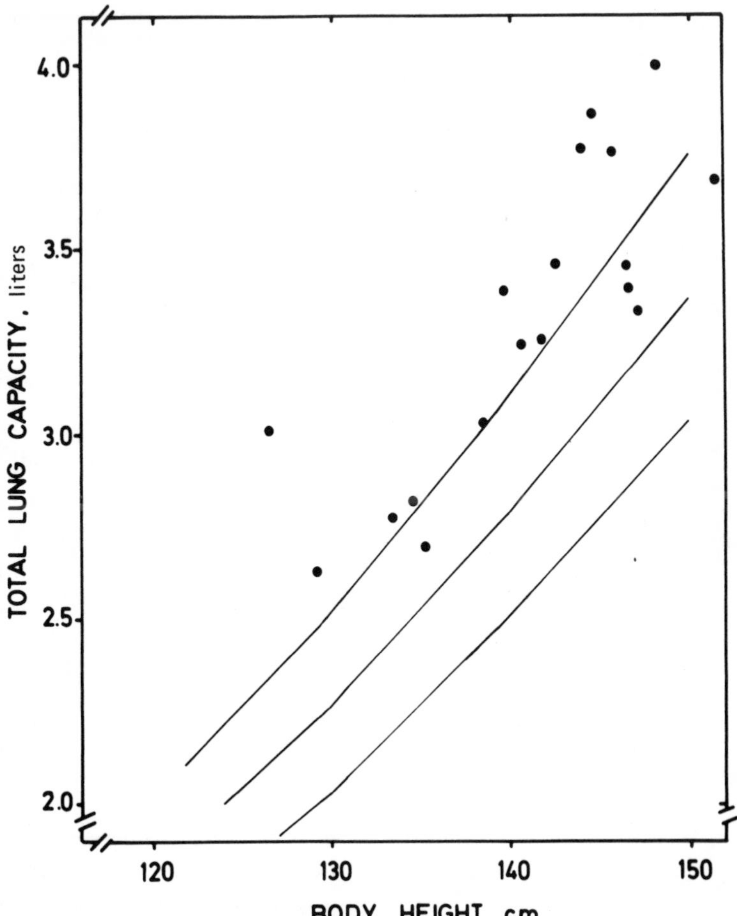


Figure 3. Individual values for total lung capacity in young boy swimmers are compared with norms for Swedish boys (±2 SD) (Engström, Karlberg, and Schwartz, 1962).

It is hard to say whether other differences in body composition and anthropological measurements indicated that the boy swimmers belonged to a select category of boys specially suited for swimming. An increased body height was found in the first report on girl swimmers (Åstrand et al., 1963). From a theoretical point of view, greater height is advantageous in swimming. Thus, increased body height might be another factor of importance in becoming a good swimmer.

The total body water/body weight ratio (TBW/BW) is said to be high in newborn babies, i.e., around 70% (Friis-Hansen, 1965), with these values decreasing with increasing age. It is not known why these 10 year old boy swimmers displayed a ratio of 75%. Their increased

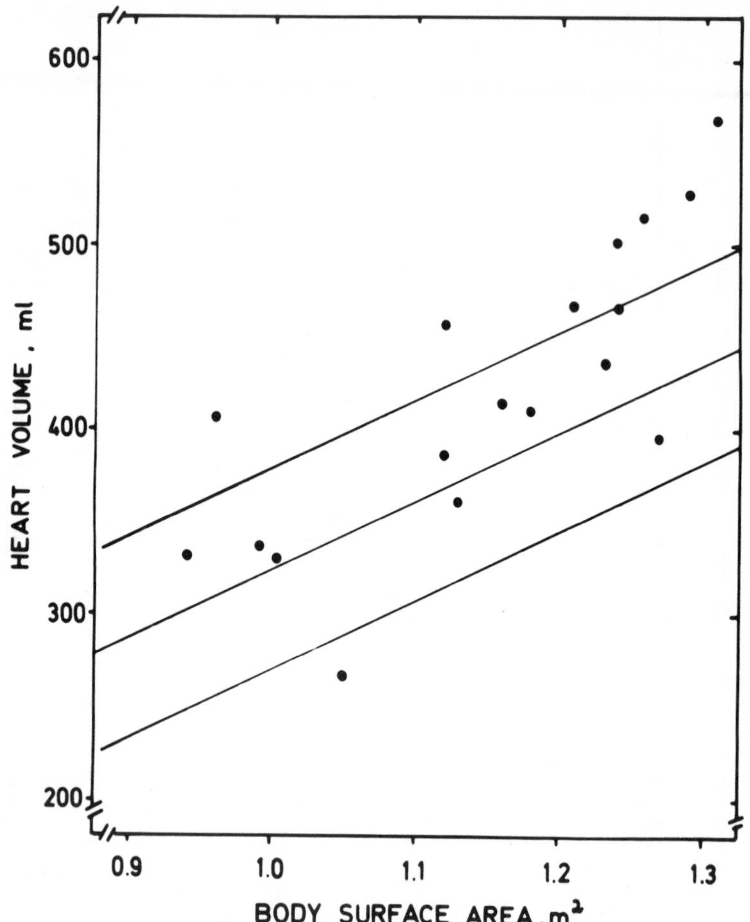


Figure 4. Individual values for heart volume in young boy swimmers are compared to norms for Swedish boys (±2 SD) (Kjellberg et al., 1954).

muscle mass may partly explain the results because muscle tissue contains much water. However, other mechanisms may have influenced this finding. It is interesting to note that increased TBW/BW ratio was also found in the longitudinal study of boys engaged in bicycle training (Berg and Bjure, 1974). Further studies are needed to explain these results fully.

Great differences are usually found when comparing the dimensions of the circulatory and respiratory organs of top athletes and normal subjects (Holmgren and Strandell, 1959; Saltin and Åstrand; 1962; Åstrand et al., 1963; Bevegård et al., 1963; Hollman, 1963; Grimby and Saltin, 1966; Magel and Andersen, 1969; Miyashita, Hayashi, and Furuhashi, 1970; Engström et al., 1971; Andrew et al., 1972). This also applies to both aerobic and anaerobic capacities. Whether these dif-

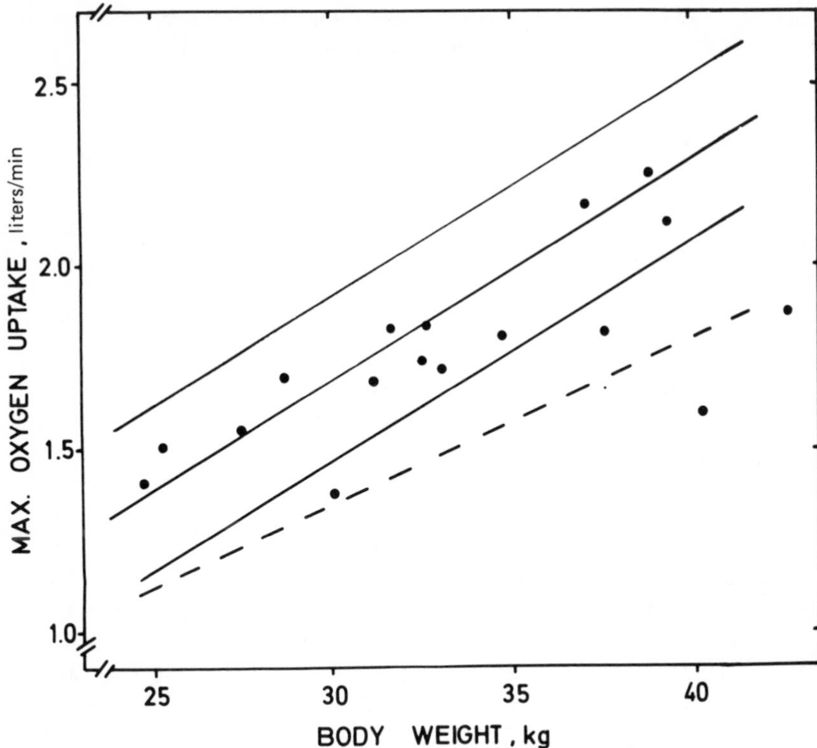


Figure 5. Individual values for maximal oxygen uptake in young boy swimmers are shown in relation to norms for Swedish boys (±2 SD) (Åstrand, 1952). A more realistic mean value for Swedish boys is also included (dotted line).

ferences can be fully explained by the effect of many years of hard training or by the possible influence of constitutional factors has been discussed (Åstrand et al., 1963).

The young boys in this study displayed only minor differences in their circulatory dimensions. Thus, both blood volume and total hemoglobin fell within the normal ranges for body size. This was also true when these dimensions per height cubed were compared with those for the 11–13 year old boys (Table 2). Heart volume per height cubed was also comparable with data for the 11–13 year old boys (Eriksson, 1972). Thus, this study found no evidence that boys with constitutionally increased circulatory dimensions become swimmers.

Conversely, values for lung volumes exceeded both normal standards (Engström, Karlberg, and Schwartz, 1962) and values for the 11–13 year old boys (Eriksson, 1972) (Table 2). It is hardly likely that the rather brief period of training in which the boys engaged caused these results. Some constitutional factor seems more likely. The special breathing problems associated with swimming, i.e., with its

Table 2. Mean values with SD for some physiological data corrected for body size in boy swimmers as compared to "normal boys" (Eriksson, 1972)

| Variable | Boy swimmers N = 18 | Normal boys N = 12 |
|---|---|---|
| Age, years | 10.1 ± 1.1 | 11.8 ± 0.8 |
| Height (H), cm | 140.8 ± 6.8 | 151.0 ± 8.1 |
| Weight (W), kg | 33.8 ± 5.5 | 44.5 ± 6.3 |
| Weight/$H^2$, kg/$m^3$ | 12.0 ± 1.2 | 13.0 ± 1.8 |
| K/$H^3$, g/$m^3$ | 27.5 ± 2.0 | 24.4 ± 2.7 |
| TLC/$H^3$, liters/$m^3$ | 1.14 ± 0.24 | 0.96 ± 0.08 |
| VC/$H^3$, liters/$m^3$ | 0.97 ± 0.06 | 0.79 ± 0.06 |
| FRC/$H^3$, liters/$m^3$ | 0.51 ± 0.07 | 0.35 ± 0.07 |
| RV/$H^3$, liters/$m^3$ | 0.21 ± 0.07 | 0.17 ± 0.04 |
| THb/$H^3$, g/$m^3$ | 109.5 ± 15.3 | 114.3 ± 13.4 |
| BV/$H^3$, liters/$m^3$ | 0.96 ± 0.45 | 0.85 ± 0.08 |
| HV/$H^3$, ml/$m^3$ | 149.9 ± 21.5 | 144.0 ± 21.6 |
| $\dot{V}_{O_2}$ max/$H^2$, liters/min × $m^2$ | 0.88 ± 0.07 | 0.82 ± 0.10 |
| $\dot{V}_{O_2}$ max/W, ml/kg × min | 52.6 ± 6.3 | 42.2 ± 6.2 |
| $\dot{V}_E$ max/$H^2$, liters/min × $m^2$ | 33.5 ± 3.9 | 23.5 ± 5.9 |
| $\dot{V}_E$ max/$\dot{V}_{O_2}$ max | 38.0 ± 3.8 | 28.4 ± 4.1 |
| HR max, beats/min | 198.6 ± 6.2 | 196.3 ± 9.4 |
| Lactate max, mmol/liter | 8.2 ± 1.6 | 7.8 ± 1.9 |

limitations on breathing rate and the very brief amount of time allowed for inspiration, may make swimming more difficult for boys with small or average-sized lungs. This hypothesis is supported by earlier results obtained with girl swimmers (Åstrand et al., 1963; Engström et al., 1971).

Aerobic capacity ($\dot{V}_{O_2}$ max) (Figure 5) did not increase when compared to the sample of Åstrand. However, Åstrand's values are the highest "normal" values in the world (Shephard, 1971; Thorén et al., 1973). His sample did not consist of normal boys and girls sampled at random (Åstrand, 1952; Åstrand, personal communication). A more truly normal value is around 45 ml/kg of body weight × min. (Shephard, 1971; Eriksson, 1972). This value is included in Figure 5 as a regression line. Compared with this last regression line, the boy swimmers had a higher value, i.e., 52.6 ml/kg × min, than what is reported to be normal (Eriksson, 1972). On the other hand, $\dot{V}_{O_2}$ max per height squared ($\dot{V}_{O_2}/H^2$) was only slightly higher than for the 11–13 year old boys (Table 2). A good correlation was found between $\dot{V}_{O_2}$ max and body potassium (Figure 6) as well as with heart volume (Figure 7). It must be remembered that during swimming it is necessary to support only a few kg and not the entire body weight (Holmér,

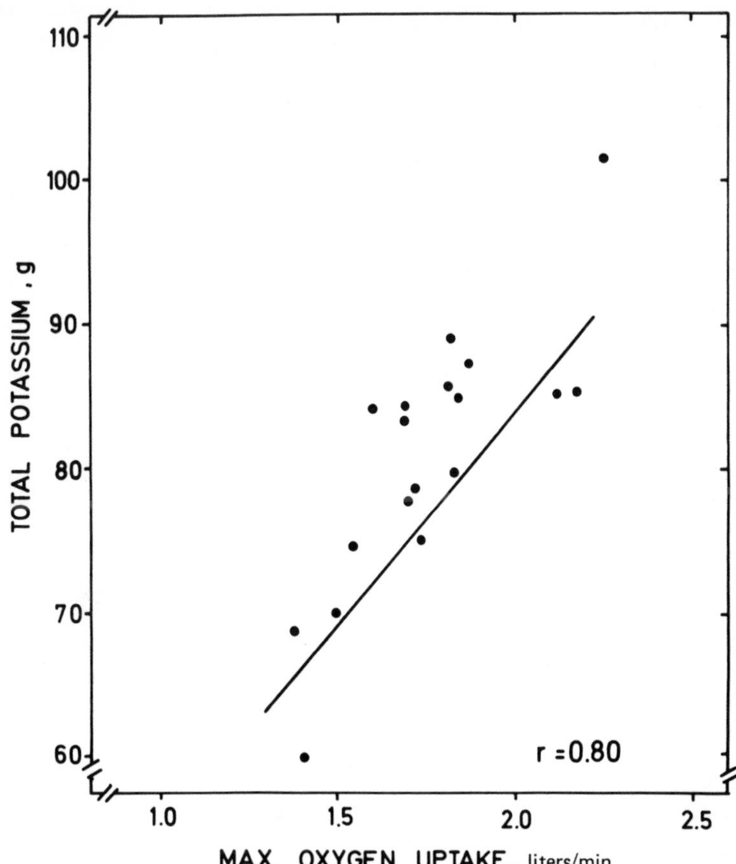


Figure 6. Individual values for maximal oxygen uptake in young boy swimmers are shown in relation to body potassium. A regression line is also included.

1974). Thus, aerobic capacity in swimmers should be expressed in absolute values, liters/min or per height squared. The increased values found indicate that increased aerobic capacity was also a criterion in selection for swimming.

It is interesting to note that anaerobic capacity, measured as maximal blood lactate concentration, did not increase in this group of boys. Because children have limited anaerobic capacity (Eriksson, Karlsson, and Saltin, 1971; Eriksson, 1972; Eriksson, Gollnick, and Saltin, 1973; Eriksson and Saltin, 1974) one would expect boys with increased anaerobic capacity to perform better and thus be selected for special training. However, this did not seem to be the case.

On the basis of this small sample of boys, it is difficult to draw any definitive conclusions regarding which factors are really characteristic

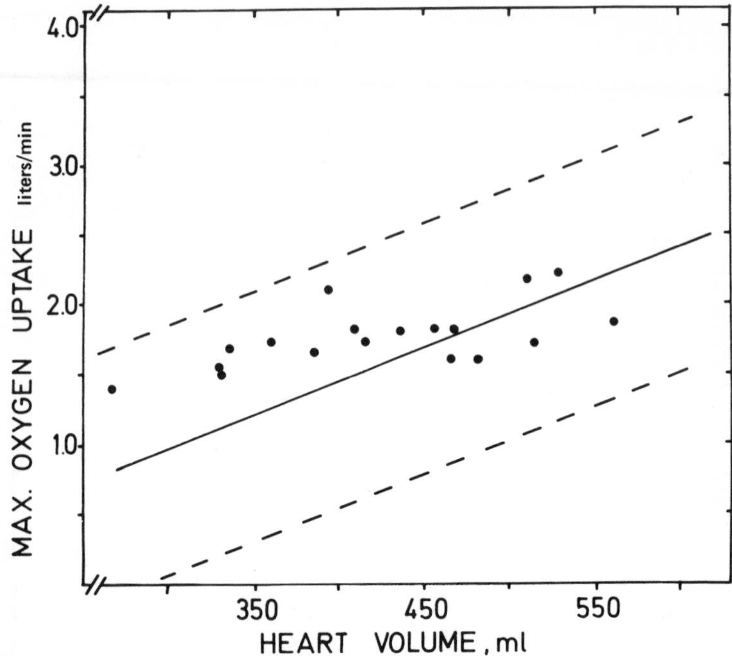


Figure 7. Individual values for maximal oxygen uptake are shown in relation to heart volume for young boy swimmers. Regression lines at ±2 SD for Swedish children are also given (Thorén, in preparation).

at this age of a potential top athlete in swimming. However, increased body height, increased muscle mass, and large lungs are believed to be of importance. A high aerobic capacity is also believed advantageous to the boys in making it possible for them to sustain hard training for a longer period of time before succumbing to fatigue. This must be of major importance to maintaining proper swimming technique. Experience has shown that the technique of a tired swimmer becomes increasingly inefficient.

## REFERENCES

Andrew, G. M., Becklake, M. R., Guleria, J. S., and Bates, D. V. 1972. Heart and lung function in swimmers and nonathletes during growth. J. Appl. Physiol. 32:245–251.

Asmussen, E., and Heeböll-Nielsen, K. 1955. A dimensional analysis of physical performance and growth in boys. J. Appl. Physiol. 7:593–603.

Åstrand, P.-O. 1952. Experimental Studies of Physical Working Capacity in Relation to Age and Sex. Munksgaard, Copenhagen.

Åstrand, P.-O. Engström, L., Eriksson, B. O., Karlberg, P., Nylander, I., Saltin, B., and Thorén, C. 1963. Girl swimmers. Acta Paediatr. Scand. (suppl. 147):1–75.

Åstrand, P.-O., and Rodahl, K. 1970. Textbook of Work Physiology. McGraw-Hill Book Company, New York.

Berg, K., and Bjure, J. 1974. Preliminary results of long-term physical training of adolescent boys with respect to body composition, maximal oxygen uptake, and lung volumes. Acta Paediatr. Belg. 38(suppl.):183–190.

Berg, K., and Isaksson, B. 1970. Adaptation in cerebral palsy of body composition, nutrition, and physical working capacity at school age. Acta Paediatr. Scand. (suppl. 204):41–52.

Bevegård, S., Holmgren, A., and Jonsson, B. 1963. Circulatory studies in well trained athletes at rest and during exercise, with special reference to stroke volume and the influence of body position. Acta Physiol. Scand. 57:26–50.

Comroe, J. H., Jr., Forster, R. E., Dubois, A. B., Briscoe, W. A., and Carlsen, E. 1967. The Lung. Clinical Physiology and Pulmonary Function Tests. 2nd Ed. Year Book Medical Publications, Chicago.

von Döbeln, W., and Eriksson, B. O. 1972. Physical training, maximal oxygen uptake, and dimensions of the oxygen transporting and metabolizing organs in boys 11–13 years of age. Acta Paediatr. Scand. 61:653–660.

Engström, I., Eriksson, B. O., Karlberg, P., Saltin, B., and Thorén, C. 1971. Preliminary report on the development of lung volumes in young girl swimmers. Acta Paediat. Scand. 60(suppl. 217):73–76.

Engström, I., Karlberg, P., and Schwartz, C. 1962. Respiratory studies in children. IX. Relation between mechanical properties of the lungs, lung volumes, and ventilatory capacity in healthy children 7–15 years of age. Acta Paediatr. Scand. 51:68–80.

Eriksson, B. O. 1972. Physical training, oxygen supply and muscle metabolism in 11–13 year old boys. Acta Physiol. Scand. Suppl. 384.

Eriksson, B. O., Engström, I., Karlberg, P., Lundin, A., Saltin, B., and Thorén, C. Long-term of intensive swim-training in girls. A 10-year follow up of the girl swimmers. Acta Paediatr. Scand. In press.

Eriksson, B. O., Engström, I., Karlberg, P., Saltin, B., and Thorén, C. 1971. Physical analysis of former girl swimmers. Acta Paediatr. Scand. (suppl. 217):68–72.

Eriksson, B. O., Engström, I., Karlberg, P., Saltin, B., and Thorén, C. Longitudinal study of the effect of intensive swim-training in young girls. In preparation.

Eriksson, B. O., Gollnick, P. D., and Saltin, B. 1973. Muscle metabolism and enzyme activities after training in boys 11–13 years old. Acta Physiol. Scand. 87:485–497.

Eriksson, B. O., Karlsson, J., and Saltin, B. 1971. Muscle metabolites during exercise in pubertal boys. Acta Paediat. Scand. (suppl. 217):154–157.

Eriksson, B. O., Lundin, A., and Saltin, B. 1975. Cardiorespiratory function in former girl swimmers and the effect of a period of physical training. Scand. J. Clin. Lab. Invest. 35:135–145.

Eriksson, B. O., and Saltin, B. 1974. Muscle metabolism during exercise in boys aged 11–16 years, compared with adults. Acta Paediatr. Belg. 28(suppl.):257–265.

Friis-Hansen, B. 1965. Hydrometry of growth and aging. In: J. Brozek (ed.), Human Body Composition, pp. 191–209. Pergamon Press, Oxford.

Frisancho, A. R., Garn, S. M., and Ascoli, W. 1970. Subperiostal and endosteal bone apposition during adolescence. Hum. Biol. 42:639–664.

Grimby, G., and Saltin, B. 1966. Physiological analysis of physically well trained middle-aged and old athletes. Acta Med. Scand. 179:513–526.

Hermansen, L. 1973. Oxygen transport during exercise in human subjects. Acta Physiol. Scand. (suppl. 399).

Hollman, W. 1963. Höchst- und Dauerleistungsfähigkeit des Sportlers. Barth, München.

Holmér, I. 1974. Physiology of swimming man. Acta Physiol. Scand. (suppl. 407).

Holmgren, A., and Strandell, T. 1959. The relationship among heart volume, total hemoglobin, and physical working capacity in former athletes. Acta Med. Scand. 163:149–160.

Karlberg, P., Klackenberg, G., Engström, I., Klackenberg-Larsson, I., Lichtenstein, H., Stensson, J., and Svennberg, I. 1968. The development of children in a Swedish urban community. A prospective longitudinal study. Acta Paediatr. Scand. (suppl. 187).

Karlberg, P., and Lind, J. 1955. Studies of the total amount of hemoglobin and the blood volume in children. I. Determination of total hemoglobin and blood volume in normal children. Acta Paediatr. Scand. 44:17–34.

Kjellberg, S., Lind, J., Lönroth, H., and Rudhe, U. 1954. Variation in heart volume in normal children of school age. Acta Radiol. 41:441–445.

Kjellberg, S. R., Rudhe, U., and Sjöstrand, T. 1949. The relation of cardiac volume to the weight and surface of the body, the blood volume, and the physical capacity for work. Acta Radiol. 31:113–122.

Magel, J. R., and Andersen, K. L. 1969. Pulmonary diffusing capacity and cardiac output in young trained Norwegian swimmers and untrained subjects. J. Med. Sci. Sport 1:131–139.

Marshall, W. A., and Tanner, J. M. 1970. Variations in pattern of pubertal changes in boys. Arch. Dis. Child. 45:13–23.

McNeill, K. G., and Grenn, R. M. 1959. Measurements with a whole body counter. Can. J. Physics 37:683–699.

Miyashita, M., Hayashi, Y., and Furuhashi, H. 1970. Maximum oxygen intake of Japanese top swimmers. J. Sports Med. 10:211–216.

Saltin, B., and Åstrand, P.-O. 1962. Maximal oxygen uptake in athletes. J. Appl. Physiol. 23:353–358.

Shephard, R. J. (ed.). 1971. The working capacity of school children. In: Frontiers of Fitness. pp. 319–344. Charles C. Thomas, Springfield.

Scholander, P. F. 1947. Analyzer for accurate estimation of respiratory gases in one-half cubic centimeter samples. J. Biol. Chem. 167:235–250.

Scholz, R., Schnitz, H., Bücher, T., and Lampen, J. O. 1959. Ueber die Wirkung von Nystatin auf Bäckerhefe. Biochem. Z. 331:71–86.

Tanner, J. M. 1962. Growth at Adolescence. Blackwell Scientific Publications, Oxford.

Tanner, J. M., and Whitehouse, R. H. 1959. Standards for Skeletal Maturity. Part I. International Children's Center, Paris.

Taranger, J. 1976. The somatic development of children in a Swedish urban community. Acta Paediatr. Scand. (suppl. 258).

Thorén, C., Seliger, V., Máček, M., Vávra, J., and Rutenfranz, J. 1973. The influence of training on physical fitness in healthy children and children with chronic diseases. In: Current Aspects of Perinatology and Physiology of Children, pp. 82–112. Springer-Verlag, Berlin.

Williams, J. A., and Fine, J. 1961. Measurement of blood volume with a new apparatus. New Engl. J. Med. 264:842–848.

# Evaluation of Some Physiological Parameters in Swimming School Students During a Two-Year Period

**P. Marconnet, W. Spinel, M. Gastaud, and J. L. Ardisson**

The lack of longitudinal studies on teenage athletes is well known. In the same way, data on the effects of training have not been commonly related either to type, intensity, and duration of work, or to the process of growth and development. The aim of this chapter is to present a longitudinal analysis of a few simple parameters in light of these special aspects.

## METHODS

### Material

The data were gathered on seven male subjects aged 13.5–15 years (mean: 14.37 ±0.4 years) who entered the swimming section of Lycée d'Antibes in September 1975.

### Training program

All the subjects selected were good swimmers who trained regularly in three to four sessions per week at their club prior to participation in this study. The training frequency was increased to daily workouts, and during the first winter the boys swam approximately 5 km/day in a 25-m swimming pool. The training consisted of long distance workout (4,000 m, 4 strokes). During the spring of 1976, it became more intensive (8 × 400 m). Beginning in February, the subjects swam in a 50-m outdoor pool. Strength training on land completed the program. The regular work was interrupted for a 2-month rest period (July 1st–September 1st). During the second winter (1976– 1977), long distance training was again included, but the volume was increased to 7 km/day in the 50-m outdoor pool.

## Procedure

Medical examinations were given three times a year—September (C+), January (C−), and June (C×) in the first year. Of the second year results, only those from the first (C +) and second (C −) examinations are available for reporting at this time. From the complete examinations, the following areas have been retained for the study: anthropometric measurements; results of cardiovascular examinations at rest, in a sitting position (index "I" = Initial); and during submaximal exercise (index "E").

The submaximal tests were given in the morning, in an 18−22°C ambient temperature, on a Monark cycloergometer at 50 rpm. The durations and loads were 6 min-450, 3 min-600, 3 min-750 kpm/mn without rest the first year, plus 3 min-900 kpm/mn the second year. Before, during and after exercise, for 5 min, the CM5 electrocardiogram lead was monitored continuously, and arterial pressure was recorded intermittently (Narco Bio System Transducers and Physiograph DPM 4B).

A few data were derived from direct measurements: the percentage of body fat (Forsyth and Sinning, 1973); the estimation of mean blood pressure (MBP) by taking one-third of pulse pressure above the diastolic pressure; the systolic tension time index (STT) (Sarnoff et al., 1958); the estimated left maximal spatial vector (A) (Liebman et al., 1966); and the $PWC_{170}$. A longitudinal analysis was conducted with the paired "t" test. One-way analysis of variance was used for cross-sectional comparisons. Statistical significance was indicated when differences had a probability of occurrence of 0.05 or less.

## RESULTS

Mean values of parameters are plotted against controls in time in Figures 1, 2 and 3. Height (H), (Figure 1a) increased from 168.36 ±9.68 to 174.71 ±6.8 cm. Weight (W), (Figure 1b) paralleled height, increasing from 58.86 ±11.38 to 65.60 ±8.58 kg, except during the first spring when it showed an insignificant decrease. Percentage of body fat (Figure 1c) was calculated from June 1976 only and showed a marked rise from 11.37 ±5.73 to 16.14 ±4.01% during the summer period when training was interrupted.

Heart rate at rest in the sitting position ($HR_I$) (Figure 2a) decreased from 83.57 ±11.57 to 70.71 ±7.61 beats/min during the first winter period. The additional decrease was not statistically significant at only 4.14 beats/min. during an entire year. Heart rate during

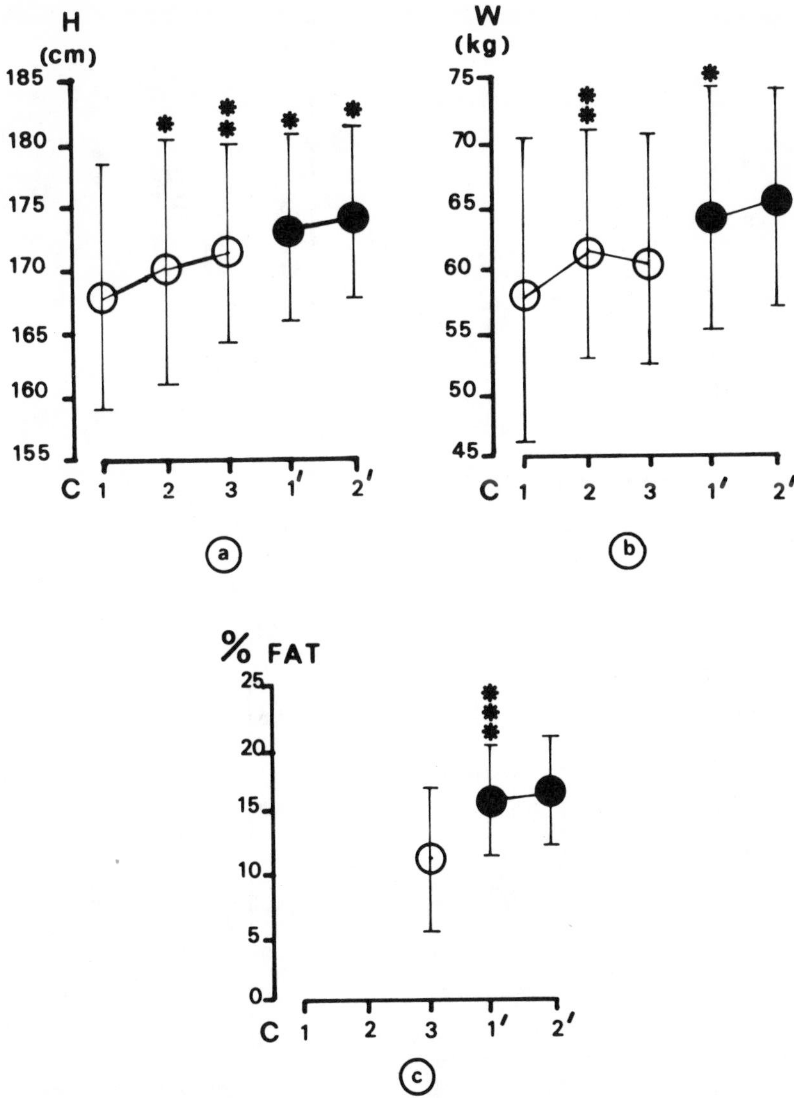


Figure 1. Biometric data from successive examinations are shown (mean ±1 SD): a shows height; b, weight; and c, percentage of body fat. Statistical differences from the preceding examination are indicated as follows: $^{*}P \leqslant 0.05$, $^{**}P \leqslant 0.01$, $^{***}P \leqslant 0.005$.

submaximal exercise ($HR_E$) (Figure 3a) also decreased significantly during the first winter at the three levels. The decrease averaged 13.12%, and there was no significant difference among the three workloads, although heart rate values changed.

The mean blood pressure at rest in the sitting position ($MBP_I$) (Figure 2c) failed to show a significant change between initial and final

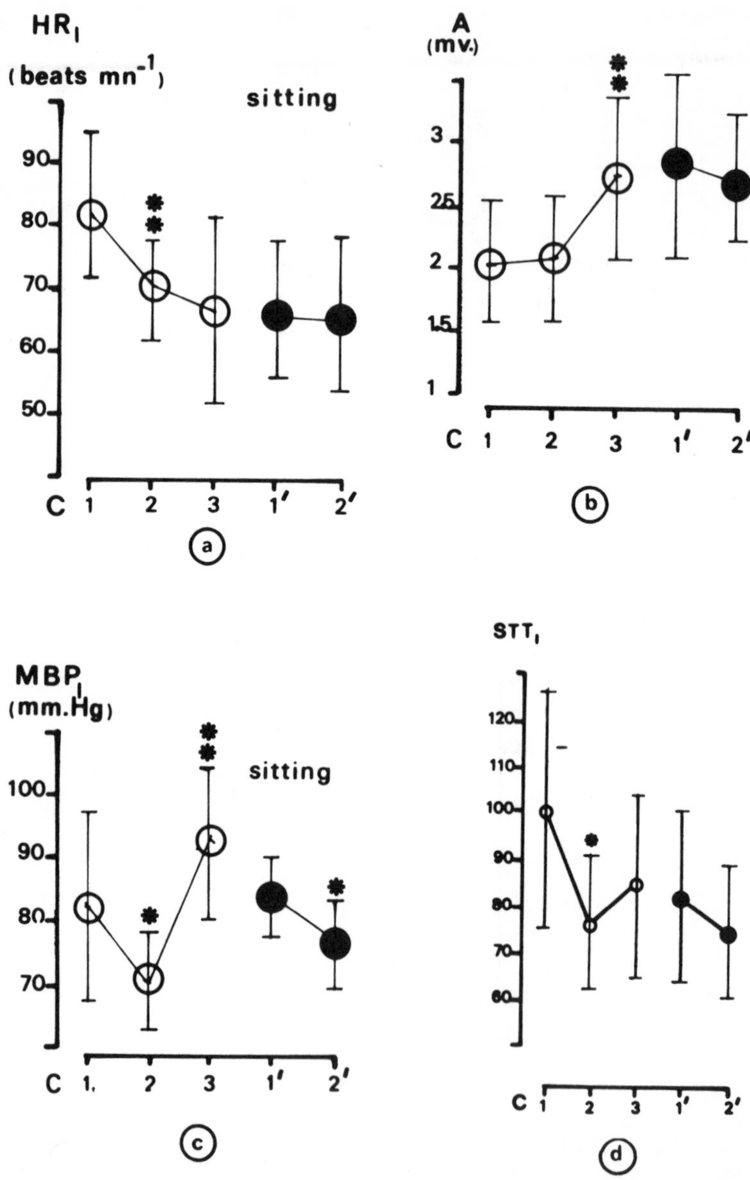


Figure 2. Cardiocirculatory parameters at rest in the sitting position are shown (mean ±1 SD): a shows heart rate; b, estimated left maximal spatial vector; c, calculated mean blood pressure; and d, systolic tension time index (divided by 100). Statistical differences from the preceding examination results are indicated as follows: $^*P \leqslant 0.05$, $^{**}P \leqslant 0.01$, $^{***}P \leqslant 0.005$.

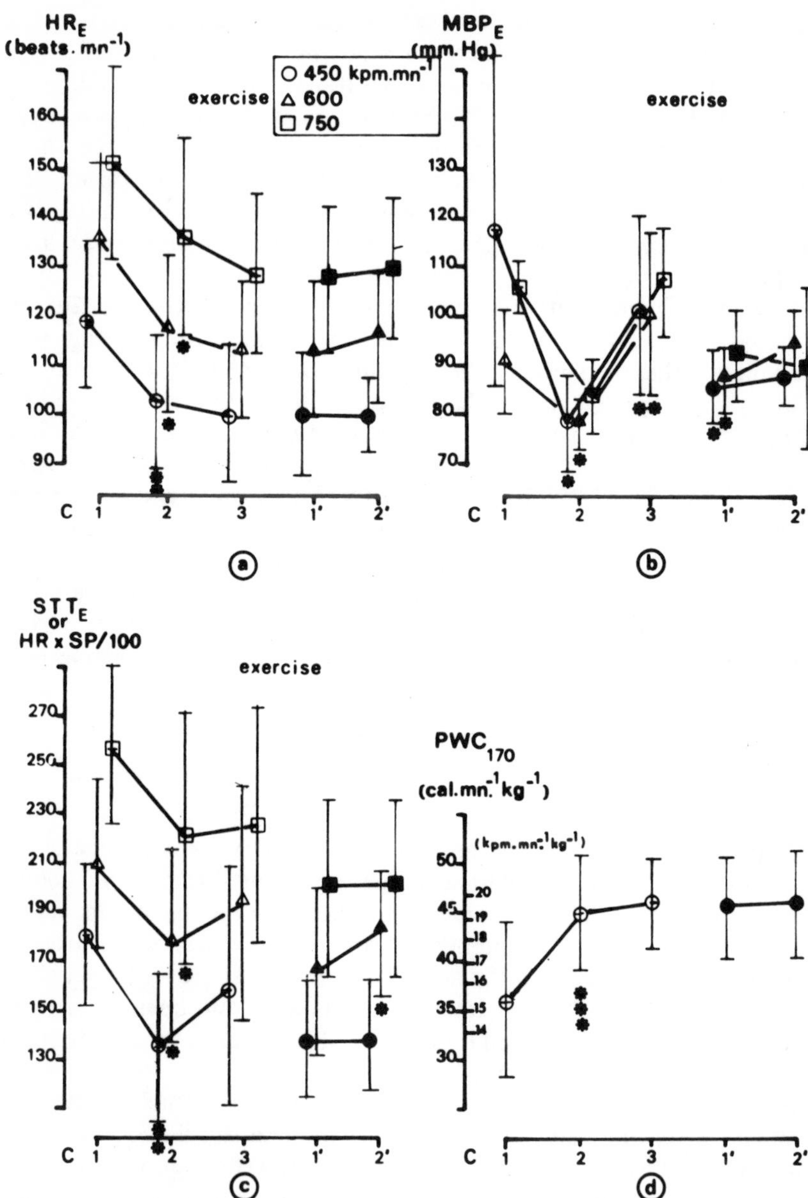


Figure 3. Cardiocirculatory parameters during submaximal exercise are shown (mean ≤1 SD): a, shows heart rate; b, calculated mean blood pressure; c, systolic tension time index; and d, PWC$_{170}$. Statistical differences from the results of the preceding examination are indicated as follows: $*P \leqslant .05$, $**P \leqslant .01$, $***P \leqslant .005$.

values (82.82 ±19.29 and 76.60 ±6.96 mm Hg, respectively), but a significant decrease, then increase, and then another decrease was noted during the first, second, and last training periods, respectively. No statistically meaningful differences existed between values of submaximal mean blood pressure ($MBP_E$) (Figure 3b) at the three workloads. The curves paralleled that of $MBP_I$, except during the second winter period. A minimum mean value of 81 ±2.88 mm Hg and maximum mean value of 103.51 ±3.55 mm Hg were obtained in January and June, respectively.

The estimated left maximal spatial vector (A) (Figure 2b) increased from 2.07 ±0.47 to 2.75 ±0.53 mV. The main variation was obtained during the spring of 1976 (from 2.09 ±0.46 to 2.76±0.61 mV). The systolic tension time index at rest in the sitting position ($STT_I$) (Figure 2d) decreased over the entire period from 100.77 ±25.23 to 75.11 ±14.47. The first period changes occurred at a very fast rate and were followed by a nonsignificant increase. The submaximal systolic tension time index ($STT_E$) (Figure 3c) demonstrated a pattern quite close to that of the resting condition; the higher the load, the higher the value became, with significant differences between each level and the next. The $PWC_{170}$ (Figure 3d) increased rapidly and significantly during the first winter from 15.38 ±3.59 to 19.39 ±2.83 kpm/min/kg, then leveled off for the remaining time.

## DISCUSSION

### Anthropometric data

Using the French INSERM growth curve chart as a reference standard, mean values for height and weight were found to be 1 SD above the normal values. That swimmers are taller than the mean population has been already been mentioned (Andrew et al., 1972). The observation period coincides with the adolescent growth spurt of the subjects and the rate of growth falls within normal limits. Consequently, growth does not seem to be affected by training. The weight changes through time were not quite as regular as were the changes in height. Initial weight gain was probably linked to sudden changes in daily activities. Increasing the intensity and volume of training during Spring, 1976 may have caused the small but nonsignificant loss of weight. The concomitant increase in weight and percentage of body fat during the summer when training was interrupted demonstrates the deviation of metabolic pathways toward the synthesis of adipose tissue.

### Heart rate

Adolescent growth spurts in all dimensions include an increase in cardiac size and stroke volume associated with decreased resting and submaximal heart rate. (Tanner, 1962; Seely, Guzman and Becklake, 1974). The decrease in resting HR for nontrained subjects has been reported to be 8.4% between 13.8 and 14.7 years of age (Seely, Guzman, and Becklake, 1974). This decrease amounted to 13.12% between 14.37 and 14.70 years in this investigation, five times greater than the decrease previously reported. Such a great change cannot be attributed to the adolescent growth spurt and must therefore be attributed to the training regimens.

Physical training induces bradycardia at rest and during submaximal exercise in children and adolescents as well as in adults. It is particularly pronounced in young swimmers (Andrew et al., 1972; Cunningham and Eynon, 1973; Shephard, Godin, and Campbell, 1974). The mechanism is still not quite clear, as stated in a recent review by Scheuer and Tipton (1977), but it is recognized that hemodynamic conditions during swimming are able to elicit the greater stroke volume associated with decreased heart rate (McArdle, Glaser, and Magel, 1971).

### $PWC_{170}$

There is a linear relationship between this parameter and: heart rate and stroke volume; and total blood volume and hemoglobin (Bevegård, Holmgren, and Jonsson, 1963; Holmgren et al., 1964). Indirect confirmation can be found here in a steep rise in $PWC_{170}$ values and a fast decrease in resting and submaximal heart rate during the first period.

### Estimation of Left Maximal Spatial Vector (A)

This parameter, selected as a criterion of cardiac hypertrophy, failed to show any increase during the first winter, while signs of cardiac dilatation rapidly settled during the same period. Conversely, the latter tapered off during the spring period as the former rose steeply. These results are in agreement with previous reports about the chronological order of cardiac adaptation to chronic exercise (Wyatt and Mitchell, 1974; Scheuer and Tipton, 1977).

### Calculated mean blood pressure

To speculate on the behavior of this parameter, one must establish some hypotheses, as follows: computation of MBP from external records gives a correct estimation of actual values; present failure of statistical differences among the three levels of submaximal exercise makes discussion of a single average value ($MBP_E$) feasible; actual variations of $MBP_E$ do not shift significantly from those reported; controls incurred at the very moment of extreme values. Previous observations about the effects of physical training on resting and submaximal arterial pressures are not in complete agreement. Increased (Bevegård, Holmgren and Jonsson, 1963; Andersen, 1968; Ekblom et al., 1968) or unchanged (Scheuer and Tipton, 1977) values for $MBP_E$ have been reported. The cyclical changes evidenced in the present study lead one to question whether $MBP_E$ is capable of ubiquitous responses to the same stress or can display specific short term responses to training programs.

### Systolic Tension Time Index

The systolic tension time index at rest and during submaximal exercise decreased steadily during the entire time except during the spring period. It can be noted that its only rise, indicating a higher myocardic oxygen consumption (Hugenholtz, 1966), coincided with signs of cardiac hypertrophy and steeply increased MBP. Provided the total peripheral resistances do not present important changes at that instant, increased MBP could be explained by a higher cardiac output resulting from a higher myocardial contractile strength and ventricular ejection. These cardiocirculatory alterations may be related to the increased intensity of training as opposite changes in hypertrophy criteria STT and MBP values may be linked to summer detraining.

## CONCLUSIONS

Important physiological alterations rapidly occur at the beginning of the first year linked to the transition from swimming clubs and family life to vigorous swimming training and boarding school life, while similar changes fail to appear the second year at the same period.

The main cause of structural and functional changes appears to be the training program, although interferences from the growing process cannot be neglected.

Cardiorespiratory adaptations can be estimated by a combined vertical and longitudinal study of quite simple parameters. Signs of adaptation are arranged in a chronological order.

## REFERENCES

Andersen, K. L. 1968. The cardiovascular system in exercise. In: H. B. Falls (ed.), Exercise Physiology, pp. 79–128. Academic Press, New York.

Andrew, G. M., Becklake, M. R., Guleria, J. S., and Bates, D. V. 1972. Heart and lung functions in swimmers and nonathletes during growth. J. Appl. Physiol. 32:245–251.

Bevegård, S., Holmgren, A., and Jonsson, B. 1963. Circulatory studies in well trained athletes at rest and during heavy exercise, with special reference to stroke volume and the influence of body position. Acta Physiol. Scand. 57:26–50.

Cunningham, D. A., and Eynon, R. B. 1973. The working capacity of young competitive swimmers, 10–16 years of age. Med. Sci. Sports 5:227–231.

Ekblom, B., Åstrand, P.-O., Saltin, B., Stenberg, J., and Wallström, B. 1968. Effect of training on circulatory response to exercise. J. Appl. Physiol. 24:518–528.

Forsyth, H. L., and Sinning, W. E. 1973. The anthropometric estimation of body density and lean body weight of male athletes. Med. Sci. Sports 5:174–180.

Holmgren, A., Mossfeldt, F., Sjöstrand, T., and Strom, G. 1964. Effect of training on work capacity, total hemoglobin, blood volume, heart volume, and pulse rate in recumbent and upright positions. In: E. Jokl and E. Simon (eds.), International Research in Sport and Physical Education, pp. 335–349. Charles C. Thomas, Springfield, Ill.

Hugenholtz, P. G. 1966. The accuracy of vectocardiographic criteria as related to the hemodynamic state. In: I. Hoffman and R. C. Taynor (eds.), Vectorcardiography, pp. 163–168. North Holland Publishing Company, Amsterdam.

Liebman, J., Romberg, H. C., Downs, T., and Agusti, R. 1966. The Frank QRS vectocardiogram in the premature infant. In: I. Hoffman and R. C. Taynor (eds.), Vectorcardiography, pp. 256–271. North Holland Publishing Company, Amsterdam.

McArdle, W. D., Glaser, R. M., and Magel, J. R. 1971. Metabolic and cardio-respiratory response during free swimming and treadmill walking. J. Appl. Physiol. 30:733–738.

Sarnoff, S. J., Braunwald, E., Welch, G., Case, R. B., Stainsby, W. N., and Macruz, R. 1958. Hemodynamic determinants of the oxygen consumption of the heart with special reference to the tension time index. Am. J. Physiol. 192:148–157.

Scheuer, J. and Tipton, C. M. 1977. Cardiovascular adaptations to physical training. Annu. Rev. Physiol. 39:221–251.

Seely, J. E., Guzman, C. A., and Becklake, M. R. 1974. Heart and lung function at rest and during exercise in adolescence. J. Appl. Physiol. 36:34–40.

Shephard, R. J. (ed.). 1971. Frontiers of Fitness. Charles C. Thomas, Springfield, Ill. p. 329.

Shephard, R. J., Godin, G., and Campbell, R. 1974. Characteristics of sprint, medium, and long distance swimmers. Eur. J. Appl. Physiol. 32:99–116.

Tanner, J. M. 1962. Growth at adolescence. 2nd Ed. Blackwell Scientific Publications, Oxford.

Wyatt, H. L., and Mitchell, J. H. 1974. Influences of physical training on the hearts of dogs. Circ. Res. 35:883–889.

# Spiroergometric Follow-up of Hungarian Swimmers—1971–1977

**P. Apor**

Publications concerning long-term following of top sportsmen are limited. According to Eriksson (1971), previously high cardio-respiratory capacities—except the heart size—returned to the sedentary levels a few years after cessation of training in top girl swimmers. Ekblom (1971) found a higher development of cardiorespiratory functions in 11 year old boys participating in endurance training over 32 months than was found in the controls. The spiroergometric results of 67 athletes hardly changed from May to October (Thomas and Reilly, 1976). Examinations, encompassing 3–6 month competitive seasons, revealed some improvement of physiological functions (e.g., Coleman et al. (1974) recorded an increase in vertical velocity of basketball players). Others observed some decrease of aerobic parameters, e.g., Hanson (1975) on Nordic skiers or Campbell (1968) on basketball players. Schmidt-Kolmer, Klimt and Schwartze (1970) noticed an improvement in the aerobic capacity of child swimmers over a 2–year period.

The progress of aerobic capacity reached the 60 ml/kg/min within 1.5–2 years, but this level was not surpassed in the following years despite increased training volume and intensity for 7–12 year old swimmers (Apor and Ölveczky, 1972). Modern pentathlon participants, retested each February and May between 1971 and 1973, did not show any improvement in aerobic capacity values in the same months of consecutive years (Apor et al., 1974).

## SUBJECTS AND PROCEDURES

Spiroergometric tests were carried out on the members of the Hungarian National Teams in May, 1971, and in the weeks following the indoor autumn seasons of consecutive years. Only the measurements overlapping the vita maxima criteria (Apor, Szabo-Wahlstab, and Miklos, 1972) were taken into account. At the beginning of 1976, the tests were performed after 7–10 days rest. The swimmers were tested on a Jaeger treadmill and a cranking ergometer and measured by a Jaeger open system Pneumotest attached on line to an Olivetti computer. BOC masks were used with valves 32 mm in diameter. The gas analyzers were checked by standard gas mixtures, and the pneumotachograph by pump before every measurement.

The annual best result in terms of the percent of the world record was designated as the swimming performance. The water $\dot{V}_{O_2}$ was calculated from the running and cranking $\dot{V}_{O_2}$ max according the formula:

$$\dot{V}_{O_2} \text{ water} = \dot{V}_{O_2} \text{ cranking} + \frac{\dot{V}_{O_2} \text{ running} - \dot{V}_{O_2} \text{ cranking}}{6}$$

Pulmonary diffusion capacity was measured by the single breath method, by 10 sec apnea (Jaeger Diffusions Test).

## RESULTS

Table 1 and Figures 1 and 2 present the measured values. Between 1971 and 1975, a significant increase was shown in the relative aerobic capacity both of male and female swimmers. During these years the members of the team were changed: the older swimmers, successful, though aerobically, not as well-trained and trained only in the short events, were replaced by swimmers from the Central Sport School (KSI; trainer, T. Széchy). Although the same boys participated in the tests in January and in December of 1976, the respectively high values at the end of 1974 were not reached again. The motivation for subjects of the tests had not changed, judged by the pH and maximal pulse.

The oxygen pulse/body weight decreased also; the change of the $O_2$-extraction was ambiguous, and its standard deviation was rather large. The individual $\dot{V}_E$ max values remained at the same levels during the examination periods. This involved the significance of the $O_2$-extraction while breathing to the changes in the aerobic capacity. To examine this, the measurement of alveolar ventilation and pulmonary diffusion was introduced. Body dimensions did not change.

In spite of the declining tendencies in aerobic parameters, Hargittay in 1975 and Verrasztó in 1976 broke the world record in 400-m medley, and Wladár broke the European record for 800 m. Hargittay had 89 and 92 ml/kg aerobic capacity values, but in 1971 and in 1976 his maximal $O_2$ uptakes were 52 and 56 ml/kg, respectively. Wladár had 65, 76, 64, 62, 69, and 55 ml/kg aerobic capacity values

Table 1. Number of persons and means of measured parameters

| Time of tests[a] | A | B | C | D | E | F | G | H | A | B | C | D | E | F | G | H |
|---|---|---|---|---|---|---|---|---|---|---|---|---|---|---|---|---|
| | Number of persons | | | | | | | | Age (years) | | | | | | | |
| Nat. team, male | 13 | | 12 | 18 | | 15 | 14 | 15 | 18.1 | | 16.1 | 16.8 | | 16.7 | 16.2 | 17.1 |
| Nat. team, female | 9 | | 10 | 13 | 13 | 13 | 12 | 9 | 18.3 | | 16.1 | 17.7 | | | | |
| Club KSI, boys | | 11 | | | 13 | | | | | 12.2 | | | 16.4 | | | |
| | Weight (kg) | | | | | | | | Height (cm) | | | | | | | |
| Nat. team, male | 69.8 | | 67.3 | 69.6 | | 67.7 | 67.7 | 68.6 | 177 | | 176 | 176 | | 177 | 177 | 177 |
| Nat. team, female | 59.9 | | 55.9 | 56.7 | | 60.8 | 53.3 | 54.7 | 166 | | 166 | 167 | | 169 | 164 | 164 |
| Club KSI, boys | | 46.6 | | | 71.3 | | | | | 159 | | | 179 | | | |
| | $\dot{V}_{O_2}$ (ml/kg × min) | | | | | | | | Oxygen pulse (ml/beat) | | | | | | | |
| Nat. team, male | 59.5 | | 70.1 | 74.1 | | 61.5 | 62.5 | 58.3 | 22.3 | | 25.3 | 25.4 | | 22.1 | 21.8 | 20.6 |
| Nat. team, female | 50.8 | | 58.5 | 62.6 | | 54.4 | 52.4 | 51.4 | 16.0 | | 16.1 | 17.5 | | 18.1 | 14.1 | 13.8 |
| Club KSI, boys | | 64.8 | | | 57.9 | | | | | 15.2 | | | 21.7 | | | |
| | $\dot{V}_E$ (liters/min) | | | | | | | | Oxygen pulse/body weight | | | | | | | |
| Nat. team, male | 137 | | 133 | 143 | | 126 | 130 | 122 | 32 | | 38 | 36 | | 33 | 32 | 29 |
| Nat. team, female | 89 | | 112 | 114 | | 112 | 94 | 90 | 26 | | 24 | 31 | | 30 | 26 | 25 |
| Club KSI, boys | | 99 | | | 139 | | | | | 33 | | | 30 | | | |
| | max $O_2$-extraction (%) | | | | | | | | Vital capacity (liters) | | | | | | | |
| Nat. team, male | 4.8 | | 3.5 | 5.4 | | 5.3 | 5.0 | 5.0 | 5.7 | | 5.5 | | | | 5.7 | 5.4 |
| Nat. team, female | 4.7 | | 4.4 | 4.6 | | 4.7 | 4.5 | 4.6 | 4.5 | | 4.6 | | | | 4.1 | 3.6 |
| Club KSI, boys | | 4.5 | | | 4.9 | | | | | 3.5 | | | | | | |

[a] Symbols: A: May, 1971—B: Jan, 1973—C: Jan, 1974—D: Jan, 1975—E: Apr, 1975—F: Jan, 1976—G: Dec, 1976—H: Apr, 1977

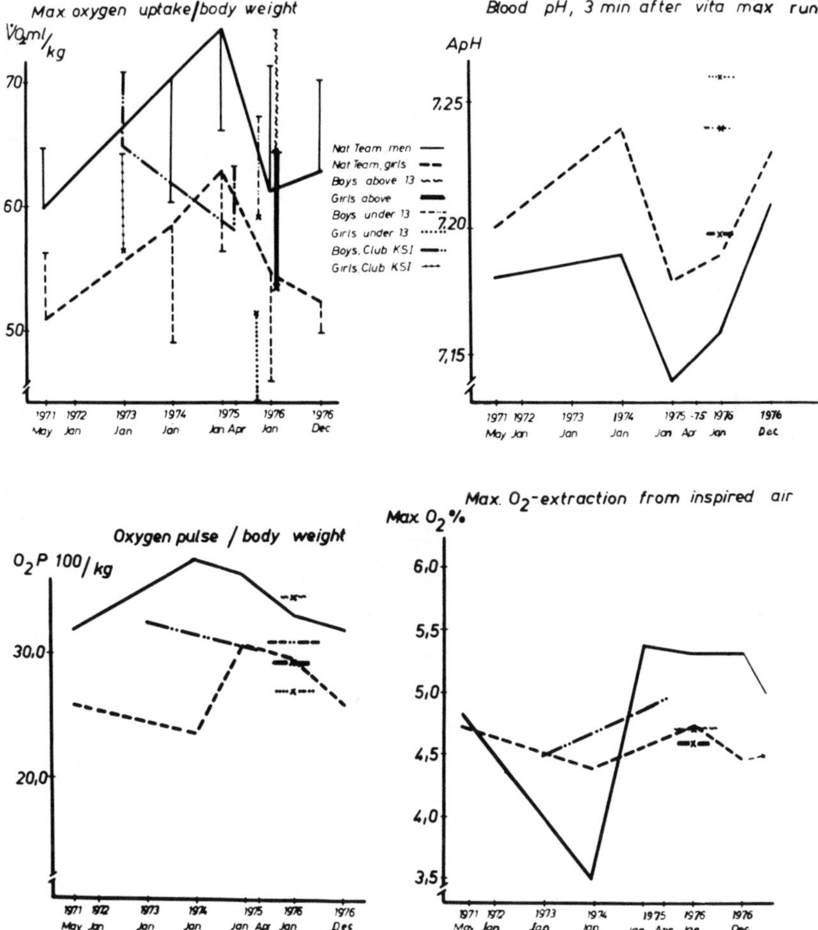


Figure 1. Vita maxima values of swimmers from the Hungarian National Team and other groups.

between 1973 and 1977, and in most of these years, he swam the 1500-m event within 16 min.

The aerobic capacity of well trained swimmers was between 55–70 ml/kg in males and between 50–60 ml/kg in females, according to several authors (Åstrand et al., 1963; Magel and Faulkner, 1967; de la Parra, 1967; Chase, 1969; McArdle, Glaser, and Magel, 1971). The measures of this study's swimmers were within these limits but changed very significantly from year to year. It was not clear whether this fluctuation depended on actual physical condition, on the differences in training methods, or on other factors. Certainly, the aerobic

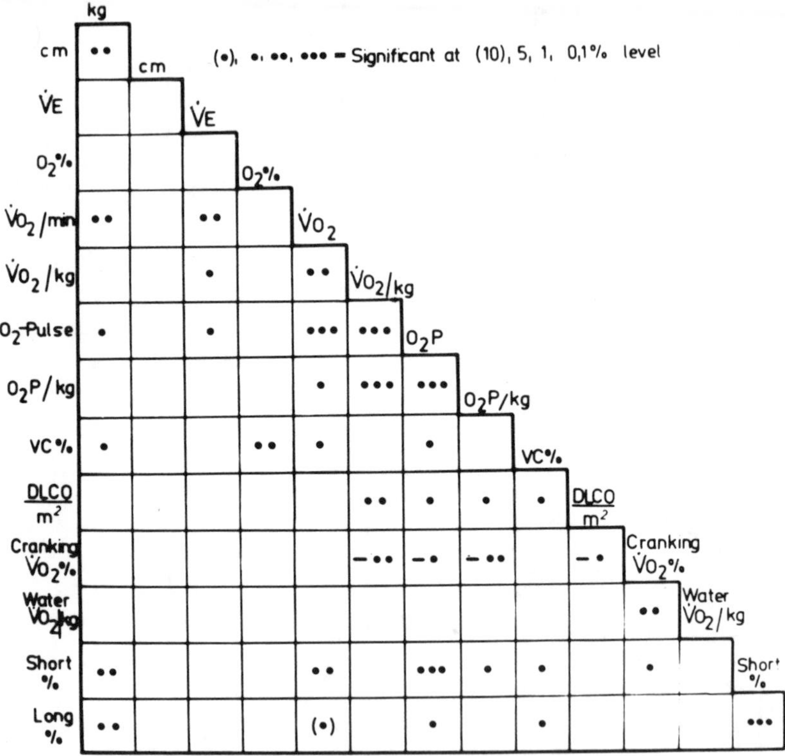


Figure 2. Correlations of physiological parameters measured on the members of the Hungarian National Teams.

capacity is not a fixed value and the acquired level can diminish in spite of continuous training.

Correlations among swimming performances and spiroergometric parameters revealed specific tendencies (Figure 3). Body weight was positively related not only to the $\dot{V}_{O_2}$ max, but also to swimming performance. A relationship existed between the resting DLCO and $\dot{V}_{O_2}$ max and max $O_2$-pulse. The cranking and running $\dot{V}_{O_2}$ max were negatively correlated. The calculated water $\dot{V}_{O_2}$ did not correlate with other parameters. The short distance performance correlated with the $\dot{V}_{O_2}$ max and in one case with the maximum oxygen pulse. The long distance performances correlated in addition with the maximum $\dot{V}_E$ and with the maximum oxygen extraction, which is the highest value measured at any time during the run. The relationship between the short distance performance and the long one is very close; the

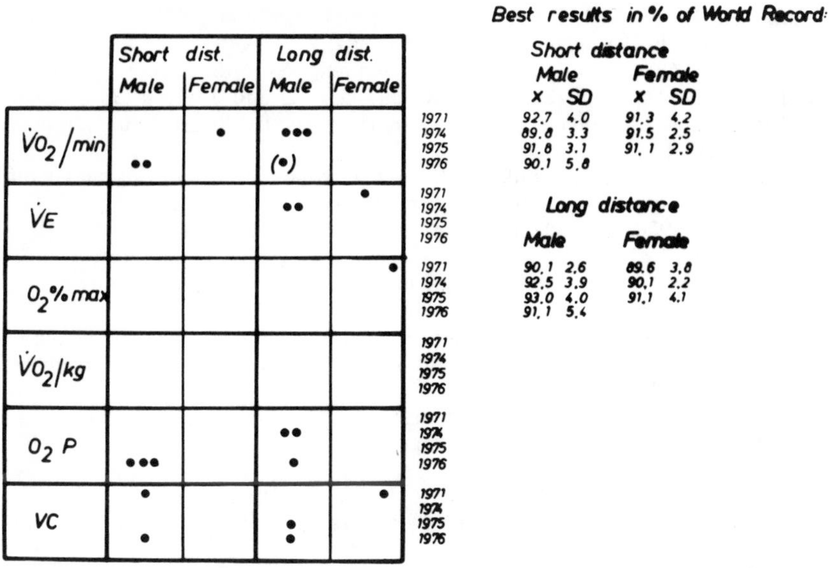

| | Short dist. | | Long dist. | | |
|---|---|---|---|---|---|
| | Male | Female | Male | Female | |
| $\dot{V}O_2$/min | •• | • | ••• (•) | | 1971 1974 1975 1976 |
| $\dot{V}_E$ | | | •• | • | 1971 1974 1975 1976 |
| $O_2$% max | | | | • | 1971 1974 1975 1976 |
| $\dot{V}O_2$/kg | | | | | 1971 1974 1975 1976 |
| $O_2$ P | ••• | | •• • | | 1971 1974 1975 1976 |
| VC | • • | | • • | • | 1971 1974 1975 1976 |

**Best results in % of World Record:**

| | Short distance | | | | Long distance | | | |
|---|---|---|---|---|---|---|---|---|
| | Male | | Female | | Male | | Female | |
| | x | SD | x | SD | | | | |
| | 92.7 | 4.0 | 91.3 | 4.2 | 90.1 | 2.6 | 89.6 | 3.8 |
| | 89.8 | 3.3 | 91.5 | 2.5 | 92.5 | 3.9 | 90.1 | 2.2 |
| | 91.8 | 3.1 | 91.1 | 2.9 | 93.0 | 4.0 | 91.1 | 4.1 |
| | 90.1 | 5.8 | | | 91.1 | 5.4 | | |

Figure 3. Correlations of performance to selected physiological parameters.

r was between 0.80 and 0.92. With only one or two tests per year, it was not possible to determine the correlation between peak form and test results.

## SUMMARY

Spiroergometric results measured in the same training period showed significant changes from year to year. Rather poor correlations were found between aerobic parameters measured in December or January, and the best swimming performance gained during the year before.

## REFERENCES

Apor, P., and Ölveczky, V. 1972. Development of physiological parameters and of athletic performance in children, p. 215. In: Sport in the Modern World. Sci. Congr. Munich, Springer-Verlag, Berlin.

Apor, P., Szabo-Wahlstab, S., and Miklos, M. 1972. Relationship between aerobic and anaerobic parameters. In: G. Hansen and H. Mellerowicz (eds.), 3rd International Seminar for Ergometry, Berlin.

Apor, P., Prónay, L., Földi, L., Dászlo, I., and Benedek, F. 1974. Two-year study on Hungarian modern pentathlonists. Testnev. Sporteü. Szemle, 14:251–259.

Åstrand, P.-O., Engström, L., Eriksson, B. O., Karlberg, P., Nylander, I., Saltin, B., and Thorén, C. 1963. Girl swimmers. Acta Paediatr. (suppl. 147):43–63.

Campbell, D. E. 1968. Heart rates of selected male college freshmen during a season of basketball. Res. Q. 39:880–887.

Chase, G. 1969. Oxygen utilization in swimming. Swimming Technique 6:2.

Coleman, A. E., Kreuzer, P., Friedrich, D. W., and Juvenal, J. P. 1974. Aerobic and anaerobic responses of male college freshmen during a season of basketball. J. Sports Med. 14:26–31.

Dixon, R. W., Jr., and Faulkner, J. 1971. Cardiac outputs during maximum effort running and swimming. J. Appl. Physiol. 30:653–656.

Dragan, I., 1970. Medical problems of swimming training. Apuntes Med. Deport 7:181–189.

Ekblom, B. 1971. Physical training in normal boys in adolescence. Acta Paediatr. Scand. (suppl. 217):60–83.

Eriksson, B., Thorén, C., Endström, I., and Karlberg, P. 1967. Influence of physical training on growth. A study on girl swimmers. Acta Paediatr. Scand. (suppl. 177):86.

Eriksson, G. 1971. Respiratory and circulatory dimensions and the functional capacity in active and postinactive girl swimmers. In: 2nd Medicoscientific Conference of FINA, Dublin.

Eriksson, B., Engström, I., Karlberg, P., Saltin, B., and Thorén, C. 1971. A physical analysis of former girl swimmers. Acta Paediatr. Scand. (suppl. 217):68–72.

Hanson, J. S. 1975. Decline of physiologic training effects during the competitive season in members of the Nordic ski team. Med. Sci. Sports 7:213–216.

Holmér, I. 1974. Physiology of swimming man. Acta Physiol. Scand. (suppl. 407).

Holmér, I., Lundin, A., and Eriksson, B. O. 1974. Maximum oxygen uptake during swimming and running by elite swimmers. J. Appl. Physiol. 36:711–714.

Magel, J., and Faulkner, J. 1967. Maximum oxygen uptake of college swimmers. J. Appl. Physiol. 22:929–938.

McArdle, W. D., Glaser, R. G., and Magel, J. R. 1971. Metabolic cardiorespiratory response during free swimming and treadmill walking. J. Appl. Physiol. 30:733–738.

de la Parra, R. 1967. Background of high performance in swimming. Rev. Chilena Educ. Fiz. Santiago 33:34–30.

Schmidt-Kolmer, E., Klimt, F., and Schwartze, P. 1970. Spiroergometric determinations of children and youth trained in swimming. Organismus of children during exercise. Berlin.

Thomas, V. and Reilly, T. 1976. Changes in fitness profiles during a season of track and field training and competition. Br. J. Sports Med. 10:217–222.

# Physiological Effects of Training in Elite Swimmers

**B. O. Eriksson, I. Holmér, and A. Lundin**

It is well known that physical training causes an increase in aerobic power. This is perhaps most marked in sedentary persons (Saltin et al., 1968; Kilbom, 1971; Eriksson, 1972). However, even well trained subjects may show an increase (Saltin et al., 1968; Ekblom, 1969). In top athletes, however, only marginal improvements following intensive physical training have been reported (for references see Åstrand and Rodahl, 1970). Thus, maximal aerobic power displays a much smaller variation than would be expected from trained swimmers' performances in competition, especially in endurance athletes.

In swimming an athlete is able to improve his swimming performance quite markedly with intensive training. Is this so because swim training in elite swimmers has a more pronounced influence on the oxygen transporting system?

Recently, some of the best swimmers in Sweden stayed at a swim center (Klippan), where they could combine their high school studies with intensive swim training. Thus, a suitable sample of top athletes living at the same place, and trained by the same coach, were available for this study. The main purpose of this study was, therefore, to analyze the interrelationships among swim training, swim performance, and maximal aerobic power.

## SUBJECTS

During the period of this study, 13 girls and 6 boys were training in the swim center. Their mean age, height, and weight are given in Table 1. All 19 were elite Swedish swimmers. Almost all of them had participated on the Swedish National Team. All 19 swimmers volunteered for this study.

---

This study was supported by the Research Council of the Swedish Sport Federation.

Table 1. Mean value with SD in 19 elite swimmers for some anthropological data and some physiological values obtained in submaximal exercise on bicycle ergometer and in submaximal swimming[a]

| Variable | Girls (N = 13) | | | Boys (N = 6) | | | Girls + Boys (N = 19) | | |
|---|---|---|---|---|---|---|---|---|---|
| | B | | A | B | | A | B | | A |
| Age, years | 16.6 | | 17.5 | 16.9 | | 17.8 | 16.7 | | 17.6 |
| SD | 1.3 | | 1.3 | 1.1 | | 1.1 | 1.2 | | 1.2 |
| Height, cm | 169.4 | n.s. | 168.9 | 180.1 | n.s. | 180.5 | 172.8 | n.s. | 172.6 |
| SD | 4.1 | | 4.1 | 6.1 | | 6.5 | 6.9 | | 7.3 |
| Weight, kg | 64.3 | n.s. | 64.7 | 71.7 | xx | 75.0 | 66.6 | n.s. | 68.6 |
| SD | 4.5 | | 5.0 | 8.1 | | 8.5 | 6.6 | | 7.5 |
| Submaximal bicycling | | | | | | | | | |
| Heart rate, beats/min | 151.7 | n.s. | 157.9 | 156.2 | n.s. | 153.2 | 153.1 | n.s. | 156.4 |
| SD | 9.4 | | 11.1 | 7.6 | | 12.1 | 8.9 | | 11.4 |
| Lactate, mmol/liter | 2.8 | n.s. | 2.6 | 2.6 | n.s. | 2.7 | 2.7 | n.s. | 2.7 |
| SD | 1.4 | | 1.1 | 1.1 | | 1.2 | 1.3 | | 1.2 |
| Submaximal swimming | | | | | | | | | |
| Heart rate, beats/min | 141.8 | n.s. | 140.1 | 150.6 | n.s. | 148.0 | 144.9 | n.s. | 142.9 |
| SD | 12.0 | | 13.0 | 10.9 | | 9.3 | 12.0 | | 12.1 |
| $\dot{V}_{O_2}$, liters/min STPD | 1.97 | n.s. | 1.86 | 2.73 | n.s. | 2.74 | 2.26 | n.s. | 2.19 |
| SD | 0.26 | | 0.20 | 0.50 | | 0.32 | 0.52 | | 0.51 |
| $\dot{V}_E$, liters/min BTPS | 45.1 | xx | 39.5 | 62.9 | n.s. | 58.4 | 51.7 | x | 46.6 |
| SD | 7.6 | | 7.3 | 15.0 | | 9.6 | 13.8 | | 12.3 |
| $\dot{V}_E/\dot{V}_{O_2}$ | 22.8 | x | 21.1 | 22.8 | n.s. | 21.2 | 22.8 | xx | 21.1 |
| SD | 2.1 | | 2.3 | 2.2 | | 1.7 | 2.1 | | 2.1 |
| R | 0.84 | n.s. | 0.83 | 0.84 | n.s. | 0.81 | 0.84 | n.s. | 0.82 |
| SD | 0.04 | | 0.05 | 0.09 | | 0.08 | 0.06 | | 0.06 |
| Oxygen pulse, ml/beat | 14.0 | n.s. | 13.3 | 19.4 | n.s. | 18.8 | 15.9 | n.s. | 15.3 |
| SD | 1.8 | | 1.2 | 3.2 | | 3.0 | 3.5 | | 3.4 |
| Lactate, mmol/liter | 1.8 | n.s. | 2.3 | 2.3 | | 1.3 | 1.9 | | 2.0 |
| SD | 0.6 | | 2.7 | 1.0 | | 0.6 | 0.8 | | 2.3 |

[a] Levels of significance between values obtained before (B) and after (A) 9 months of intensive training are designated by xxx = $P \leqslant 0.001$, xx = $P \leqslant 0.01$, x = $P \leqslant 0.05$, n.s. = $P > 0.05$.

## METHODS

Body height and body weight were carefully measured using a standardized technique. Bicycle exercise was performed on a mechanically braked ergometer (Monark) at a pedal rate of 50 rpm. Heart rate was monitored from ECG tracings. Blood lactate concentration was obtained from blood drawn from a prewarmed fingertip and analyzed with a colorimetric method (Barker and Summersson, 1941).

Running was performed on a treadmill that was capable of both increased velocity and inclination (Åstrand, 1952). Oxygen uptake and external ventilation were measured with the Douglas bag technique. The volumes of the bags were measured in a balanced Tissot spirometer and gas analyses were made with a modified Haldane technique.

Physiological measurements during swimming were performed in the swimming flume (Åstrand and Englesson, 1972). Thus, measurements of oxygen uptake, ventilation, heart rate, and blood lactate concentration were taken during swimming at a predetermined, constant swimming speed. For further details see Holmér (1974).

## PROCEDURES

The entire group of swimmers was examined in Stockholm during the last days of September in 1971 (Study 1). At that time only two weeks of swim training in Klippan had elapsed. The second examination (Study 2) was performed during the last days of May in 1972, i.e., at the end of the school year. At these two examinations, all 19 swimmers underwent the same program.

They reported to the laboratory at eight o'clock in the morning. Height and weight were measured, followed by 6 min submaximal exercise on a bicycle ergometer. The rate of work on the ergometer was chosen in order to obtain a heart rate of 150–170 beats/min. Heart rates were checked every min. Blood for lactate analysis was obtained immediately after the work period.

The swimmers were then divided into two groups. One group performed a running exercise on the treadmill while the other group performed swim tests in the flume. After a pause for lunch and a rest of 1 hr, the groups changed places.

The design of the treadmill exercise was the following. The subject started with a 5 min warm-up at a moderate speed. Guided by the estimated maximal aerobic power from the bicycle ergometer test, a suitable velocity and inclination were then chosen for the maximal running exercise (Hermansen and Saltin, 1969). If the subject was not exhausted within 4–5 min, the inclination was increased until exhaustion was obtained. Expired air was collected during the last min of exercise. Two bags of at least 30–40 s each were obtained for every subject. Maximal oxygen uptake was defined using the levelling off criterion (Åstrand, 1952). Heart rate was monitored at 1 min intervals and continuously during the last min to ensure obtaining the peak value. Blood lactate assays were obtained immediately after and 3–4 min after the exercise.

The swimming test was preceded by a period suitable for the swimmer to become acquainted with the test situation. None of the subjects had any special problems with performing the test. This started with some 5 min of warm-up with "loose" swimming. The subject then swam for 6 min at a submaximal swimming speed of 0.8 or 1.0 m/s. The swimmers performed in their best swimming style with the exception of the butterfly swimmers, who swam the front crawl; the methodological problems associated with obtaining measurements during butterfly swimming had not been satisfactorily solved at the time of this investigation. Thus, 12 subjects swam the crawl, four swam the breast stroke, and two swam the backstroke. Expired air was collected during the last 2 min of swimming. Heart rate was measured every min with a telemetric technique, and blood lactate assay was taken immediately after the submaximal test.

After some min of rest, the subject performed the maximal swimming exercise. This was started with a 2 min warm-up at a submaximal velocity, immediately followed by the maximal velocity. The swimming performance and the heart rate response to the submaximal swimming were used as guidelines when choosing the maximal velocity (Holmér, 1974). If the subject was not exhausted within 4–5 min of exercise (excluding the warm-up period), a further increase was made in water velocity in the flume. Thus, each swimmer performed maximal swimming to complete exhaustion within 8–10 min. Mean time for maximal swimming time was 4.85 min (range: 2.35–7.65 min) during Study 1 and 5.01 min (range: 3.35–9.60 min) during Study 2. Velocity during maximal crawl swimming was, on an average, 1.22 m/sec (range: 1.10–1.30 m/sec) for the girls and 1.38 m/sec (range: 1.30–1.50 m/sec) for the boys. The three male breaststrokers swam at 1.10 m/sec and the one female swam at 1.05 m/sec during Study 1. All the breaststrokers swam at 1.10 m/sec during Study 2. Each of the two backstrokers swam at the same speed in both studies, i.e., 1.20 m/sec for the girl and 1.30 m/sec for the boy.

The swim training performed between Studies 1 and 2 was of the interval type and included 100-, 200-, and 400-m intervals at high work intensity and with several repetitions. However, rather long distances were also covered. All swimmers trained two times a day, 5–7 days a week, and the mean training distance per day was between 10,000 and 15,000 m. Each swimmer maintained a training diary, in order to evaluate and control the quality and quantity of the training.

## RESULTS

Individual values for Studies 1 and 2 are given in Figures 1–4 and mean values with SD in Tables 1 and 2.

No increase was found in height, while the boys showed an increase in weight of 3.3 kg. This increase could be attributed to an increase in muscle mass because skinfold measurements did not indicate any increase in subcutaneous fat.

At maximal work on the bicycle ergometer, no statistical differences were found in heart rate and blood lactate concentration between Studies 1 and 2 (Table 1).

During maximal running, mean heart rate was 203 beats/min; blood lactate concentration, 12.0 mmol/liter; $\dot{V}_E$, 130.1 liters/min; $\dot{V}_{O_2}$, 3.90 liters/min; and $\dot{V}_E/\dot{V}_{O_2}$, 33.4 in Study 1. $\dot{V}_E$ and $\dot{V}_E/\dot{V}_{O_2}$ were sig-

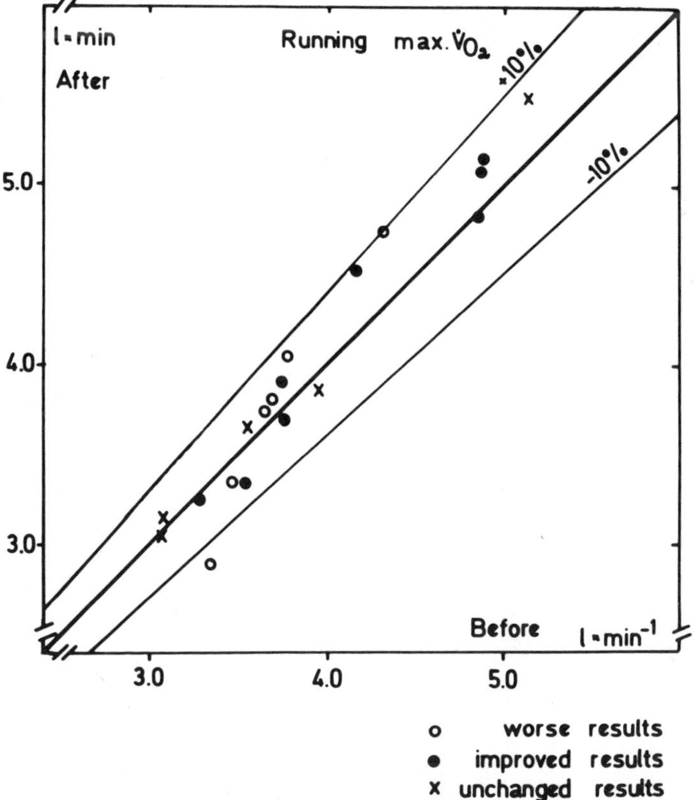


Figure 1. This graph shows individual values for maximal oxygen uptake in elite swimmers during running before and after 9 months of intensive swimming training. Also included with different symbols are those subjects who showed improved, unchanged, and poorer swimming performances, close to the examination period. The 45° identification line with lines indicating ±10% are drawn.

Table 2. Mean values with SD for some physiological values obtained at maximal running and maximal swimming in 19 elite swimmers[a]

| Variable | Girls (N = 13) | | | Boys (N = 6) | | | Girls + Boys (N = 19) | | |
|---|---|---|---|---|---|---|---|---|---|
| | B | | A | B | | A | B | | A |
| **Maximal running** | | | | | | | | | |
| Heart rate, beats/min | 201.9 | n.s. | 201.7 | 203.7 | n.s. | 203.8 | 202.5 | n.s. | 202.4 |
| SD | 9.5 | | 6.8 | 9.8 | | 11.5 | 9.4 | | 8.3 |
| $\dot{V}_{O_2}$ max, liters/min STPD | 3.54 | n.s. | 3.51 | 4.70 | xx | 4.96 | 3.90 | n.s. | 3.97 |
| SD | 0.27 | | 0.37 | 0.37 | | 0.35 | 0.63 | | 0.77 |
| $\dot{V}_E$ max, liters/min BTPS | 117.8 | x | 125.5 | 156.6 | x | 167.4 | 130.1 | xx | 138.7 |
| SD | 10.9 | | 16.6 | 5.0 | | 10.6 | 20.7 | | 24.8 |
| $\dot{V}_E$ max/$\dot{V}_{O_2}$ max | 34.8 | xx | 35.9 | 33.5 | n.s. | 33.8 | 33.4 | xx | 35.2 |
| SD | 9.6 | | 4.4 | 2.2 | | 2.3 | 2.7 | | 3.9 |
| R | 1.09 | n.s. | 1.10 | 1.10 | n.s. | 1.07 | 1.09 | n.s. | 11.4 |
| SD | 0.05 | | 0.05 | 0.04 | | 0.05 | 0.05 | | 0.05 |
| Lactate, mmol/liter | 11.1 | n.s. | 11.0 | 13.8 | n.s. | 12.4 | 12.0 | n.s. | 11.4 |
| SD | 1.8 | | 2.1 | 1.9 | | 1.0 | 2.2 | | 1.9 |
| **Maximal swimming** | | | | | | | | | |
| Heart rate, beats/min | 185.7 | n.s. | 187.7 | 190.8 | n.s. | 192.0 | 187.1 | n.s. | 189.4 |
| SD | 11.9 | | 9.4 | 7.8 | | 7.0 | 11.2 | | 8.9 |
| $\dot{V}_{O_2}$ max, liters/min STPD | 3.25 | x | 3.37 | 4.45 | n.s. | 4.68 | 3.62 | xx | 3.78 |
| SD | 0.27 | | 0.26 | 0.45 | | 0.62 | 0.66 | | 0.74 |
| $\dot{V}_E$ max, liters/min BTPS | 91.7 | n.s. | 96.7 | 137.2 | n.s. | 135.6 | 106.1 | n.s. | 109.0 |
| SD | 15.4 | | 15.1 | 20.7 | | 20.4 | 27.4 | | 25.7 |
| $\dot{V}_E$ max/$\dot{V}_{O_2}$ max | 28.2 | n.s. | 28.7 | 32.8 | xxx | 28.9 | 29.0 | n.s. | 28.8 |
| SD | 3.5 | | 4.1 | 10.6 | | 2.0 | 3.4 | | 3.5 |
| R | 1.04 | n.s. | 1.02 | 1.08 | n.s. | 1.06 | 1.05 | n.s. | 1.03 |
| SD | 0.07 | | 0.06 | 0.04 | | 0.06 | 0.07 | | 0.06 |
| Lactate, mmol/liter | 8.6 | n.s. | 9.7 | 9.4 | n.s. | 9.5 | 8.8 | n.s. | 9.6 |
| SD | 2.4 | | 1.4 | 1.9 | | 1.6 | 2.2 | | 1.4 |

[a] Levels of significance between values obtained before (B) and after (A) 9 months of intensive training are designated by xxx = $P \leqslant 0.001$, xx = $P \leqslant 0.01$, x = $P \leqslant 0.05$, n.s. = $P > 0.05$.

nificantly higher in Study 2. The six boys increased their $\dot{V}_{O_2}$ max significantly from a mean value of 4.70 to 4.96 liters/min (Table 2 and Figure 1).

With submaximal swimming, significantly lower values were found for $\dot{V}_E$ and $\dot{V}_E/\dot{V}_{O_2}$ after training, while only a minor decrease was found for $\dot{V}_{O_2}$, from 2.26 to 2.19 liters/min (Table 1).

During maximal swimming, no differences were found in mean heart rates, $\dot{V}_E$, $\dot{V}_E/\dot{V}_{O_2}$, R, and blood lactate concentration (Table 2). $\dot{V}_{O_2}$ max increased from 3.62 to 3.78 liters/min ($P < 0.01$) (Figure 3).

The ratios of values obtained during maximal swimming and maximal running were all below 1.0. The girls showed a significantly higher ratio for maximal oxygen uptake in swimming and running, 0.96 in Study 1 compared with 0.92 in Study 2 (Figure 4). For the group as a whole, no significant differences were obtained when comparing Studies 1 and 2 with the exception of the lower $\dot{V}_E/\dot{V}_{O_2}$ after training.

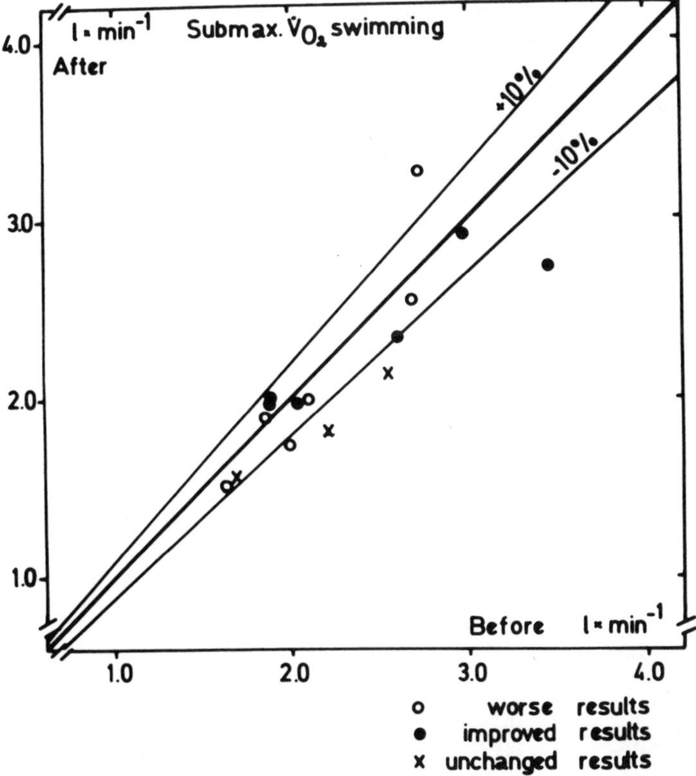


Figure 2. Individual values for oxygen uptake in elite swimmers during swimming at the same submaximal water speed in the flume before and after 9 months of intensive training are shown here.

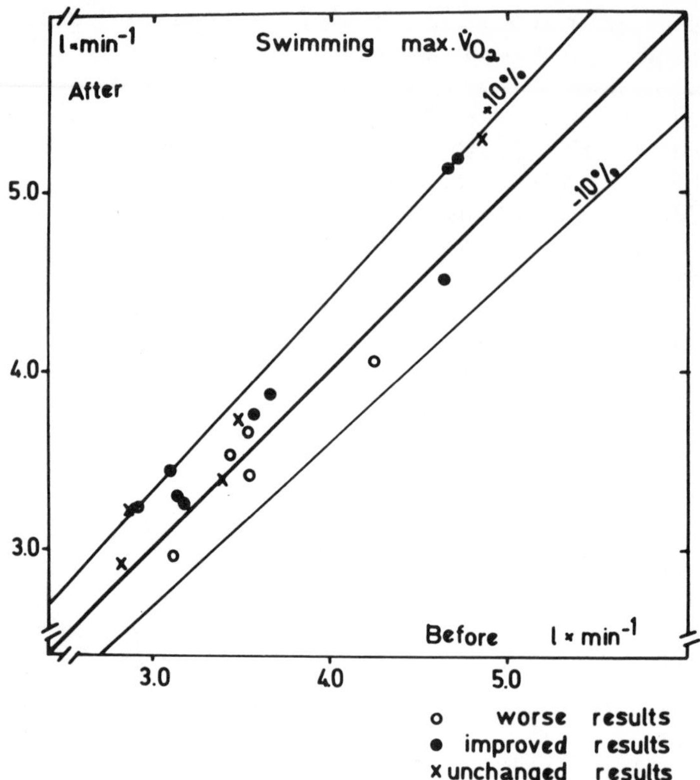


Figure 3. Individual values for maximal oxygen uptake during swimming in 19 elite swimmers are given. Values obtained before and after 9 months of intensive training are indicated.

During the training period (September to May), nine of the swimmers improved their results, four had mainly unchanged results, and the remaining six swimmers showed slightly impaired results (Figures 1–4).

## DISCUSSION

This group of 19 girls and boys constituted a good sample of elite Swedish swimmers. All of them performed in a controlled and intensive swim training. Only nine of the swimmers improved their performances during the course of this study. Thus, it was not possible to demonstrate that this type of training was beneficial to swimmers. This is also emphasized by the rather moderate, although statistically significant, increase in $\dot{V}_{O_2}$ max during swimming for the group as a whole

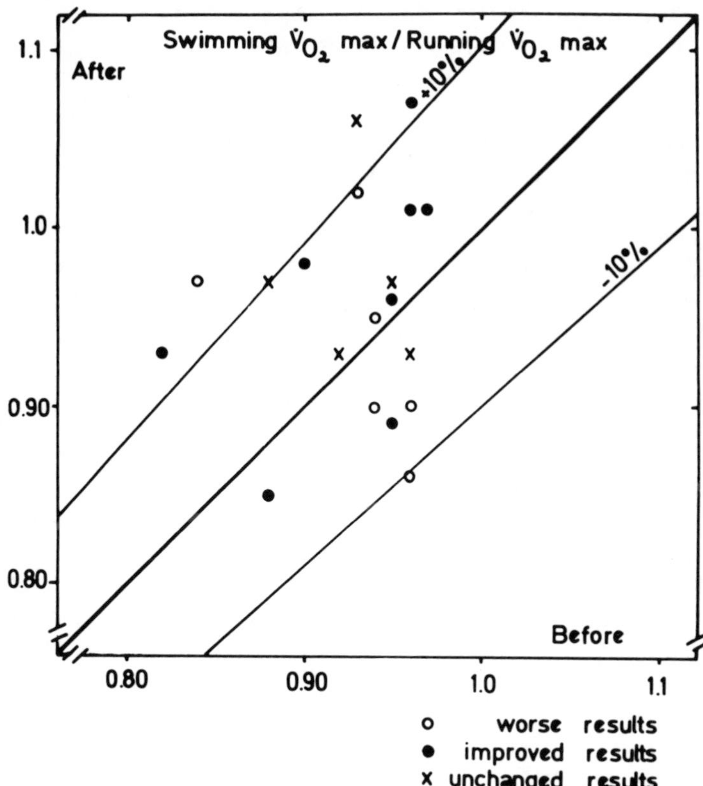


Figure 4. This graph shows individual values for the ratios between maximal oxygen uptake during swimming and maximal oxygen uptake while running in 19 elite swimmers before and after 9 months of intensive swimming training.

and the fact that four swimmers actually obtained lower swimming $\dot{V}_{O_2}$ max during Study 2 (Figure 3).

Because only half of the group showed improved swimming performances and the other half exhibited unchanged or poorer results, an opportunity arose to determine whether these differences in competitive performances were related to the physiological variables measured. As can be seen in Figure 3, a rather firm relationship between swimming performances and $\dot{V}_{O_2}$ max during swimming was substantiated; seven of the nine swimmers with improved results also demonstrated an increase in maximal $\dot{V}_{O_2}$ during swimming. On the other hand, $\dot{V}_{O_2}$ max during running did not show the same correlation (Figure 1). Thus, the data further emphasize that the effects of swim training should be measured during swimming, as has been clearly evidenced by previous investigations (Holmér and Åstrand, 1972;

Holmér, Eriksson, and Lundin, 1974; Magel et al., 1974). In general, exercise tests for evaluation of the effects of physical training should imitate as closely as possible the type of exercise used for training.

For the total group, an increase of 4.4% in swimming $\dot{V}_{O_2}$ max was obtained, while running $\dot{V}_{O_2}$ max was unchanged. The increase in swimming $\dot{V}_{O_2}$ max was achieved despite unchanged total ventilation. This is interesting because both total ventilation and $\dot{V}_E/\dot{V}_{O_2}$ were lower in swimming than in running or bicycling (Åstrand et al., 1963; Holmér, 1974). Alveolar ventilation was sufficient to saturate the blood in the lung capillaries with oxygen even at maximal swimming (Holmér, 1974). The increase in $\dot{V}_{O_2}$ max was probably caused by increased arteriovenous oxygen difference, or increased cardiac output, or both. The relatively pronounced hyperventilation seen at maximal running was not seen in swimming and was evidently not necessary during maximal work. Although respiration in swimming was characterized by a shortened inspiration phase and increased resistance because of the water, ventilation did not constitute a limiting factor for swimming $\dot{V}_{O_2}$ max.

Energy cost during swimming at a given submaximal velocity can be regarded as a measure of swimming efficiency. However, a true calculation of the propulsive efficiency also requires that the water resistance for the individual swimmer be known. Assuming that the water resistance was unchanged during the elapsed time of this study, determination of oxygen uptake at a given submaximal velocity would give direct information about swimming technique. However, water resistance may vary as a consequence of, for example, changes in body constitution and stroke mechanics. A lowered water resistance then contributes to increased efficiency and to conservation of energy. The significance of these factors has not yet been quantified.

In this group of elite swimmers, no decrease in submaximal oxygen uptake was found (Figure 2). This could be taken as an indication that only minor improvements in swimming technique were obtained during the training period. This is not surprising because swimming technique usually is established at an earlier age. In addition, an elite swimmer very seldom reaches his position with a poor technique, i.e., a technique that can readily be improved.

The main purpose of this investigation was to determine whether improvements in swimming performance can be predicted from physiological measurements. The results obtained indicate that the measurement of $\dot{V}_{O_2}$ max during swimming gives an indication of swimming performance even in elite swimmers. This contrasts to the poor predictive value of running $\dot{V}_{O_2}$ max for the swimmer's performance.

## REFERENCES

Åstrand, P.-O. 1952. Experimental Studies of Physical Working Capacity in Relation to Sex and Age. Munksgaard, Copenhagen.

Åstrand, P.-O. and Englesson, S. 1972. A swimming flume. J. Appl. Physiol. 33:514.

Åstrand, P.-O., Engström, L., Eriksson, B. O., Karlberg, P., Nylander, I., Saltin, B. and Thorén, C. 1963. Girl swimmers. Acta Paediat. Scand. (suppl. 147):1–75.

Åstrand, P.-O. and Rodahl, K. 1970. Textbook of Work Physiology McGraw-Hill Book Company, New York.

Barker, S. B. and Summersson, W. H. 1941. The colorimetric determination of lactic acid in biological materials. J. Biol. Chem. 138:535–554.

Ekblom, B. 1969. Effect of physical training on oxygen transport in man. Acta Physiol. Scand. (suppl. 328).

Eriksson, B. O. 1972. Physical training, oxygen supply, and muscle metabolism in 11–13 year old boys. Acta Physiol. Scand. (suppl. 384).

Hermansen, L. and Saltin, B. 1969. Oxygen uptake during maximal treadmill and bicycle exercise. J. Appl. Physiol. 26:31–37.

Holmér, I. 1974. Physiology of swimming man. Acta Physiol. Scand. (suppl. 407).

Holmér, I. and Åstrand, P.-O. 1972. Swimming training and maximal oxygen uptake. J. Appl. Physiol. 33:510–513.

Holmér, I., Eriksson, B. O., and Lundin, A. 1974. Maximal oxygen uptake during swimming and running by elite swimmers. J. Appl. Physiol. 36:711–714.

Kilbom, Å. 1971. Physical training in women. Scand. J. Clin. Lab. Invest. 28(suppl. 119).

Magel, J. R., Foglig, G. F., McArdle, W. D., Gutin, B., Pechar, G. S., and Katch, F. I. 1974. Specificity of swim training on maximum oxygen uptake. J. Appl. Physiol. 38:151–155.

Saltin, B., Blomqvist, G., Mitchell, J. H., Johnsson, R. L., Jr., Wildenthal, K. and Chapman, C. B. 1968. Response to exercise after bed rest and training. Circulation. 38(suppl. 7).

Saltin, B., Hartley, L. H., Kilbom, Å., and Åstrand, I. 1971. Physical training in sedentary middle-aged and older men. II. Oxygen uptake, heart rate, and blood lactate concentrations at submaximal and maximal exercise. Scand. J. Clin. Lab. Invest. 24:323–334.

# Somatotyping of Top Swimmers by the Heath-Carter Method

C. G. S. Araújo

Somatotyping was first described by Sheldon, Stevens, and Tucker (1940). This method has since been modified; the modification introduced by Heath and Carter (1967) has been extensively utilized by this author and by other investigators. Heath and Carter defined a somatotype as "a description of present morphological conformation."

Body type is always represented by a three-numeral rating in which each number represents the evaluation of one of the primary components of physique. The first component (endomorphy) is related to the amount of body fat. The second component (mesomorphy) represents the musculoskeletal development per unit of height. The third component (ectomorphy) indicates the linearity of the individual. (DeGaray, Levine, and Carter, 1974).

In this study, the Heath-Carter anthropometric somatotyping method was chosen because of its simple execution and high reproducibility as well as the existence of considerable data on reference populations prepared with this method, mainly from the Mexico City Olympic Games (DeGaray, Levine, and Carter, 1974). Moreover, the Heath-Carter method has been utilized in all functional evaluations of Brazilian top sportsmen over the past 2 years.

The purposes of this study were to assess the similarities in Heath-Carter anthropometric somatotypes among top swimmers of Brazil and other countries and to determine the validity of somatotype determinations for swimmers.

## METHODS

A total of 65 swimmers, 46 males and 19 females, from the Brazilian (N = 44) and Indiana University (N = 21) swimming teams participated in

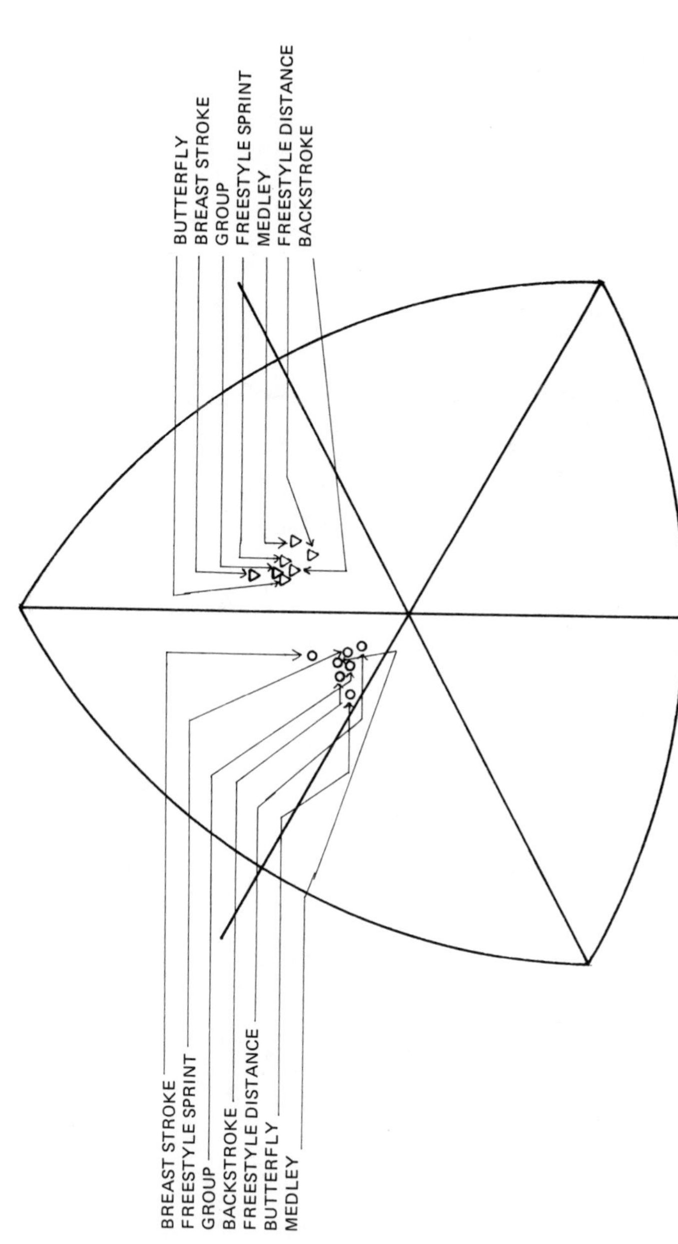


Figure 1. This somatochart classifies Brazilian male swimmers and female swimmers in group and subgroup somatoplots.

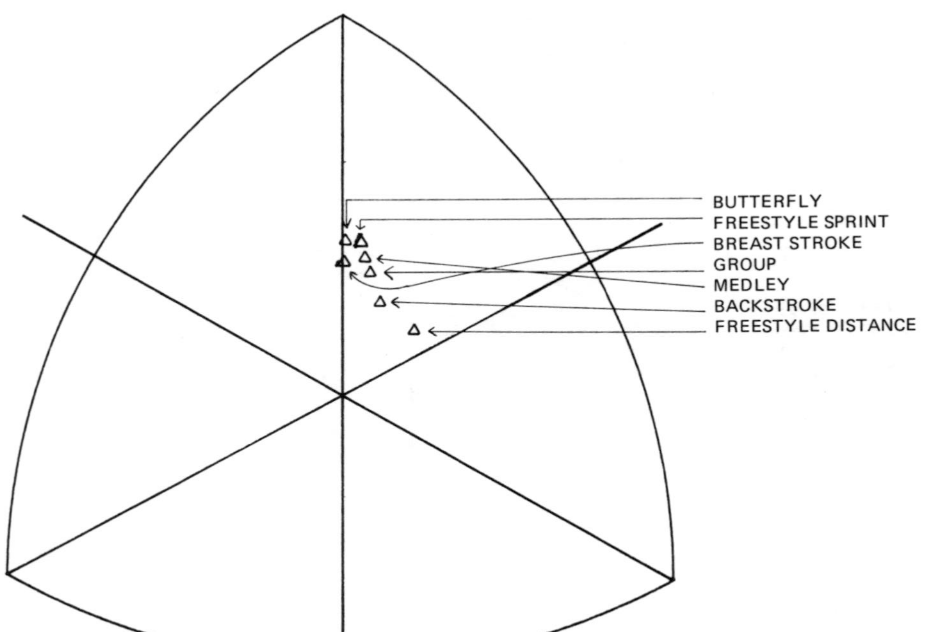


Figure 2. This somatochart classifies Indiana University male swimmers in group and subgroups somatoplots.

this study. The Brazilian swimmers were measured during the trials for the 1975 world swimming championships at Cali, Colombia, and in the functional evaluation of the Brazilian swimming team prior to the 1975 Pan-American Games. A less endomorphic measurement was chosen for this study because it correlated better with the best performance and with a higher degree of training. The Indiana University (IU) swimmers were measured in December 1976, during their visit to Rio de Janeiro, Brazil.

Measurements were obtained as follows: skinfolds with a Harpender skinfold caliper; bone diameter with a Martin anthropometer; girths with a flexible steel metric tape; and weight and height with a calibrated balance and scale. All measurements were calculated to the accuracy of one decimal place using the reference units of the International Standardization for Physical Fitness Tests.

The swimmers were divided in six subgroups: freestyle sprint (100–200 m); freestyle distance (400–1500m); backstroke; breast stroke; butterfly; and individual medley. It was possible to categorize each of the swimmers in one or more of the subgroups, depending on their specialties; the Brazilian ranking and the coaches' opinions were the criteria utilized for this division.

The researcher utilized regression equations developed by him to calculate the Heath-Carter somatotype ratings, so that the components were each calculated to the nearest hundredth of a unit (Araújo and Gomes, 1977). The somatotype dispersion distance (SDD) and somatotype dispersion index (SDI), as described by Ross and Wilson (1973), along with the mean and standard deviations were the statistical procedures utilized for the analysis of groups and subgroups. Comparisons were made among Brazilian (BR), Indiana University (IU), and Mexico City Olympic (MC) male swimmers, and between Brazilian and Mexico City Olympic female swimmers.

## RESULTS

Tables 1, 2, and 3 show the results of BR and IU swimmers. The tables present the number of cases, ages, heights, weights, endomorphy, mesomorphy, ectomorphy (mean ±SD), and the SDI for the whole group and for the subgroups. Tables 4, 5, and 6 present the SDD between the whole group and subgroups, and the SDD between subgroups.

Finally, Tables 7 and 8 make comparisons among Brazilian, Indiana University, and Mexico City Olympic swimmers. The criteria utilized in this study were the same as those used by Hebbelinck, Carter, and DeGaray (1975) to analyze somatotype dispersion. A SDD of 2.00 is the equivalent of the change by one component rating of 1

Table 1. Characteristics of male Brazilian swimmers (N = 25)

| Event[a] | N | Age (years) | Height (cm) | Weight (kg) | Endomorphy | Mesomorphy | Ectomorphy | SDI |
|---|---|---|---|---|---|---|---|---|
| SWM | 25 | 18.60 ± 2.58 | 178.29 ± 5.78 | 71.70 ± 7.12 | 2.20 ± 0.89 | 4.49 ± 0.68 | 2.85 ± 0.66 | 2.38 |
| FRS | 14 | 18.21 ± 2.36 | 179.68 ± 6.27 | 72.75 ± 7.72 | 2.07 ± 0.72 | 4.46 ± 0.66 | 2.95 ± 0.54 | 2.13 |
| FRD | 6 | 17.00 ± 1.67 | 177.88 ± 8.94 | 69.17 ± 10.13 | 2.22 ± 0.93 | 4.06 ± 0.73 | 3.17 ± 0.58 | 2.47 |
| BKS | 6 | 18.50 ± 2.17 | 181.87 ± 2.47 | 75.08 ± 6.07 | 2.20 ± 0.69 | 4.35 ± 0.73 | 2.98 ± 0.67 | 2.36 |
| BRS | 6 | 19.50 ± 3.73 | 176.68 ± 5.94 | 70.42 ± 7.00 | 2.07 ± 0.51 | 4.65 ± 0.84 | 2.74 ± 0.64 | 2.11 |
| BUT | 11 | 18.18 ± 1.99 | 177.59 ± 4.99 | 70.55 ± 6.61 | 2.27 ± 1.08 | 4.52 ± 0.74 | 2.89 ± 0.78 | 2.60 |
| MED | 10 | 18.20 ± 1.93 | 179.15 ± 4.65 | 70.78 ± 7.22 | 1.92 ± 0.52 | 4.22 ± 0.65 | 3.15 ± 0.53 | 1.88 |

[a] SWM, swimmers; FRS, freestyle sprint; FRD, freestyle distance; BKS, backstroke; BRS, breast stroke; BUT, butterfly; MED, medley.

Table 2. Characteristics of male Indiana University swimmers (N = 21)

| Event[a] | N | Age (years) | Height (cm) | Weight (kg) | Endomorphy | Mesomorphy | Ectomorphy | SDI |
|---|---|---|---|---|---|---|---|---|
| SWM | 21 | 19.52 ± 1.33 | 183.59 ± 6.17 | 77.28 ± 6.52 | 2.55 ± 0.92 | 4.62 ± 0.70 | 2.96 ± 0.77 | 2.71 |
| FRS | 7 | 20.43 ± 0.98 | 186.13 ± 6.27 | 81.78 ± 7.37 | 2.80 ± 1.24 | 4.82 ± 0.65 | 2.86 ± 0.65 | 3.07 |
| FRD | 3 | 18.33 ± 0.58 | 183.27 ± 7.24 | 72.42 ± 7.55 | 2.52 ± 0.72 | 3.99 ± 0.84 | 3.65 ± 0.14 | 1.64 |
| BKS | 5 | 19.60 ± 1.52 | 182.12 ± 6.34 | 73.26 ± 5.37 | 2.64 ± 1.26 | 4.42 ± 1.11 | 3.37 ± 0.66 | 3.27 |
| BRS | 10 | 19.60 ± 1.65 | 181.48 ± 6.46 | 75.98 ± 4.59 | 2.42 ± 1.09 | 4.77 ± 0.65 | 2.81 ± 0.78 | 2.78 |
| BUT | 11 | 19.82 ± 1.25 | 183.90 ± 6.05 | 79.46 ± 6.66 | 2.63 ± 1.10 | 4.85 ± 0.67 | 2.66 ± 0.64 | 2.69 |
| MED | 9 | 19.00 ± 1.41 | 180.89 ± 5.40 | 74.09 ± 5.57 | 2.58 ± 1.16 | 4.73 ± 0.63 | 2.85 ± 0.70 | 2.75 |

[a] SWM, swimmers; FRS, freestyle sprint; FRD, freestyle distance; BKS, backstroke; BRS, breast stroke; BUT, butterfly; MED, medley.

Table 3. Characteristics of female Brazilian swimmers (N = 19)

| Event[a] | N | Age (years) | Height (cm) | Weight (kg) | Endomorphy | Mesomorphy | Ectomorphy | SDI |
|---|---|---|---|---|---|---|---|---|
| SWM | 19 | 15.84 ± 1.68 | 165.00 ± 4.37 | 58.75 ± 4.22 | 3.43 ± 0.84 | 3.63 ± 0.59 | 2.48 ± 0.73 | 2.52 |
| FRS | 14 | 16.00 ± 1.84 | 166.71 ± 3.02 | 59.72 ± 4.28 | 3.32 ± 0.83 | 3.65 ± 0.63 | 2.63 ± 0.64 | 2.55 |
| FRD | 9 | 16.22 ± 1.30 | 166.39 ± 3.10 | 58.68 ± 4.05 | 3.34 ± 1.07 | 3.58 ± 0.73 | 2.75 ± 0.67 | 2.96 |
| BKS | 9 | 16.22 ± 2.28 | 165.94 ± 3.93 | 59.80 ± 4.95 | 3.49 ± 0.79 | 3.80 ± 0.63 | 2.48 ± 0.45 | 2.21 |
| BRS | 4 | 15.00 ± 1.15 | 160.75 ± 5.56 | 55.75 ± 3.30 | 2.91 ± 0.75 | 3.82 ± 0.48 | 2.20 ± 1.18 | 2.66 |
| BUT | 7 | 16.43 ± 1.81 | 166.79 ± 3.62 | 61.57 ± 4.06 | 3.62 ± 0.79 | 3.62 ± 0.45 | 2.32 ± 0.53 | 1.86 |
| MED | 9 | 15.33 ± 1.00 | 163.94 ± 5.28 | 58.03 ± 4.23 | 3.28 ± 0.85 | 3.68 ± 0.61 | 2.40 ± 0.94 | 2.70 |

[a] SWM, swimmers; FRS, freestyle sprint; FRD, freestyle distance; BKS, backstroke; BRS, breast stroke; BUT, butterfly; MED, medley.

Table 4. Somatotype Dispersion Distance (SDD) among Brazilian male swimmers (N = 25)

| Swimming stroke | Freestyle sprint | Freestyle distance | Back-stroke | Breast stroke | Butterfly | Medley |
|---|---|---|---|---|---|---|
| Group | 0.40 | 1.31 | 0.47 | 0.56 | 0.07 | 1.15 |
| Freestyle sprint | — | 1.18 | 0.42 | 0.69 | 0.45 | 0.81 |
| Freestyle distance | — | — | 0.84 | 1.83 | 1.28 | 0.80 |
| Backstroke | — | — | — | 0.99 | 0.45 | 0.79 |
| Breast stroke | — | — | — | — | 0.62 | 1.48 |
| Butterfly | — | — | — | — | — | 1.17 |
| Medley | — | — | — | — | — | — |

Table 5. Somatotype Dispersion Distance (SDD) among Indiana University swimmers (N = 21)

| Swimming stroke | Freestyle sprint | Freestyle distance | Back-stroke | Breast stroke | Butterfly | Medley |
|---|---|---|---|---|---|---|
| Group | 0.66 | 1.27 | 1.06 | 0.58 | 0.95 | 0.39 |
| Freestyle sprint | — | 2.85[a] | 1.63 | 0.66 | 0.43 | 0.37 |
| Freestyle distance | — | — | 1.23 | 2.81[a] | 3.22[a] | 2.67[a] |
| Backstroke | — | — | — | 1.59 | 1.99 | 1.44 |
| Breaststroke | — | — | — | — | 0.63 | 0.35 |
| Butterfly | — | — | — | — | — | 0.56 |
| Medley | — | — | — | — | — | — |

[a] Significant difference (>2.00).

unit. The empirical value of 2.00 was then used for estimating the significance of the differences between the mean somatoplots of groups and subgroups.

## Male Swimmers

The mean somatotypes for the Brazilian and IU swimmers were 2.20-4.49-2.95, and 2.55-4.62-2.96, respectively. Each group's SDI was approximately the same (2.38 and 2.71), indicating a similarity of distribution in the two samples.

The breast stroke swimmers were more mesomorphic than freestyle distance swimmers, but freestyle distance swimmers and backstrokers were more ectomorphic than the other swimmers, whether Brazilian or from IU. The first component, endomorphy, was

Table 6. Somatotype Dispersion Distance (SDD) among Brazilian female swimmers (N = 19)

| Swimming stroke | Freestyle sprint | Freestyle distance | Back-stroke | Breast stroke | Butterfly | Medley |
|---|---|---|---|---|---|---|
| Group | 0.45 | 0.68 | 0.30 | 1.25 | 0.61 | 0.35 |
| Freestyle sprint | — | 0.33 | 0.62 | 1.18 | 1.06 | 0.47 |
| Freestyle distance | — | — | 0.92 | 1.47 | 1.25 | 0.79 |
| Backstroke | — | — | — | 1.04 | 0.60 | 0.23 |
| Breaststroke | — | — | — | — | 1.60 | 0.90 |
| Butterfly | — | — | — | — | — | 0.82 |
| Medley | — | — | — | — | — | — |

Table 7. Comparisons among Brazilian, Indiana University, and Mexico City Olympic male swimmers

| Swimming stroke | BR/IU | BR/MC | IU/MC |
|---|---|---|---|
| Group | 0.46 | 1.10 | 1.44 |
| Freestyle sprint | 1.42 | — | — |
| Freestyle distance | 0.97 | — | — |
| Backstroke | 0.70 | 0.73 | 1.12 |
| Breast stroke | 0.52 | 1.12 | 1.34 |
| Butterfly | 1.15 | 1.83 | 1.74 |
| Medley | 1.79 | 2.73 | 2.17 |

almost constant for all styles, but breast stroke swimmers had the smallest values when all subjects were considered collectively.

The freestyle distance swimmers were younger and lighter than the others; BR breast stroke swimmers and IU freestyle sprinters were older than other members of their respective groups. The breast stroke swimmers were also shorter than the other swimmers.

### Female Swimmers

The female swimmers presented a mean endomorph-mesomorph somatotype of 3.43-3.63-2.48. The subgroups do not differ from each other on mesomorphy and ectomorphy, but in the endomorphy, the breast stroke swimmers had a lesser index than did the whole group and the other subgroups.

The breast stroke swimmers were shorter, lighter, and younger than the other competitive swimmers. On the other hand, the butterfly swimmers were taller, heavier, and older than the swimmers in the other subgroups.

## DISCUSSION

The BR and IU male swimmers demonstrated similar patterns of somatotype distribution. Most of the swimmers belonged to an ecto-

Table 8. Comparison between Brazilian and Mexico City Olympic female swimmers

| Swimming stroke | BR/MC |
|---|---|
| Group | 1.57 |
| Backstroke | 1.55 |
| Breast stroke | 1.71 |
| Medley | 0.24 |

mesomorph somatotype. The mean values for the whole group had a nonsignificant SDD (0.46). When compared with Olympic swimmers, the somatotype dispersion distance was also nonsignificant.

The small differences in the endomorphic component between Brazilian and American swimmers may be attributable to differing stages of training at the time of measurement. Perhaps during the "tapering-off" period, the IU swimmers would be slimmer than on the occasion on which they were measured. It must be remembered that at time of assessment the Brazilian swimmers were at the end of preparation for important competitions. Intrasubgroup differences were more pronounced in the IU swimmers. The freestyle sprint/distance, freestyle distance/breast stroke and freestyle distance/backstroke comparisons were significantly different (more than 2.00 SDD units). Similar tendencies were seen in the BR swimmers, although values observed were not significant (< 2.00).

The major difference between the subgroups (BR/IU) occurred in the medley swimmers (SDD: 1.79), probably because the IU medley swimmers were mostly breast stroker specialists: this was not true of the BR swimmers. A division on medley events (200- and 400-m) using somatotype classification might eliminate this difference between the groups of medley swimmers.

The less mesomorphic value for freestyle distance swimmers might indicate small necessity for musculoskeletal development or it might have been attributable to the younger ages of those swimmers. The linearity component seemed to be important principally for freestyle distance and backstroke competitors. When the Brazilian, Indiana University, and Mexico City swimmers were compared, there were no significant differences except among individual medley swimmers.

The female swimmers were of the endomorph-mesomorph type. All of the intragroup comparisons showed nonsignificant differences; as in the males, one of higher differences in the females was in the freestyle distance/breast stroke comparison (SDD: 1.47). The other high value was in the breast stroke/butterfly (SDD: 1.60). In the comparisons performed, no significant differences were found between the BR and MC female swimmers; this comparison was incomplete, however, because there were no butterfly swimmers in the MC group.

Unfortunately, Hebbelinck, Carter, and DeGaray (1975) did not divide the freestyle competitors into sprint and distance swimmers. This writer considers such a division very useful because more significant differences appeared when this separation was employed.

An interesting observation made in this analysis was that the BR and IU breast stroke swimmers tended to be less endomorphic and less ectomorphic than the other subgroups of swimmers. This point needs further study to determine whether it is of importance. Perhaps there is a relationship with lesser buoyancy that is characteristic of the breast stroke style.

Another point of uncertainty involves the extent to which the differences in performances between men and women could be attributed to somatotype differences.

This writer suggests that a SDD of 2.00 or fewer units is compatible with a good swimming performance. SDD values of 4.00 or more should be called to the attention of the team physician or swimming coach who should attempt to determine the reason for this deviation, and to ascertain whether it is possible to orient the training to correct this deficiency. The competitive swimming training did not seem to be specific enough to induce significant differences in somatotype ratings between competitive styles.

The mean somatotypes presented must be close to the present ideal values. With the advancement of research, swimming types will probably drop out and other ideal somatotypes will arise.

## CONCLUSIONS

The following conclusions were drawn based on the results of this study:

1. Somatotype seems to be an important factor in swimming performance
2. Top Brazilian swimmers had similar mean somatotypes to those of the Indiana University and the Mexico City Olympic swimmers
3. The characteristics of height, weight, and age may vary widely between groups of top swimmers

## ACKNOWLEDGMENTS

The author thanks Dr. James Counsilman and Jan Prints, Head and Assistant swimming coach, respectively, at Indiana University, Bloomington, Ind., for their cooperation. Prof. José Ney Ferraz Guimarães and Claudio Abtibol Neto for their assistance in the collection of data. A special thanks is extended to Dr. Mauricio Leal Rocha, Head of Laboratório de Fisiologia do Exercício for his indefatigable and kindly help. Finally, the swimmers that participated in this study are to be thanked for their cooperation and motivation.

## REFERENCES

Araújo, C. G. S., and Gomes, P. S. C. 1977. Regression equations for the Heath-Carter anthropometric somatotype calculations. Paper presented at the 6th Brazilian Congress on Sports Medicine, April 25, Recife, Brazil.

DeGaray, A. L., Levine, L., and Carter, J. E. L. (eds.). 1974. Genetic and Anthropological Studies of Olympic Athletes. Academic Press, New York.
Heath, B. H., and Carter, J. E. L. 1967. A modified somatotype method. Am. J. Phys. Anthrop. 27:57–74.
Hebbelinck, M., Carter, J. E. L., and DeGaray, A. L. 1975. Body build and somatotype of Olympic swimmers, divers, and waterpolo players. In: L. Lewillie and J. P. Clarys (eds.), Swimming II: International Series on Sport Sciences, Vol. 2., pp. 285-305. University Park Press, Baltimore.
Ross, W. D., and Wilson, B. D. 1973. A somatotype dispersion index. Res. Q. 44:372.
Sheldon, W. H., Stevens, S. S., and Tucker, W. B. 1940. Varieties of Human Physique. Harper Brothers, New York.

# Unexpected Cardiovascular Parameters in Olympic Athletes

**M. O'Brien and D. E. FitzGerald**

The purpose of this investigation was to determine the effects of rapid forward whole body tilting on a group of top class athletes and to determine whether their cardiovascular responses to tilting differed from those of nonathletic subjects (Brew and FitzGerald, 1977).

## METHODS

Ten males of an Olympic rowing squad and one male Olympic swimmer took part. Their ages ranged from 17–29 years. The control group consisted of nine nonathletic males in the same age group. The maximum $\dot{V}_{O_2}$ values of the athletes were predicted by their submaximal performances on a Monark bicycle ergometer using Åstrand's method (Åstrand and Rhyming, 1954).

Conditions were standardized. On each occasion, the subjects were tested in the afternoon at approximately the same time. First they were tilted and then their maximum $\dot{V}_{O_2}$ values were predicted from their performances on the bicycle ergometer. The Cattell Personality 16PF Test was administered to both groups.

The subjects were placed on a tilting table, with their shoulders against a padded board. The foot piece was adjustable so that it rested lightly against the sole of the foot. The subjects were placed in the horizontal plane for 5 min prior to the tilt. They were then tilted rapidly forward through 45° (i.e., so that their feet were dependant). On each occasion, two tilts lasting 2 min each were performed, with an interval of 5 min between each tilt and after the last tilt.

Blood pressure was measured automatically at 1 min intervals, using a Roche Arterio-Sonde 1217, and manually just before, during, and after the tilt. Heart rate was measured continuously from an ECG signal using standard chest electrodes.

Transit time was the time, measured in msec, for the transmission of a pulse pressure wave along a selected segment of an artery, using Doppler Flow ultrasound. In these experiments, the velocity of the red cells passing through a continuous beam of ultrasound was calculated. The continuous wave was produced by a piezoelectric crystal, which had a positive wave on one side and a negative wave on the other. When the charges were oscillated electrically, the crystal moved backward and forward, producing low energy ultrasound with a penetration of 10 cm. Ultrasound must go through a fluid medium because it is poorly conducted through air or bone.

Transit time varies with the distance between the probes and with the state of the vessel wall. If the wall stiffens, transit time shortens; conversely, transit time lengthens if the walls soften. If the vessel is obstructed, transit time is longer, but there is a different wave formation (FitzGerald and Carr, 1977). If the pressure inside the vessel rises, this stiffens the wall. Normally, upon tilting a subject, blood pressure rises locally in the feet because of gravity, the arterial wall stiffens, and the transit time shortens.

In these experiments, transit time was taken as the time between 50% of the rising slope of the R wave on the ECG signal and the arrival of the pulse pressure wave at the posterior tibial artery at the ankle. This was monitored using a 10 megahertz transcutaneous ultrasound flowmeter (Parks, Model 806). The chart recorder was a Hewlett Packward, 7700 Model.

Eleven Olympic athletes were tested, five of them on two occasions. The swimmer was examined on three occasions. Because each session consisted of two tilts, the data consisted of a total of 36 tilts. The control group consisted of nine subjects who were tilted four times each, a total of 36 tilts.

## RESULTS

All the controls showed a pattern consistent with that previously reported in normal subjects (FitzGerald, Gosling, and Woodcock, 1971). Upon tilting, blood pressure rose, heart rate increased, and transit time shortened for the period of the tilt. In 32 of the tilts, the athletes followed a pattern that was consistently different from that found in the controls; in four tilts, the response was similar to that of the controls. The transmission of the pulse pressure wave along the arterial system in the lower limbs was shorter in the athletes than in the controls at rest. The transit time, in response to rapid, whole body tilting through 45°, was shorter in the athletes than in the controls, but there was a greater difference in the response to the tilting in the controls than in the athletes.

Table 1. Transit time (msec)[a]

| | Athletes (N = 11) | Controls (N = 9) |
|---|---|---|
| Resting | 337 ± 40 | 385 ± 31 |
| Mean tilt | 315 ± 34 | 351 ± 32[b] |
| First minute of tilt | 299 ± 32 | 351 ± 32 |
| Second minute of tilt | 330 ± 36[b] | 351 ± 32 |

[a] Values are given as mean ± SD
[b] $p \leqslant 0.01$

In the first minute of the tilt, the actual change in transit time was the same in both groups, but the time for the athletes was shorter. During the second minute of the tilt, there was a considerable recovery or lengthening of the transit time in the athletes. This did not occur in the controls (Table 1).

It was found that the average systolic and diastolic blood pressure of the athletes at the time of examination on the tilting table was higher than that of the controls. The blood pressure of the athletes rose during the first minute of the tilt but dropped during the second minute, unlike the controls, whose blood pressure remained the same during the period of the tilt. Subsequent examination of the blood pressure of the athletes a few days later, gave much lower values than those recorded when they were on the tilting table (Table 2).

There was no significant difference in the heart rates of the two groups (Table 3).

The predicted $\dot{V}_{O_2}$ max of the athletes was greater than 70 ml/$O_2$/kg, except in the two who had responses similar to those of the controls. One was a rower with a $\dot{V}_{O_2}$ max of 58 ml/$O_2$/kg. The other was the swimmer, during his first test.

Table 2. Blood pressure (mm Hq)[a]

| | Athletes (N = 11) | | Controls (N = 9) | |
|---|---|---|---|---|
| | Systolic | Diastolic | Systolic | Diastolic |
| Resting | 123 ± 12 | 95 ± 14 | 106 ± 5 | 75 ± 5 |
| Mean tilt | 126 ± 16 | 99 ± 12 | 111 ± 6 | 81 ± 6[b] |
| First minute of tilt | 130 ± 13 | 100 ± 10 | 111 ± 6 | 81 ± 6 |
| Second minute of tilt | 122 ± 15[b] | 99 ± 6 | 111 ± 6 | 81 ± 6 |

[a] Values are given as mean ± SD
[b] $p \leqslant 0.01$

Table 3. Heart rate (at 6 pm)[a]

| | Athletes (N = 11) | Controls (N = 9) |
|---|---|---|
| Resting | 57 ± 8 | 51 ± 3 |
| Mean tilt | 64 ± 7[c] | 60 ± 4[c] |
| First minute of tilt | 62 ± 7 | 60 ± 4 |
| Second minute of tilt | 67 ± 7[b] | 60 ± 4 |

[a] Values are given as mean ± SD.
[b] $p \leq 0.01$.
[c] $p \leq 0.001$.

## DISCUSSION

These results show that the responses of the athletes to tilting were markedly different from those of the controls (Table 4). The transit time was shorter in the athletes at rest, and, when tilted, their transit time shortened still further during the first minute, but lengthened during the second minute. This occurred only in the athletes with a high level of fitness.

The athletes approached the examination in a state of physical awareness unlike that of the controls. The resting values of the athletes on the table were in fact as high as the controls' values were while tilted. Blood pressure in both groups rose when they were tilted. This

Table 4. Changes when tilted

| | Athletes (N = 11) | Controls (N = 9) |
|---|---|---|
| Δ BPS | 3 ± 4 | 5 ± 3 |
| Δ BPS 1st min | 7 ± 3 | 5 ± 3 |
| Δ BPS 2nd min | −1 ± 5[a] | 5 ± 3 |
| Δ BPD | 4 ± 7 | 6 ± 5 |
| Δ BPD 1st min | 5 ± 10 | 6 ± 5 |
| Δ BPD 2nd min | 4 ± 6 | 6 ± 5 |
| Δ HR | 7 ± 4[a] | 9 ± 4[a] |
| Δ HR 1st min | 5 ± 4 | 9 ± 4 |
| Δ HR 2nd min | 10 ± 6 | 9 ± 4 |
| Δ TT | −22 ± 9[a] | −34 ± 9[a] |
| Δ TT 1st min | −38 ± 9 | −34 ± 9 |
| Δ TT 2nd min | −8 ± 9 | −34 ± 9 |

[a] $p \leq 0.001$.

condition remained steady for the period of the tilt in the controls; the blood pressure of the athletes dropped during the second minute of the tilt. This could explain the lengthening of transit time during the second minute of the tilt in the athlete.

These results raise a question: Do the athletes react in a similar manner to the everyday challenges of life and, if so, will this reaction have a beneficial or detrimental effect on their immediate training program or on their long-term state of health? This question remains to be answered.

## REFERENCES

Åstrand, P.-O., and Rhyming, I. 1954. A nomogram for the calculation of aerobic capacity (physical fitness) from pulse rate during submaximal work. J. Appl. Physiol. 7:218.

Brew, K. and FitzGerald, D. E. 1977. Transcutaneous assessment of arterial elasticity. Ultrasound in Med. and Biol. 2:263–270.

FitzGerald, D. E., and Carr, J. 1977. Peripheral arterial disease: Assessment by arteriography and alternative noninvasive measures. Am. J. Roentgenol. 128:385–388.

FitzGerald, D. E., Gosling, R. G., and Woodcock, J. P. 1971. Grading dynamic capability of arterial collateral circulation. Lancet 9:66–67.

O'Brien, M., FitzGerald, D. E., Rodahl, A. et al. 1976. Cardiovascular responses to whole body tilting in athletes and controls. Irish J. Med. Sci. 145(9):310.

# Metabolism

# Metabolic Responses to Exercise, with Special Reference to Training and Competition in Swimming

**M. E. Houston**

## RESYNTHESIS OF ATP IN THE MUSCLE CELL

For the contractile proteins of muscle to interact in their unique and specific way, and thus to do work, an immediate source of energy must always be available. Energy for the contractile proteins is made available during the hydrolysis of the terminal phosphate group of ATP (adenosine triphosphate molecule), catalyzed by specific components of the myosin molecule having ATPase activity. The hydrolysis products of ATP in this reaction are ADP (adenosine diphosphate) and Pi (inorganic phosphate). For muscle to continue contracting, a continual resynthesis of ATP must occur because the actual intramuscular concentration of ATP is quite low (Karlsson, Diamant, and Saltin, 1971; Harris, Hultman, and Nordesjö, 1974). Despite the low concentration of ATP in muscle (4–6 mmoles $\times$ $kg^{-1}$ wet weight), the level of ATP in human muscle has not been observed to fall below 60% of the rest value no matter how intense or prolonged the muscle contractions (Hultman, Karlsson, Diamant, and Saltin, 1967; Diamant et al., 1971; Sahlin, Harris, and Hultman, 1975).

To maintain the ATP concentrations close to rest levels despite hard or prolonged contractions involves a number of carefully coordinated, quickly responding metabolic reactions (Figure 1). These systems for ATP resynthesis operate in skeletal muscle. Two of these can function for short periods without oxygen (anaerobic alactic and anaerobic lactic), while the third system is precisely integrated with oxygen utilization in the mitochondria (Table 1). The anaerobic systems operate essentially in the cytoplasm (sarcoplasm) of the muscle

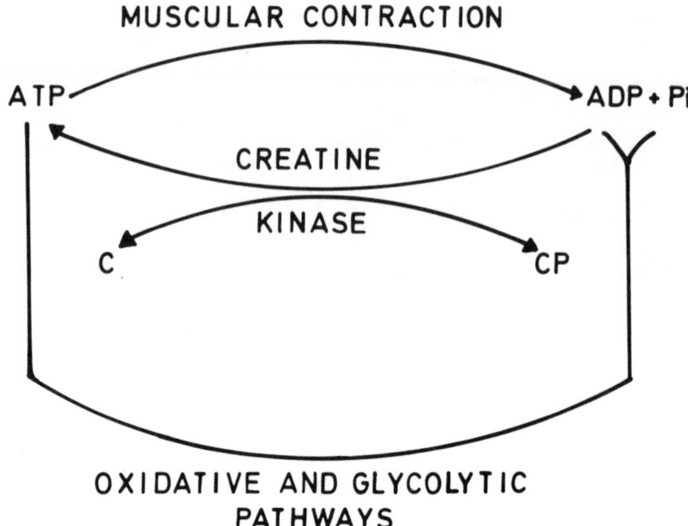


Figure 1. An overview of the breakdown and resynthesis of ATP in the muscle cell is depicted here.

cell, whereas the oxidation of carbohydrate-derived pyruvate, fatty acids, and ketone bodies occurs in the muscle mitochondria. It should also be pointed out that the metabolism of muscle is vastly more complicated than indicated here. However, for the present discussion this approach is satisfactory. McGilvery (1975), in a recent article, has provided a more comprehensive view of muscle metabolism.

## EXERCISE METABOLISM

### Fuels for Muscular Work

The immediately available phosphagen stores in muscle (ATP and CP) can provide the energy for all-out muscular work for about 4–5 sec

Table 1. Major systems for ATP resynthesis in the muscle cell[a]

| |
|---|
| *Anaerobic alactic* |
| ADP + CP (creatine phosphate) ↔ ATP + C (creatine) |
| *Anaerobic lactic (glycolysis)* |
| Glycogen/Glucose + ADP + Pi → Lactate + ATP |
| *Aerobic (oxidative)* |
| Carbohydrate (pyruvate) + $O_2$ + ADP + Pi → $CO_2$ + $H_2O$ + ATP |
| Fat (fatty acids, ketone bodies) + $O_2$ + ADP + Pi → $CO_2$ + $H_2O$ + ATP |

[a] No attempt has been made to chemically balance the equations.

only (Saltin, 1973a). This means that glycolytic or oxidative processes must be turned on rapidly. Margaria, Cerretelli, and Mangili (1964) originally proposed that the phosphagen stores of muscle had to be markedly depleted before glycolysis was activated. However, Saltin et al. (1971) have shown that after just 10 sec of maximal bicycle exercise the metabolites (glucose, glucose-6-phosphate, and lactate) had increased above rest values in the exercising muscle, and muscle glycogen concentration was reduced. Furthermore, the ATP and CP values were higher after 10 sec than after 20 sec of work at the same workload. These data reveal that there is a prompt glycolytic response very early in exercise, and that glycolysis is initiated before the phosphagen levels are maximally depleted. In the same study, blood gas measurements pointed to a very early increase in oxygen uptake in the exercising muscle, suggesting that the onset of oxidative metabolism is also quite rapid. McGilvery (1975) arrived at similar conclusions from theoretical considerations.

Obviously, fuels other than the phosphagens are rapidly utilized very early in exercise, and, because of the limited phosphagen stores, these fuels must be available readily and in sufficient quantity to sustain working muscles for many hours. During muscular work, fuel may be utilized from within the working muscle itself, as well as from stores outside the muscle. As the data in Table 2 indicate, the energy stores for man are quite large, even excluding potential protein sources. However, this apparent surfeit of available energy is misleading because a number of factors (Table 3) can alter the metabolism of muscle,

Table 2. Approximate energy stores of a sedentary young male in the postprandial state

| Energy source | Concentration or quantity available | Total energy equivalent (kilojoule) |
|---|---|---|
| Intramuscular | | |
| ATP | 5 mmoles × $kg^{-1}$ (wet weight) | 5.5 |
| CP | 18 mmoles × $kg^{-1}$ (wet weight) | 22.8 |
| Glycogen | 80 mmoles glucose units × $kg^{-1}$ (wet weight) | $6.7 \times 10^3$ |
| Triglyceride | 65 mmoles × $kg^{-1}$ (wet weight) | $6.2 \times 10^4$ |
| Extramuscular | | |
| Glucose | 10 g | 167 |
| Liver glycogen | 70 g | $1.2 \times 10^3$ |
| Triglyceride | 6 kg | $2.2 \times 10^5$ |

[a] Based on data from Saltin (1973a), Essén et al. (1975b), Hultman and Nilsson (1975), McGilvery (1975), Womersley et al. (1976), and Green, Houston, and Thomson (unpublished data).

Table 3. Factors influencing sources and proportions of fuels utilized in working skeletal muscle

1. Relative intensity of muscular work: load and frequency of contractions
2. Duration of work
3. Quantity of substrate stores available
4. Type of contractions: dynamic, static
5. Manner in which the work is performed: continuous, intermittent
6. Size of the working muscle mass
7. Duration of work and rest periods (intermittent exercise)
8. Environmental factors: altitude, temperature, relative humidity

forcing a primary reliance on selected substrates such as intramuscular phosphagens and glycogen. Constraints placed on fuel utilization can result in situations where fatigue is directly attributable to a lack of specific intramuscular or extramuscular carbohydrate. Before discussing fuel utilization and exercise, however, it is necessary to review some important characteristics of human muscle.

## Human Muscle Fiber Types

In recent years, human skeletal muscle has been classified into two major populations of fibers based on the histochemically demonstrated myofibrillar ATPase reaction (Padykula and Herman, 1955; Engel, 1962). Those fibers that stain dark following alkaline preincubation are designated Type II (fast twitch or FT) and those that stain light under these conditions, Type I (slow twitch or ST). Saltin (1973a) has reviewed some of the characteristics of Type I (ST) and Type II (FT) fiber types in man. Brooke and Kaiser (1970) have demonstrated that Type II fibers can be separated into three subgroups based on differential pH and temperature sensitivities to the preincubation medium of the histochemical ATPase reaction. These subgroups have been identified as Types II-A, II-B, and II-C. Ordinarily, the proportion of Type II-C fibers in mature human muscle is rather low (ca. 1%); thus a three-fiber nomenclature is preferable. More detailed studies on the three fiber types have recently been reported (Essén et al., 1975a; Saltin et al., 1971), suggesting that the adoption of a three-fiber nomenclature system, as opposed to a two-fiber system, is preferable for studies in exercise physiology.

## Intramuscular Substrates and Exercise

The intramuscular energy sources are composed of the phosphagens, glycogen, and triglyceride (Table 2), and all of these may contribute to the energy requirements of the contracting muscle fiber. The relative contribution of these energy sources depends to a great extent on the factors outlined in Table 3.

The fibers of any muscle are enervated by specific alpha-motoneurons; the muscle fibers plus the motoneuron are collectively called a motor unit. Within any muscle, hundreds of motor units are available for activation during muscular contractions. The kind of motor units, the number of motor units, and the frequency with which the motor units are activated can vary enormously depending upon the type, intensity, and duration of work that the muscle is required to do (Burke and Edgerton, 1975; Edgerton, 1976). Although the muscle fibers within a motor unit seem to have similar characteristics, the motor units themselves have a range of properties such as time to peak tension and twitch and tetanic tensions, as well as metabolic properties, e.g., endurance (Edgerton, 1976).

In terms of phosphagen concentrations in working muscles, Karlsson (1971) has shown that there is an inverse relationship between phosphagen levels and relative work intensity. This is particularly noticeable with CP, which fell linearly from rest values (ca. 16 mmoles $\times$ kg$^{-1}$ wet weight) to approximately 3 mmoles $\times$ kg$^{-1}$ at a work intensity of 100% of $\dot{V}_{O_2}$ max. The decline in ATP concentration was much less apparent, and, during maximal work, the ATP concentration was still approximately 70% of the rest value (Karlsson, 1971). When work is performed intermittently, the levels of ATP and CP at the end of each work bout are inversely related to the length of the work period (Saltin and Essén, 1971).

Associated with vigorous muscular contractions is an increase in lactate concentration in both working muscles and blood (Gollnick and Hermansen, 1973). Lactate is a product of glycolysis, and, being a small and easily diffusible molecule, may be found in all the water compartments of the body except cerebrospinal fluid (Hermansen, 1971) in concentrations related to its rate of formation. Lactate is formed in the sarcoplasm of muscle as a reduction product of glycolytically generated pyruvate. Its concentration in both muscle and blood during exercise is regarded as an index of anaerobic ATP production (Gollnick and Hermansen, 1973). Hermansen (1971) has shown that there is an exponential increase in blood lactate concentration as the relative workload is increased to 100% of $\dot{V}_{O_2}$ max. This holds true for both trained and untrained subjects, although Hermansen's data (Figure 2) show that the blood lactate level at any relative workload is lower for trained subjects.

The rate at which ATP can be generated through glycolysis in muscle greatly exceeds that produced through oxidative metabolism (McGilvery, 1975). As a result, near the beginning of exercise, when

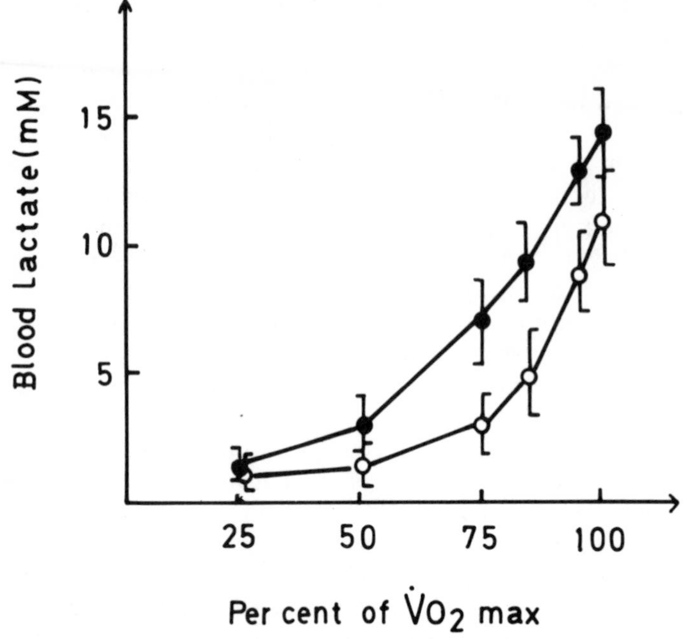


Figure 2. The concentration of blood lactate in trained (open circles) and untrained subjects is shown as a function of relative work intensity. Values are means ± SD (Hermansen, 1971).

mitochondrial oxygen consumption is not optimal, and during very intense exercise, when pyruvate production exceeds the mitochondrial capacity to oxidize it, lactate accumulates in the muscle cell. For very severe work intensities or when blood flow to muscle is partially or wholly occluded, muscle and blood lactate levels may reach very high values (Gollnick and Hermansen, 1973; Sahlin, Harris, and Hultman, 1975). Under continuous work conditions, the increase in blood lactate levels lags behind that of muscle lactate (Gollnick and Hermansen, 1973), the two becoming equal some 7 min after exercise. However, when repeated bouts of severe intermittent exercise are performed, the muscle lactate reaches its maximal or nearly maximal levels after one or two work bouts, whereas the blood lactate levels increase with each succeeding work period, eventually plateauing at a level approximately equal to that of the muscle (Saltin and Essén, 1971; Green, Houston, and Thomson, unpublished observations). The increase in lactate concentration in exercising muscle is associated with a proportionate increase in the production of hydrogen ions. Furthermore, the decrease in muscle pH during severe exercise has been shown to be linearly related to the intramuscular pyruvate plus lactate concentrations. The relationship of the increase in muscle $H^+$ concentration (decrease in pH) to fatigue in the muscle has been recently discussed (Sahlin, Harris, and Hultman, 1975; Sahlin et al., 1976; Wenger and Reed, 1976).

The importance of muscle glycogen as a fuel for muscular exercise has been demonstrated in a large number of studies (Hultman, 1967; see Bergström and Hultman, 1972, for a summary of earlier work). The earlier studies demonstrated that work time was positively related to muscle glycogen content, and that prior diet and exercise could influence the content of muscle glycogen stores (Hultman, 1967). The primacy of glycogen as a fuel during many work situations is related to the fact that at workloads greater than 85–90% of $\dot{V}_{O_2}$ max, carbohydrate becomes the exclusive fuel for working muscle (Bergström and Hultman, 1972). Because the major carbohydrate stores of the body are found in muscle and are immediately available for muscular work, the essential role for muscle glycogen is rather obvious. For very low submaximal workloads, glycogen depletion is rather low, but as the intensity of work increases to supramaximal levels, the rate at which muscle glycogen is consumed increases in an exponential fashion (Saltin and Karlsson, 1971).

More recent experiments have examined the depletion of glycogen in specific muscle fiber types in order to understand fiber recruitment during exercise. Based on the intensity of the periodic acid Schiff (PAS) histochemical stain, the quantity of glycogen in specific fibers can be assessed. By comparing the intensity of the PAS staining in specific fibers before, during, and after exercise, an appreciation of the order and extent of fiber recruitment during specific exercise situations can be obtained. Results from experiments using dynamic exercise have revealed that during submaximal exercise ST (Type I) fibers were the first to lose their glycogen, and the FT (Type II) fibers were recruited during submaximal exercise when the ST fibers were depleted or during work requiring an intensity greater than $\dot{V}_{O_2}$ max (Costill et al., 1973; Gollnick et al., 1973a; Gollnick et al., 1973b; Gollnick, Piehl, and Saltin, 1974). It has also been demonstrated that exercising muscle may take up and utilize lactate (Jorfeldt, 1970), and that the lactate molecule, although an end product of glycolytic metabolism, may actually serve as a carbohydrate substrate for the more oxidative ST (Type I) fibers when the muscle glycogen concentration is very low (Essén et al., 1975b).

Glycogen depletion studies in man have now been extended using the three fiber types of human skeletal muscle, that is, looking at the preferential glycogen depletion (recruitment) of the II-A and II-B subgroups of the FT fibers. Results from submaximal dynamic exercise indicate that the order of fiber recruitment is Type I, Type II-A, and then Type II-B (Andersen and Sjøgaard, 1975; Thomson, Green, and Houston, 1976). For supramaximal dynamic exercise and maximal static contractions, the extent of glycogen depletion is reversed, that is Type II-B > Type II-A > Type I (Secher and Nygaard, 1976; Thomson, Green, and Houston, 1976). Although glycogen depletion data can reveal which fibers have been involved in different types of work, the fact that glycogen can be metabolized both aerobically and anaerobically suggests that some caution must be exercised in the interpretation of the depletion data in terms of revealing the extent to which different fibers have been involved in the work.

The intramuscular supply of triglyceride is potentially capable of fueling working muscle for many hours, neglecting the contribution from other sources. That it does make some contribution as an energy source is based on observations showing a decline in intramuscular triglyceride with prolonged skiing (Fröberg and Mossfeldt, 1971) and with shorter periods of continuous and intermittent exercise (Carlsson, Ekelund and Fröberg, 1971). However, definitive conclusions based on these observations must be viewed with caution because muscle has the capacity to take up and esterify plasma free fatty acids (FFA). The actual decrease in muscle triglyceride with exercise may thus be more indicative of an imbalance between hydrolysis of intramuscular triglyceride and esterification of absorbed plasma FFA, with the actual source of the oxidized fatty acids being in doubt (Zierler, 1976).

### Extramuscular Energy Sources

The contribution of extramuscular carbohydrate and lipid to muscle metabolism has been well documented for a variety of exercise conditions in man, including continuous, submaximal leg exercise (Pernow and Saltin, 1971; Ahlborg et al., 1974), intermittent exercise (Keul, Haralambie, and Trittin, 1974), as well as forearm (Hagenfeldt and Wahren, 1971; Hagenfeldt and Wahren, 1972) and arm exercise (Karlsson et al., 1975). The contribution of the various substrates to energy release in the working muscles has been assessed using arterial and venous catheters (Keul, Haralambie, and Trittin, 1974) and radioactive-labeled substrates (Hagenfeldt and Wahren, 1972; Ahlborg et al., 1974). Also, factors regulating the release and uptake of extramuscular substrates have been studied using specific blocking agents (Pernow and Saltin, 1971; Galbo et al., 1976). Respiratory quotients and exchange ratios may provide an overall picture of the proportion of lipid and carbohydrate utilization during exercise, but unless these measurements are associated with changes in intramuscular energy stores, they cannot differentiate between intra- and extramuscular energy contributions.

Results from glycogen depletion studies and studies where the lipid contribution to exercise is determined show that at low work intensities, and especially if the work is prolonged, lipid is the preferred fuel for muscular exercise. As the work intensity is increased or if the work time is brief, carbohydrate takes an increasingly greater role as a fuel, up to nearly 90% or even more of $\dot{V}_{O_2}$ max, when carbohydrate is the exclusive fuel for working muscle (Bergström and Hultman, 1972). The greater reliance on lipid at low work intensities and the increasing importance of carbohydrate at higher workloads can be accounted for from a number of perspectives. For example, from a teleological viewpoint, the quantitatively greater stores of body fat compared with carbohydrate (Table 2) and coupled with the fact that certain tissues such as the central nervous system and red blood cells have an obligatory requirement for glucose, make the sparing of carbohydrate, where possible, an important metabolic adjustment. Thus, for low to moderate workloads, there is a recruitment of higher oxidative Type I fibers, and blood FFA levels increase while insulin concentration decreases (Ahlborg et al., 1974). For heavier workloads, there is a greater reliance on high threshold, low oxidative motor units. Under these conditions blood lactate levels increase and FFA levels decrease as carbohydrate becomes the predominant fuel (Figure 3).

However, in addition to the arguments based on fiber recruitment, fuel utilization within individual muscle fibers is precisely controlled by the intracellular levels of certain metabolities that can activate and inhibit certain regulatory enzymes, and thus control substrate flux through the degradative pathways (Newsholme and Start, 1973; Crabtree and Newsholme, 1975; McGilvery, 1975; Ramaiah, 1976). Briefly, the intensity of contractile activity as well as time can influence the intracellular concentration of such metabolites as ATP, ADP, AMP, acetyl CoA, glucose-6-phosphate, and citrate. These metabolites, in addition to other factors, can modulate the activity of such regulatory enzymes as phosphorylase (ATP, AMP), hexokinase (glucose-6-phosphate), phosphofructokinase (ATP, ADP, AMP, and citrate) and pyruvate dehydrogenase (acetyl CoA and ATP). Hence the uptake of substrate, the mobilization of substrate, and the type of substrate being metabolized can be controlled in the muscle cell. In summary, the specific demands of exercise can effect the motor unit recruitment pattern as well as metabolite levels, and these in turn can control substrate utilization.

The previous arguments have focused on factors controlling the type of fuel utilized, with no distinction being made between the source of these substrates, i.e., blood glucose versus muscle glycogen and blood-borne FFA versus intramuscular triglyceride. Blood glucose has been shown to be a quantitatively important substrate for exercising

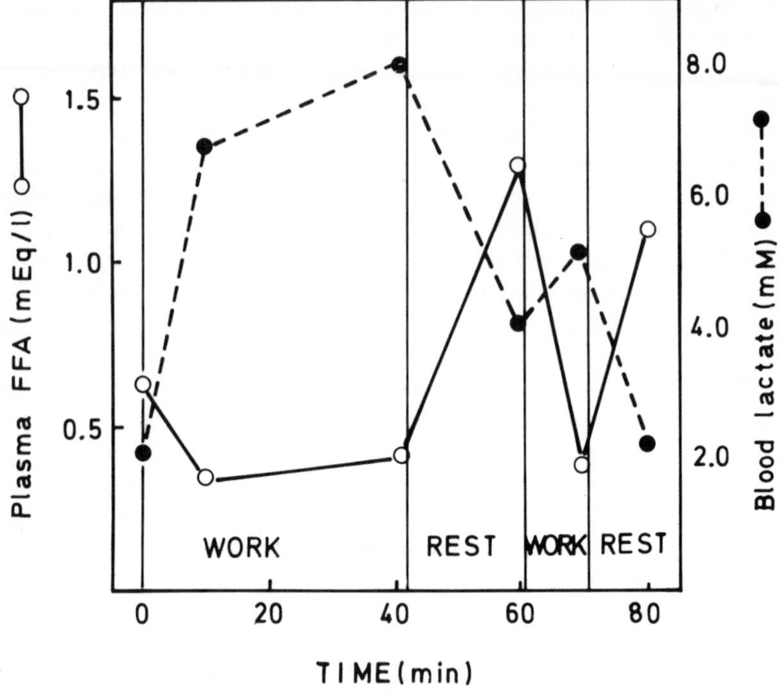


Figure 3. This graph demonstrates the reciprocal relationship between blood lactate and FFA concentrations for one subject during work (86% of $\dot{V}_{O_2}$ max) and rest periods (Pruett, 1970).

muscle in both diabetic (Wahren, Hagenfeldt, and Felig, 1975; Mæhlum, Jervell, and Pruett, 1976) and nondiabetic subjects (Wahren et al., 1971; Ahlborg et al., 1972). Glucose release from the liver as a result of enhanced glycogenolysis and gluconeogenesis may increase by up to eight times resting values during hard exercise (Hultman and Nilsson, 1975). Despite both the increased release of glucose from the liver and falling insulin levels in the blood, there is an enhanced uptake of glucose by the muscle with time, resulting in falling arterial glucose values during prolonged submaximal exercise (Ahlborg et al., 1974). Even during shorter periods of more intense continuous exercise (Wahren et al., 1971) or during maximal intermittent exercise glucose oxidation may represent from 11% to 37% of the total oxidized substrate. Saltin (1975) has proposed that the glucose uptake by skeletal muscle increases as the concentration of muscle glycogen decreases, and he has suggested that the release of inhibition of hexokinase secondary to a reduced production of glucose-6-phosphate from glycogenolysis may be a major factor in regulating the uptake of blood glucose by exercising muscle.

The uptake of blood borne FFA by exercising skeletal muscle is determined by the blood FFA levels and the blood flow through the working muscle (Ahlborg et al., 1974), that is, a mass action effect. The plasma FFA concentration during exercise is positively related to the duration of work and the intensity of work for low to moderate workloads (Pruett, 1970). For near maximal, maximal, and supramaximal workloads, i.e., loads requiring a preponderance of carbohydrate as a fuel, FFA concentrations decrease with time. This decline in plasma FFA levels at higher workloads is related to the rising blood lactate levels (Fredholm, 1971), and under these conditions a reciprocal relationship between blood lactate and FFA levels can be demonstrated (Figure 3). During prolonged continuous exercise (Ahlborg et al., 1974) or during more intense intermittent exercise (Keul, Haralambie, and Trittin, 1974) oxidation of plasma FFA may account for a major fraction of the oxidized substrate. Where FFA mobilization is impaired by nicotinic acid (Pernow and Saltin, 1971; Galbo et al., 1976) or with a beta-adrenergic blocking agent (Galbo et al., 1976), performance time is decreased.

## SWIMMING METABOLISM

### Energy Requirements

To understand the metabolic requirements of swimming during competition and training, published data on swimming as well as other forms of exercise can be used. Unfortunately, there is a paucity of information available on such factors as substrate utilization and fiber recruitment during training and competition in swimming. Data are available on oxygen costs and hemodynamic responses during tethered swimming (Magel and Faulkner, 1967; Magel et al., 1974), free swimming (McArdle, Glaser, and Magel, 1971), and swimming in a flume (Holmér, 1972; Holmér and Åstrand, 1972; Holmér, Lundin, and Eriksson, 1974; Holmér et al., 1974) for trained and untrained swimmers. Those studies, however, have not focused on metabolism, nor have they in fact used swimming speeds comparable with those swum during world class competition.

In view of the limited data available on the metabolism of swimming, a judicious degree of speculation and application of known requirements for related activities must be used. Before attempting this, it should be stressed that previous swimming studies have shown that at higher swimming velocities, $\dot{V}_{O_2}$ (Holmér, 1972), and caloric costs

(Karpovich and Millman, 1944) increase at a faster rate than swimming speed. This is related to the fact that water drag is approximately proportional to the square of the swimming speed (Holmér, 1974); drag may be even greater for velocities approaching 2 m $\times$ $sec^{-1}$.

In an attempt to put the requirements of competitive swimming in a meaningful metabolic perspective, the total energy costs and the proportion of aerobic and anaerobic metabolism during freestyle swimming at world record speeds has been estimated for a male swimmer having a $\dot{V}_{O_2}$ max of 5.0 liters $\times$ $min^{-1}$ and a maximal oxygen debt capacity of 12 liters of oxygen (Table 4). The basis for these estimates is the assumption that the maximal oxygen debt capacity would be utilized completely in events up to and including the 400-m distance. Thus, for all the swimming distances shown in Table 4, the anaerobic component has been predicted first. The aerobic component was then included, assuming that both the 800- and 1500-m events would be swum at speeds requiring at least 100% of $\dot{V}_{O_2}$ max. Because Hermansen (1969) has shown that small increments in near maximal swimming speed produce correspondingly larger increases in oxygen debt, and because events such as 100-m freestyle swimming and 400-m running at racing paces result in very large oxygen debts (Hermansen, 1969), the underlying basis for these estimates seems justified.

The predictions in Table 4 also indicate that, for maximal swimming velocities for the various distances, there is an exponential increase in total energy requirements as the swimming speed increases. Moreover, these estimates also show that a major reliance on anaerobic processes is a prerequisite for maximal 100- and 200-m swimming speeds. Because more than 75% of the Olympic swimming events for both men and women involve 100- or 200-m distances, great attention must be directed to the anaerobic component of metabolism during training. Thus, on the basis of these estimates, an improved anaerobic capacity would result in a greater improvement in 100-m and 200-m swim performances than would a comparable improvement in $V_{O_2}$ max, all other factors being similar.

### Substrate Utilization During Swimming

On the basis of the earlier discussion concerning substrate utilization during such activities as bicycle exercise and treadmill running, as well as the estimations of energy costs during competitive swimming, it is proposed that the energy supply to swimming muscles during competition is derived from phosphagen stores, glycolysis, and carbohydrate oxidation. Lipid oxidation is thus assumed to have a negligible role. The maximal capacities of phosphagen stores and glycolytic metabolism can provide approximately 1 liter and 5–10 liters of oxygen

Table 4. Relative contribution of anaerobic and aerobic metabolism to total energy requirements during freestyle swimming at world record speeds (July, 1976) for men

| Freestyle distance (m) | Swimming speed (percent of 100-m speed) | Total energy requirements (liters of $O_2$) | Energy output (liters of $O_2$) | | Relative contribution (percent) | |
|---|---|---|---|---|---|---|
| | | | Anaerobic metabolism | Aerobic metabolism | Anaerobic metabolism | Aerobic metabolism |
| 100 | 100.0 | 15.0 | 12.0 | 3.0 | 80 | 20 |
| 200 | 90.7 | 20.0 | 12.0 | 8.0 | 60 | 40 |
| 400 | 86.2 | 30.0 | 12.0 | 18.0 | 40 | 60 |
| 800 | 83.1 | 47.0 | 8.0 | 39.0 | 17 | 83 |
| 1500 | 83.1 | 82.0 | 8.0 | 74.0 | 10 | 90 |

as energy equivalents, respectively (Karlsson, 1971; Saltin, 1973b). Therefore, as the competitive swimming distance increases, the contribution of carbohydrate oxidation to the overall energy yield increases, and for 800-m and 1500-m races, dominates the energy picture. Conversely, for the shorter competitive distances of 100- and 200-m, energy derived from phosphagen depletion and glycolysis predominates.

In swimming training, a much more complicated energy picture presents itself, because vast differences in total training distances, interval distances, swimming intensities, and recovery times can occur at various times in a training year. For example, during 'volume' training, distances of up to 20 km per day may be swum in two training sessions of 5–6 hours' total duration. At other times of the year, much less total distance is swum, but the swimming speed is comparatively much faster. By necessity, the metabolic demands during these contrasting training modes would be different.

To gain further insight into the metabolism during swim training, glycogen depletion in the deltoid muscle was studied in two young swimmers during two different types of training on successive days. Following a day without training, muscle biopsies were taken before and after a 2.5 hr training session in which the emphasis was on low intensity, repeated intervals of 50–400 m duration with short rest periods. The next day, following a warm-up of five relatively low intensity 200-m intervals, fast repeats of 25–100 m were swum at near maximal to maximal speed; rest pauses between intervals were correspondingly longer. In both training situations, the front crawl was used, except for 1000 m during Day 1 and 700 m during Day 2 of flutter kicking intervals. During training on Day 1, 6.1 km of freestyle swimming was performed, and on Day 2, the distance was 2.15 km. Histochemistry was performed on a portion of each muscle sample for the determination of fiber types (Brooke and Kaiser, 1970) and PAS staining. The glycogen content before and after training was assessed on the basis of the PAS staining intensity (Gollnick, Piehl, and Saltin, 1974) in the Type I and Type II-A fibers (no II-B fibers were found in these histochemical sections). In addition, the total glycogen content in the remaining portion of the muscle samples was measured (Gollnick et al., 1973a).

Resting muscle glycogen content was rather high before training on both days, although the pretraining value on Day 2 was still 19% lower than the corresponding value for Day 1, which had been preceded by a day without training (Table 5). In view of the fact that only 6.1 km of front crawl swimming had been performed, and this in only one training session, the possibility that muscle glycogen levels could limit training performance during more prolonged training with two training sessions a day on successive days seems likely. This observation suggests that considerable attention should be paid to the carbohydrate intake in the diet of swimmers. The data in Table 5 also reveal that when training intensity is high, the glycogen depletion per km of swimming is increased. Furthermore, it must be noted that over 40% of the front crawl swimming on Day 2 was a low intensity warm-up; this suggests that if the duration of fast swimming had been greater, a much more marked depletion of glycogen would have resulted.

The pattern of PAS staining (Figure 4) indicates that while both Type I and Type II-A fibers were involved in the training on Day 1, the more completely and partially depleted fibers were Type I. On Day 2, both Types I and II-A fibers were equally depleted of glycogen. Because the glycolytic potential of the Type II-A fibers, and hence the rate at which glycogen can be utilized, is greater than that of Type I fibers (Essén et al., 1975a) it is evident that considerable Type I fiber recruitment occurred during the more intense swimming.

The contribution of lipid oxidation to fuel the energy demand for the two days of swimming was calculated using the glycogen depletion data, the estimated contribution from glucose taken up by the blood, and the energy cost per km swum for the two subjects (300 kcal $\times$ km$^{-1}$ for Day 1; 320 kcal $\times$ km$^{-1}$, Day 2). A problem arises, however, in the estimations of the total muscle mass involved during front crawl swimming. If for the purposes of this calculation it is assumed that 15 kg of muscle is involved in front crawl swimming, having a mean glycogen depletion as represented by the deltoid muscle, the total glycogen contribution from this muscle mass may be determined. On this basis, of the 2,130 kcal of energy expended on Day 1, 46% was derived from lipid sources. For Day 2, the energy expenditure was 912 kcal, of which 34% came from fat. These figures are rather crude because it is difficult to predict the muscle involved in this type of activity, particularly because it has been shown with electromyography (Ikai, Ishii, and Miyashita, 1964) that rather large variations in muscle involvement may occur in different swimmers swimming the same

Table 5. Mean glycogen and relative glycogen utilization in deltoid muscle of two swimmers during low intensity and high intensity front crawl swim training

| Swimming intensity | Glycogen concentration (mmoles glucose units $\times$ kg$^{-1}$ (w.w.) | | Distance swum freestyle (km) | Relative glycogen depletion (mmoles glucose $\times$ kg$^{-1}$ $\times$ km$^{-1}$) |
|---|---|---|---|---|
| | Before | After | | |
| Low | 140.0 | 48.0 | 6.10 | 15.1 |
| High | 113.5 | 68.5 | 2.15 | 20.9 |

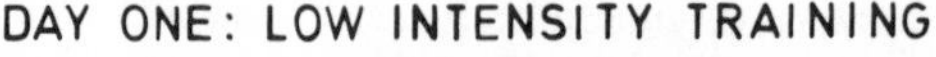


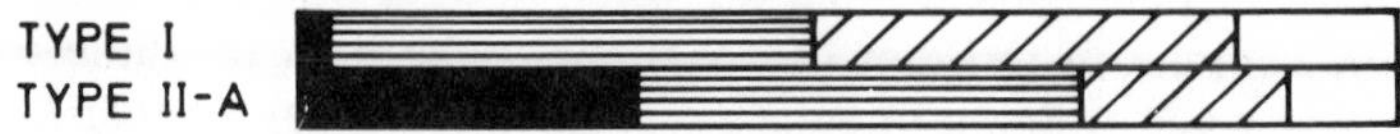




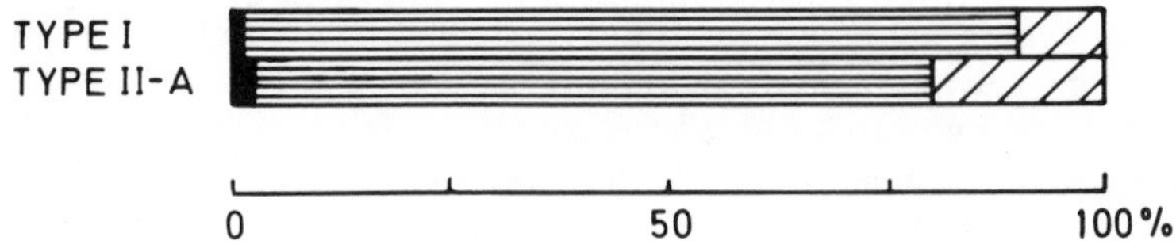


Figure 4. This figure provides a summary of the PAS staining in Type I and II-A fibers of the deltoid muscle after low and high intensity swim training. Before training, all fibers were rated as dark staining.

stroke. Nonetheless, an attempt such as this clearly indicates that a great deal more attention must be given to the study of swimming metabolism and substrate utilization. Finally, in contrast to competition swimming, lipid substrates are used to a considerable extent during training.

## TRAINING FOR MAXIMAL SWIM PERFORMANCE

### Characteristics of Swimmers

One of the unique characteristics of swimming, compared with running and cycling, is that trained swimmers can achieve a higher percent of their treadmill $\dot{V}_{O_2}$ max while swimming than can trained subjects or untrained persons (Holmér; 1972; unpublished observations). Furthermore, at any swimming speed, the $\dot{V}_{O_2}$ for swimmers is less than that of trained individuals or untrained persons (Figure 5). There are a number of explanations for these findings and these have been previously discussed (Holmér, 1972; Holmér et al., 1974; Magel et al., 1974). Briefly, the major reliance on muscles of the upper body, in addition to the more complex movements mechanics of swimming, account for the major differences between swimming and running-and-cycling $\dot{V}_{O_2}$

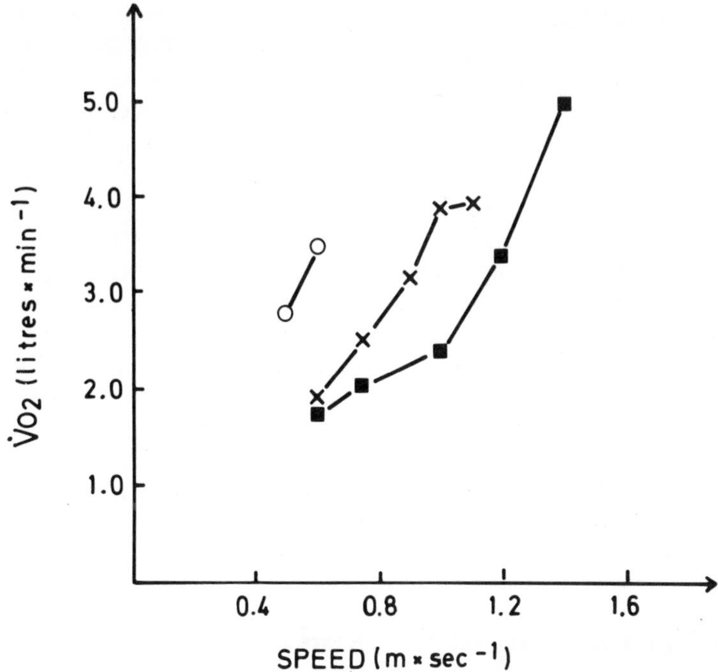


Figure 5. This graph shows oxygen uptake as a function of swim speed during front crawl swimming for a subject not trained in swimming (○), a subject trained in swimming (X), and an elite swimmer (■) (Holmér, (1972).

measures. Thus, the unique and specific demands imposed by swimming are reflected in these observations.

As a group, swimmers can be classified as endurance athletes. This classification is supported by data showing that well trained swimmers are characterized by high $\dot{V}_{O_2}$ max values (Magel and Faulkner; Gollnick et al., 1972; Holmér, 1972; Holmér, Lundin, and Eriksson, 1974) and large maximal cardiac outputs, measured during both swimming and running (Dixon and Faulkner, 1971; Saltin, 1973b). In addition, the characteristics of skeletal muscle from trained swimmers, such as the activity of the oxidative enzyme succinate dehydrogenase (Gollnick et al., 1972; Nygaard and Nielsen, pp. 282–293) and muscle capillary supply are indicative of a high oxidative metabolic capacity.

These indices of superior endurance capacity in swimmers should not be particularly surprising, considering the great volume of training swimmers perform. Because 12–16 km per day of swim training is not unusual, and may indeed be a norm, adaptations in circulatory and skeletal muscle parameters consistent with high endurance capacity would be expected. In fact, compared with the training distances reported for elite distance runners (Costill, Fink, and Pollock, 1976) and for extremely well trained orienteers (Jansson and Kaijser, 1977), swimmers are preeminent in terms of training volume. However, in view of the fact that the majority of competitive swimming distances have a performance time of approximately 2 min or less, and, further, require a greater proportion of anaerobic as opposed to aerobic metabolism, the necessity for great training distances for swimmers may be questioned. One obvious answer to such a question is that world records in all swimming events have a very short lifetime: swimming performances continually and consistently improve with time. That steady improvement in swimming performance has been a norm for a number of years cannot be denied. However, many factors may be suggested to account for this improvement in addition to the fact that swimmers are training harder now. Such factors as new swimming suits, faster pools, improvements in stroke techniques, as well as an exponential increase in the number of young swimmers, are each responsible in part for improved performances.

## Training for Optimal Metabolic Response

It is not enough just to look at swimmers and swimming today. Rather, the perspective should be one of assessing the requirements for world class performances in the years ahead, and beginning to adapt today's swimmers to these future demands. From a physiological viewpoint, three metabolic aspects must be considered: oxidative metabolism, glycolytic rate, and glycolytic capacity. (Although muscular strength is undoubtedly important, it is not included here because of the metabolic perspective.) All three metabolic parameters are, to varying degrees, necessary for optimal performance in the different swimming events. Swimmers today, as previously mentioned, are characterized as having skeletal muscle characteristics, enzyme activities, and circulatory dimensional and functional capacities similar to those of athletes involved in activities requiring much longer endurance. Apparently, current training techniques have resulted in impressive adaptations for optimal oxidative metabolism. Furthermore, for the present discussion, it is assumed that, at least early in a swimmer's career, considerable attention should be devoted to the aerobic aspects of swimming. This means that many repeats of lower intensity distances should be swum both to improve aerobic performance and to produce a foundation for tolerating more intense swimming later.

Because glycolytic metabolism has been previously shown to be a major component for energy supply in distances up to and including 400 m (Table 4), training to improve this energy system is of great importance. There are two aspects of glycolytic or anaerobic lactic metabolism to consider. Glycolytic rate refers to the rate of substrate flux and hence the rate of ATP generation through this cytoplasmic sequence of reactions. Glycolytic capacity means the ability of the glycolytic reactions to continue functioning in the face of a rapid intracellular accumulation of end products, particularly the lactate and hydrogen ions. It has been previously demonstrated that the decrease in muscle pH following hard dynamic exercise is linearly related to the muscle content of pyruvate and lactate, two glycolytic products (Sahlin et al., 1976). An increase in intramuscular $H^+$ ion (decrease in muscle pH) has been shown to inhibit the activity of the key regulatory enzyme of glycolysis, phosphofructokinase (Trivedi and Danforth, 1966). There would then seem to be an indirect feedback mechanism inhibiting the glycolytic resynthesis of ATP via an accumulation of the products lactate and pyruvate in the muscle cell. Moreover, the increase in intramuscular $H^+$ ions has also been shown to alter the equilibrium of the creatine kinase reaction (Sahlin, Harris, and Hultman, 1975), to interfere with calcium ion binding by troponin (Fuchs, Reddy, and Briggs, 1970), and to increase the calcium binding capacity of sarcoplasmic reticulum (Nakamura and Schwartz, 1972). All of these effects could account for a decrease in muscle performance at severe workloads.

It would thus seem that limitations imposed by key biochemical reactions preclude improvements in the rate and capacity of glycolytic processes in muscle. Yet athletes engaged in short-term activities such as 400- and 800-m running and 100- and 200-m swimming events can produce very large maximal oxygen debts (Hermansen, 1969), suggesting that training can definitely influence anaerobic processes. Furthermore, short-term sprint training (Thorstensson, Sjödin, and Karlsson, 1975) and longer duration, high intensity anaerobic training (Houston and Thomson, 1977) can produce significant gains in anaerobic performance. Unfortunately, there is no documentation of the effects of prolonged, intense anaerobic training on such human skeletal muscle parameters as lactate efflux from muscle during work, intramuscular buffering capacity, phosphofructokinase activity, and overall glycolytic flux rate. The fact that anaerobic metabolism seems to be a reasonably adaptable system would suggest that one or more of these factors could be modified through the proper training.

It is a well known fact that a large proportion of competitive swimmers employ dry land resistance training (strength training) as a supplement to water training. What is not known is the exact role that resistance training plays in improving swim performance. Resistance training may be performed in a number of ways, depending on the primary challenge desired for the working muscles. For example, low repetition, high load exercise primarily taxes the contractile proteins, whereas, at the other extreme, lighter loads and more and faster repetitions place the greatest demands on anaerobic energy delivery systems. As a group, athletes involved in such strength activities as weight lifting and track and field throwing events are characterized by large Type II fibers (Edström and Ekblom, 1972; Gollnick et al., 1972; Costill et al., 1976; Prince, Hikida, and Hagerman, 1976), as well as low activities for oxidative enzymes (Gollnick et al., 1972; Costill et al., 1976). These characteristics are considerably different from those previously discussed for swimmers: the effects of the low repetition, high load training of the strength athletes serves to increase contractile protein concentrations, thereby diluting the mitochondrial proteins on the basis of muscle weight. This type of training and the resulting adaptations do not seem suitable for optimal swimming performance. However, the use of lower resistance coupled with many fast repetitions could result in advantageous adaptations to anaerobic alactic and lactic energy systems. Furthermore, this type of training could recruit Type II fibers more effectively than could faster swimming repetitions, at least based on the glycogen depletion data previously discussed. Although there is a scarcity of reliable data on the metabolic consequences of resistance training for swimmers, the use of low load, high repetition training using movements simulating actual stroke mechanics would, theoretically, provide a useful adjunct to typical swimming training, and in addition to stressing the glycolytic energy systems, would undoubtedly increase muscular strength.

To illustrate how swimming training can be employed so that a primary challenge can be imposed on specific metabolic aspects previously discussed, a general training protocol is shown in Table 6. Training to improve oxidative metabolism in such endurance athletes as cross-country skiers, runners, bicyclists, and orienteers has generally involved prolonged continuous work (Saltin, Essén, and Pedersen, 1976). In contrast, swimmers generally employ interval training with short rest pauses. In view of the highly developed aerobic capacities of even young swimmers, the endurance training methods of swimmers seem to be quite suitable.

The rate of glycolytic metabolism should be maximally stressed when maximal exercise is extended beyond 5–10 sec. Thus maximal speed swimming, with or without added resistance in the form of hand paddles or extra swim suits and when performed for up to 25 sec, should severely tax the lactic ATP resynthesis reactions. Full recovery rest pauses should be allowed so that each repeat can be performed at maximal swimming speed. To challenge the glycolytic capacity fully, near maximal speed intervals should be swum for a period of

Table 6. Training to optimize specific metabolic responses for swimming competition

| Metabolic parameter | Desired physiological response | Training conditions |
|---|---|---|
| Oxidative metabolism | To increase oxygen delivery to muscle; to improve muscle capillarization; to increase the number and size of muscle mitochondria and increase oxidative enzyme activities | Continuous and intermittent swimming at submaximal intensity; longer duration swimming intervals with short rest periods |
| Glycolytic rate | To increase the flux of substrates through the glycolytic reactions and thus the rate of lactic ATP resynthesis | Short duration (10–25 sec) maximal speed swimming intervals with or without added resistance (e.g., hand paddles); high speed, high repetition (20–30 repetitions) resistance training |
| Glycolytic capacity | To maintain optimal glycolytic flux despite rising end product accumulation and falling muscle pH; to enhance muscle buffering capacity | Repeated intervals of 1–3 min duration at fast pace, with less than full recovery rest pauses |

sufficient length that a large accumulation of glycolytic products occurs in the muscle cell. Repeated intervals should be performed without rest allowances sufficient to provide full recovery so that a continued increase in muscle lactate, pyruvate, and $H^+$ occurs. This type of training is very demanding, and should be gradually introduced, reaching a peak some time before major competitions.

The extent to which oxidative and glycolytic metabolism is trained should be related to specific swimming events for each swimmer. Obviously, 1500-m swimmers will require more aerobic training, 100- and 200-m specialists more anaerobic training. "Hypoxic training," i.e., swimming with less than optimal ventilation through voluntary breath holding, is used to varying degrees in training (Kedrowsky, 1976). Hypoxic training may be useful from the perspective of forcing a greater reliance on anaerobic as opposed to oxidative processes during swimming, but this can also be done without breath holding, as has been previously discussed. In fact, unless hypoxic swimming is performed at high speed, there will not be a sufficient challenge to the glycolytic rate. Furthermore, hypoxia is not considered a stimulus for increases in the activities of oxidative enzymes because brief and prolonged exposures to hypoxia in animals have resulted in lowered concentrations of mitochondrial proteins (Hallman, 1971; Kinnula, 1976; Kinnula and Hassinen, 1977).

## REFERENCES


Ahlborg, G., Felig, P., Hagenfeldt, L., Hendler, R., and Wahren, J. 1974. Substrate turnover during prolonged exercise in man. Splanchnic and leg metabolism of glucose, free fatty acids, and amino acids. J. Clin. Invest. 53:1080–1090.

Andersen, P., and Sjøgaard, G. 1975. Selective glycogen depletion in the subgroups of Type II muscle fibres during intense submaximal exercise in man. Acta Physiol. Scand. 96:26A.

Bergström, J., and Hultman, E. 1972. Nutrition for maximal sports performance. JAMA 221:999–1006.

Brooke, M. H., and Kaiser, K. K. 1970. Muscle fibre types: How many and what kind? Arch. Neurol. (Chicago). 23:369–379.

Burke, R. E., and Edgerton, V. R. 1975. Motor unit properties and selective involvement in movement. In: J. H. Wilmore (ed.), Exercise and Sport Sciences Reviews, Vol. 3, pp. 31–81. Academic Press, New York.

Carlson, L. A., Ekelund, L.-G., and Fröberg, S. O. 1971. Concentrations of triglycerides, phospholipids, and glycogen and of free fatty acids and β-hydroxybutyric acid in blood in man in response to exercise. Eur. J. Clin. Invest. 1:248–254.

Costill, D. L., Daniels, J., Evans, W., Fink, W., Krahenbuhl, G., and Saltin, B. 1976. Skeletal muscle enzymes and fiber composition in male and female track athletes. J. Appl. Physiol. 40:149–154.

Costill, D. L., Fink, W. J., and Pollock, M. L. 1976. Muscle fiber composition and enzyme activities of elite distance runners. Medi. Sci. Sports 8:96–100.

Costill, D. L., Gollnick, P. D., Jansson, E., Saltin, B., and Stein, E. 1973. Glycogen depletion pattern in human muscle fibres during distance running. Acta Physiol. Scand. 89:374–383.

Crabtree, B., and Newsholme, E. A. 1975. Comparative aspects of fuel utilization and metabolism by muscle. In: P. N. R. Usherwood (ed.), Insect Physiology, pp. 405–500. Academic Press, New York.

Dixon, R. W., Jr., and Faulkner, J. A. 1971. Cardiac output during maximum effort running and swimming. J. Appl. Physiol. 30:653–656.

Edgerton, V. R. 1976. Neuromuscular adaptation to power and endurance work. Can. J. Appl. Sport Sci. 1:49-58.

Edström, L., and Ekblom, B. 1972. Differences in sizes of red and white muscle fibres in vastus lateralis of musculus quadriceps femoris of normal individuals and athletes. Relation to physical performance. Scand. J. Clin. Lab. Invest. 30:175–181.

Engel, W. K. 1962. The essentiality of histo- and cytochemical studies of skeletal muscle in investigation of neuromuscular disease. Neurology. 12:778–794.

Essén, B., Jansson, E., Henriksson, J., Taylor, A. W., and Saltin, B. 1975a. Metabolic characteristics of fiber types in human skeletal muscle. Acta Physiol. Scand. 95:153–165.

Essén, B., Pernow, B., Gollnick, P. D., and Saltin, B. 1975b. Muscle glycogen content and lactate uptake in exercising muscles. In: H. Howald and J. R. Poortmans (eds.), Metabolic Adaptation to Prolonged Physical Exercise, pp. 130–134. Birkhäuser Verlag, Basel.

Fredholm, B. B. 1971. Fat mobilization and blood lactate concentration. In: B. Pernow and B. Saltin (eds.), Muscle Metabolism During Exercise, pp. 249–255. Plenum Press, New York.

Fröberg, S. O., and Mossfeldt, F. 1971. Effect of prolonged strenuous exercise on the concentration of triglycerides, phospholipids, and glycogen in muscle of man. Acta Physiol. Scand. 82:167–171.

Fuchs, F., Reddy, V., and Briggs, F. N. 1970. The interaction of cations with the calcium-binding site of troponin. Biochim. Biophys. Acta. 221:407–409.

Galbo, H., Holst, J. J., Christensen, N. J., and Hilsted, J. 1976. Glucagon and plasma catecholamines during beta-receptor blockage in exercising man. J. Appl. Physiol. 40:855–863.

Gollnick, P. D., Armstrong, R. B., Saubert, C. W., IV. Piehl, K., and Saltin, B. 1972. Enzyme activity and fiber composition in skeletal muscle of untrained and trained men. J. Appl. Physiol. 33:312–319.

Gollnick, P. D., Armstrong, R. B., Saubert, C. W., IV, Sembrowich, W. L., Shepherd, R. E., and Saltin, B. 1973a. Glycogen depletion patterns in human skeletal muscle during prolonged work. Pflügers Arch. 344:1–12.

Gollnick, P. D., Armstrong, R. B., Sembrowich, W. L., Shepherd, R. E., and Saltin, B. 1973b. Glycogen depletion pattern in human skeletal muscle fibers after heavy exercise. J. Appl. Physiol. 34:615–618.

Gollnick, P. D., and Hermansen, L. 1973. Biochemical adaptations to exercise: Anaerobic metabolism. In: J. H. Wilmore (ed.), Exercise and Sport Sciences Reviews, Vol. 1, pp. 1–43. Academic Press, New York.

Gollnick, P. D., Piehl, K., and Saltin, B. 1974. Selective glycogen depletion pattern in human muscle fibers after exercise of varying intensity and at varying pedalling rates. J. Physiol. 241:45–57.

Hagenfeldt, L., and Wahren, J. 1971. Metabolism of free fatty acids and ketone bodies in skeletal muscle. In: B. Pernow and B. Saltin (eds.), Muscle Metabolism During Exercise, pp. 153–163. Plenum Press, New York.

Hagenfeldt, L., and Wahren, J. 1972. Human forearm muscle metabolism during exercise. VII. FFA uptake and oxidation at different work intensities. Scand. J. Clin. Lab. Invest. 30:429–436.

Hallman, M. 1971. Changes in mitochondria and respiratory chain proteins during prenatal development. Evidence of the importance of environmental $O_2$ tensions. Biochim. Biophys. Acta. 253:360–372.

Harris, R. C., Hultman, E., and Nordesjö, L.-O. 1974. Glycogen, glycolytic intermediates, and high energy phosphates determined in biopsy samples of musculus quadriceps femoris of man at rest. Methods and variance of values. Scand. J. Clin. Lab. Invest. 19:56–66.

Hermansen, L. 1969. Anaerobic energy release. Med. Sci. Sport 1:32–38.

Hermansen, L. 1971. Lactate production during exercise. In: B. Pernow and B. Saltin (eds.), Muscle Metabolism During Exercise, pp. 401–407. Plenum Press, New York.

Holmér, I. 1972. Oxygen uptake during swimming in man. J. Appl. Physiol. 33:502–509.

Holmér, I. 1974. Physiology of swimming man. Acta Physiol. Scand. (suppl. 407).

Holmér, I., and Åstrand, P.-O. 1972. Swim training and maximal oxygen uptake. J. Appl. Physiol. 33:510–513.

Holmér, I., Lundin, A., and Eriksson, B. O. 1974. Maximum oxygen uptake during swimming and running by elite swimmers. J. Appl. Physiol. 36:711–714.

Holmér, I., Stein, E. M., Saltin, B., Ekblom, B., and Åstrand, P.-O. 1974. Hemodynamic and respiratory responses compared in swimming and running. J. Appl. Physiol. 37:49–54.

Houston, M. E., and Thomson, J. A. 1977. The response of endurance-adapted adults to intense anaerobic training. Eur. J. Appl. Physiol. 36:207–213.

Hultman, E., Bergström, J., and Anderson, N. McL. 1962. Breakdown and resynthesis of phosphorylcreatine and adenosine triphosphate in connection with muscular work in man. Scand. J. Clin. Lab. Invest. 19:56–66.

Hultman, E. 1967. Studies on muscle metabolism of glycogen and active phosphate in man with special reference to exercise and diet. Scand. J. Clin. Lab. Invest. 19(suppl. 94).

Hultman, E., and Nilsson, L. H:son 1975. Factors influencing carbohydrate metabolism in man. Nutr. Metab. 18(suppl. 1):45–64.

Ikai, M., Ishii, K., and Miyashita, M. 1964. An electromyographic study of swimming. Res. J. Phys. Educ. 7:47–62.

Jansson, E., and Kaijser, L. 1977. Muscle adaptation to extreme endurance training in man. Acta Physiol. Scand. In press.

Jorfeldt, L. 1970. Metabolism of L(+)–lactate in human skeletal muscle during exercise. Acta Physiol. Scand. (suppl. 338).

Karlsson, J. 1971. Lactate and phosphagen concentrations in working muscles of man. Acta Physiol. Scand. 82(suppl. 358).

Karlsson, J., Bonde-Petersen, F., Henriksson, J., and Knuttgen, H. G. 1975. Effect of previous exercise with arms or legs on metabolism and performance in exhaustive exercise. J. Appl. Physiol. 38:763–767.

Karlsson, J., Diamant, B., and Saltin, B. 1971. Muscle metabolites during submaximal and maximal exercise in man. Scand. J. Clin. Lab. Invest. 26:385–394.

Karpovich, P. V., and Millman, N. 1944. Energy expenditure in swimming. Am. J. Physiol. 142:140–144.

Kedrowsky, G. V. 1976. Hypoxic training. Swimming Technique 13:55–62.

Keul, J., Haralambie, G., and Trittin, G. 1974. Intermittent exercise: Arterial lipid substrates and arteriovenous differences. J. Appl. Physiol. 36:159–162.

Kinnula, V. L. 1976. Mitochondrial cytochrome concentrations in rat heart and liver as a consequence of different hypoxic periods. Acta Physiol. Scand. 96:417–421.

Kinnula, V. L., and Hassinen, I. 1977. The effects of hypoxia on mitochondrial mass and cytochrome concentrations in rat heart and liver during postnatal development. Acta Physiol. Scand. 99:462–466.

Mæhlum, S., Jervell, J., and Pruett, E. D. R. 1976. Arterial-hepatic vein glucose differences in normal and diabetic man after a glucose infusion at rest and after exercise. Scand. J. Clin. Lab. Invest. 36:415–422.

Magel, J. R., and Faulkner, J. A. 1967. Maximum oxygen uptakes of college swimmers. J. Appl. Physiol. 22:929–938.

Magel, J. R., Foglia, G. P., McArdle, W. D., Gutin, B., Pechar, G. S., and Katch, F. I. 1974. Specificity of swim training on maximum oxygen uptake. J. Appl. Physiol. 38:151–155.

Margaria, R., Cerretelli, R., and Mangili, F. 1964. Balance and kinetics of anaerobic energy release during strenuous exercise in man. J. Appl. Physiol. 19:623–628.

McArdle, W. D., Glaser, R. M., and Magel, J. R. 1971. Metabolic and cardiorespiratory response during freestyle swimming and treadmill walking. J. Appl. Physiol. 30:733–738.

McGilvery, R. W. 1975. The use of fuels for muscular work. In: H. Howald and J. R. Poortmans (eds.), Metabolic Adaptations to Prolonged Physical Exercise, pp. 12–30. Birkhäuser Verlag, Basel.

Nakamura, Y., and Schwartz, S. 1972. The influence of hydrogen ion concentration on calcium binding and release by skeletal muscle sarcoplasmic reticulum. J. Gen. Physiol. 59:22–32.

Newsholme, E. A., and Start, C. 1973. Regulation in Metabolism. John Wiley and Sons, London.

Padykula, H. A., and Herman, E. 1955. The specificity of the histochemical method for adenosine triphosphatase. J. Histochem. Cytochem. 3:170–195.

Pernow, B., and Saltin, B. 1971. Availability of substrates and capacity for prolonged heavy exercise in man. J. Appl. Physiol. 31:416–422.

Prince, F. P., Hikida, R. S., and Hagerman, F. C. 1976. Human muscle fiber types in power lifters, distance runners, and untrained subjects. Pflügers Arch. 363:19–26.

Pruett, E. D. R. 1970. FFA mobilization during and after prolonged severe muscular work in men. J. Appl. Physiol. 29:809–815.

Ramaiah, A. 1976. Regulation of glycolysis in skeletal muscle. Life Sci. 19:455–466.

Sahlin, K., Harris, R. C., and Hultman, E. 1975. Creatine kinase equilibrium and lactate content compared with muscle pH in tissues obtained after isometric exercise. Biochem. J. 152:173–180.

Sahlin, K., Harris, R. C., Nylind, B., and Hultman, E. 1976. Lactate content and pH in muscle samples obtained after dynamic exercise. Pflügers Arch. 367:143–149.

Saltin, B. 1973a. Metabolic fundamentals in exercise. Med. Sci. Sports 5:137–146.

Saltin, B. 1973b. Oxygen transport by the circulatory system during exercise in

man. In: J. Keul (ed.), Limiting Factors in Physical Performance, pp. 235–252. Thieme, Stuttgart.
Saltin, B. 1975. Adaptive changes in carbohydrate metabolism with exercise. In: H. Howald and J. R. Poortmans (eds.), Metabolic Adaptation to Prolonged Physical Exercise, pp. 94–100. Birkhäuser Verlag, Basel.
Saltin, B., and Essén, B. 1971. Muscle glycogen, lactate, ATP, and CP in intermittent exercise. In: B. Pernow and B. Saltin (eds.), Muscle Metabolism During Exercise, pp. 419–424. Plenum Press, New York.
Saltin, B., Essén, B., and Pedersen, P. K. 1976. In: E. Jokl (ed.), Advances in Exercise Physiology, Medicine and Sport, Vol. 9, pp. 23–51. S. Karger, Basel.
Saltin, B., Gollnick, P. D., Piehl, K., and Eriksson, B. 1971. Metabolic and circulatory adjustments at onset of exercise. In: A. Gilbert and P. Guille (eds.), Onset of Exercise, pp. 63–76. University of Toulouse.
Saltin, B., Henriksson, J., Nygaard, E., and Andersen, P. 1977. Fiber types and metabolic potentials of skeletal muscle in sedentary men and endurance runners. Ann. N.Y. Acad. Sci. In press.
Saltin, B., and Karlsson, J. 1971. Muscle glycogen utilization during work of different intensities. In: B. Pernow and B. Saltin (eds.), Muscle Metabolism During Exercise, pp. 289–299. Plenum Press, New York.
Secher, N. H., and Nygaard, E. 1976. Glycogen depletion pattern in Types I, II-A, and II-B muscle fibres during maximal voluntary static and dynamic exercise. Acta Physiol. Scand. (suppl. 440):100.
Thomson, J. A., Green, H. J., and Houston, M. E. 1976. Glycogen depletion in human muscle as a function of four fiber types. Paper presented at the International Congress of Physical Activity Sciences, Quebec City.
Thorstensson, A., Sjödin, B., and Karlsson, J. 1975. Enzyme activities and muscle strength after "sprint training" in man. Acta Physiol. Scand. 94:313–318.
Trivedi, B., and Danforth, W. H. 1966. Effect of pH on the kinetics of frog muscle phosphofructokinase. J. Biol. Chem. 241:4110–4112.
Wahren, J., Felig, P., Ahlborg, G., and Jorfeldt, L. 1971. Glucose metabolism during leg exercise in man. J. Clin. Invest. 50:2715–2725.
Wahren, J., Hagenfeldt, L., and Felig, P. 1975. Splanchnic and leg exchange of glucose, amino acids, and free fatty acids during exercise in diabetes mellitus. J. Clin. Invest. 55:1303–1314.
Wenger, H. A., and Reed, A. T. 1976. Metabolic factors associated with muscular fatigue during aerobic and anaerobic work. Can. J. Appl. Sport Sci. 1:43–48.
Womersley, J., Durin, J. V. G. A., Boddy, K., and Mahaffy, M. 1976. Influence of muscular development, obesity, and age on the fat free mass of adults. J. Appl. Physiol. 41:223–229.
Zierler, K. L. 1976. Fatty acids as substrates for heart and skeletal muscle. Circ. Res. 38:459–463.

# Adaptations in Skeletal Muscle During Training for Sprint and Endurance Swimming

**D. L. Costill**

By today's standards and current swimming records, I find it a bit embarrassing to admit that I swam competitively. The mention of my best collegiate performances in the late 1950's is always good for a few laughs and some outright demeaning remarks from today's breed of swimmers. But then, I can always shock them by providing some details about swimming training during that period. Most of the listeners are surprised to find out that I didn't drown during a race with so little preparation.

Certainly, changes in training methods and volume must be credited with a large part in the improved swimming performances produced by today's competitors. For a moment, however, let us compare the swimming records of today with the best performances of 20 years ago. Figure 1 is based on past and current American records (short course) for freestyle events of 50–1640-yards (45.7–1500-m). The obvious improvements in maximal swimming velocities are shown in the upper panel of this figure. If it is assumed that the best time posted for 50 yards (45.7 m) represents the maximal velocity ($V_{max}$) attainable by swimmers in 1957 and 1977, then it is possible to compute the percentage of $V_{max}$ averaged during record performances in the longer events (91–1500-m). These relative velocities have been plotted in the lower panel of Figure 1.

This method of representing the best performances from 1957 and 1977 offers two interesting points. First, the percentage of $V_{max}$ is identical for events of 91- and 183-m (100- and 200-yards). This is interpreted to mean that sprint swimmers in 1957 were capable of main-

The findings reported in this paper were the result of research supported by grants from the National Institutes of Health (HL 20408-01) and Lumex, Inc.

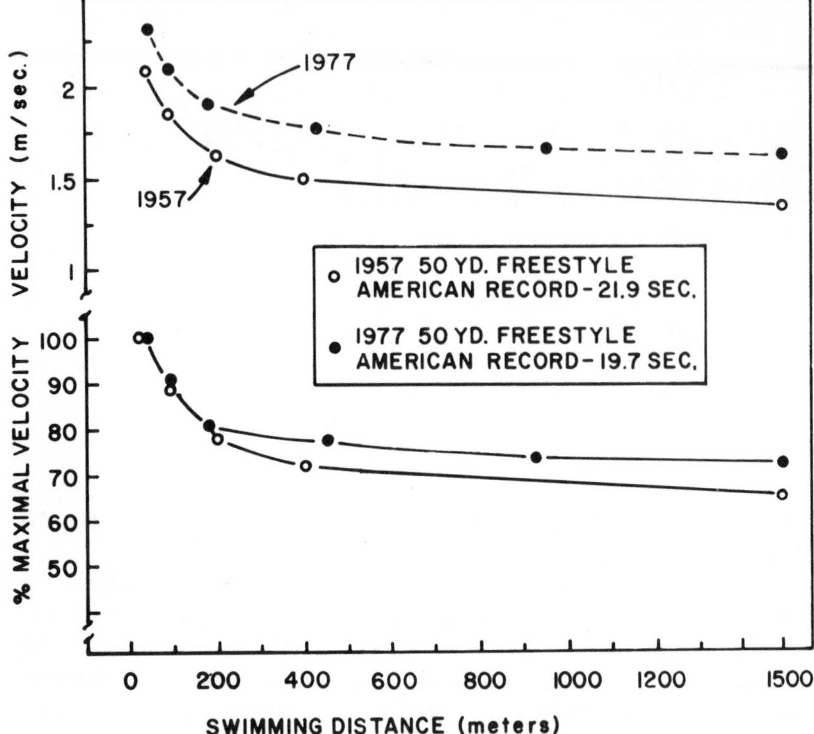


Figure 1. Swimming velocities averaged during the performance of American freestyle records in 1957 and 1977 are shown in the upper panel. In the lower panel, the American record for 50 yards (45 m) is assumed to represent the maximal velocity attainable for swimmers and was used to compute the percentage of maximal velocity averaged during the longer freestyle events.

taining the same percentage of $V_{max}$ through 200 m as their 1977 counterparts. Thus, improvements in these shorter events are the result of an increase in $V_{max}$. Because $V_{max}$ is to a large degree dependent on the swimmer's power, the faster freestyle sprint times must be attributable to a greater strength component in the swimming musculature.

The second point of interest in Figure 1 (lower panel) is that 1977 American freestyle record performances show a higher "relative" velocity at distances of 400 m or more. These intermediate distance events stress the aerobic mechanisms for energy production significantly more than do the 45.7–183-m events (Gollnick and Hermansen, 1973). Thus, it might be postulated that the great volume of work performed by today's swimmers results in an enhanced capacity for oxidative metabolism and the ability to maintain a higher relative velocity in these predominantly aerobic events.

Simply stated, the rapid improvements in swimming records are the combined result of the greater muscular strength and aerobic capacities of today's swimmers. Because both of these qualities are adaptable with training, an examination of the biochemical changes that occur in skeletal muscle during strength and endurance training follows. Perhaps in this way the capacity of the swimmer's skeletal muscle to modify its powers and to achieve more fully its ultimate potential will be better understood.

## ANAEROBIC POWER TRAINING

Repeated maximal contraction of skeletal muscle requires the breakdown and rapid resynthesis of adenosine triphosphate (ATP). In competitive events lasting only a few seconds, most of the energy demands of the contractile filaments can be satisfied by the muscle's available ATP and creatine phosphate (CP). This system of providing energy anaerobically comes under the direct influence of several enzymes, as shown in Figure 2. These enzymatic reactions of myokinase (MK) and creatine phosphokinase (CPK), however, do not limit the rate of ATP resynthesis. Saltin (1973) has suggested that the phosphagen stores in muscle may last for only 4–5 sec in sprint events. Thus, high swimming velocities can only be maintained for longer periods through the continuous glycolytic resynthesis of ATP and CP (Figure 2). In this anaerobic system there are two enzymes that limit the rate of ATP formation: phosphorylase and phosphofructokinase (PFK).

In an effort to assess the effects of strength/speed training on the ATP-CP and glycolytic systems of energy production, a recent study focused on men who trained one leg with repeated 6-sec exercise bouts. Each subject's other leg was trained with an equal volume of work ($\sim$1650 kg $\times$ m/day) performed in 30-sec interval bouts, 4 days per week for 7 weeks. All leg training (knee extension) was conducted isokinetically as shown in Figure 3. Each maximal contraction was isolated to an angular velocity of 3.14 rad/sec. Work bouts of 6 and 30 sec were selected to stress the ATP-CP and glycolytic systems, respectively. Measurement of muscle and blood lactate after repeated maximal isokinetic contractions revealed little, if any, stimulation of glycolysis with exercise of 6 sec or less (Costill, Benham, and Lesmes, 1977). On the other hand, 30 sec of maximal effort caused a 10- to 15-fold increase in muscle lactate, indicating a high rate of glycolysis.

Both training programs produced similar gains in knee extension strength at angular velocities equal to or slower than the velocity used in training (3.14 rad/sec). At high velocities, however, there was no change in maximal angular force (torque). These findings suggest that

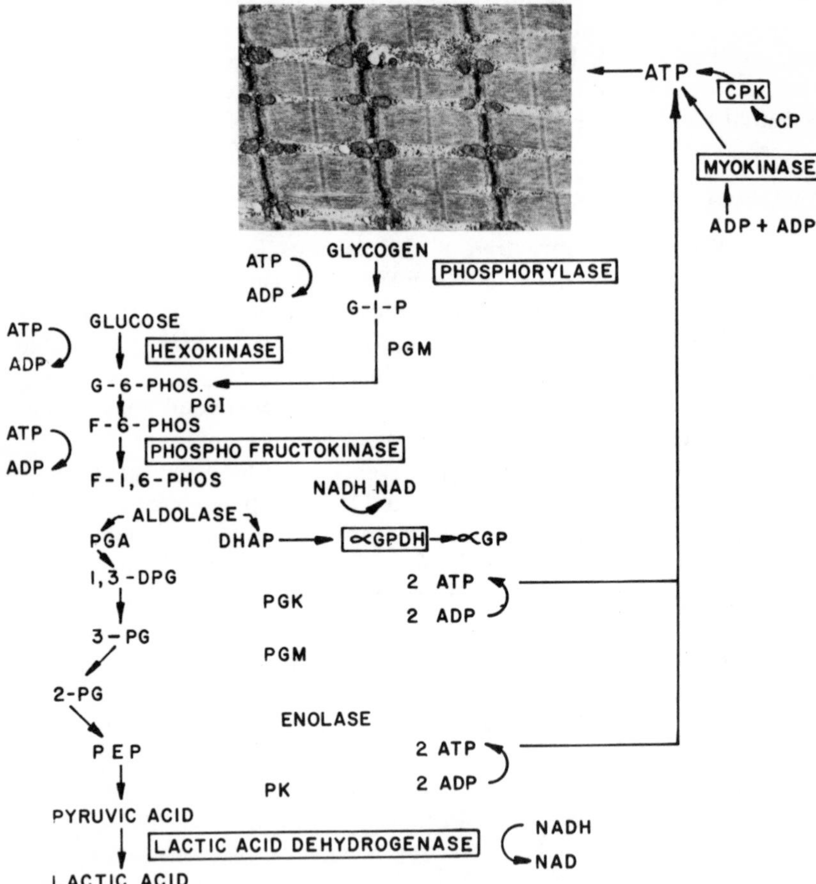


Figure 2. Schematic representation of anaerobic energy sources used principally during events of 50–200 yards (45.7–183m).

strength training benefits may be limited to speeds used during training and to slower velocities. Because more swimmers supplement their swimming training with weight lifting and isokinetic training, it seems appropriate that such strength developing programs be performed at speeds equal to or faster than the limb actions used in competitive swimming. This finding also suggests that anticipated power gains achieved during swimming may be specific to the swimmer's training velocity. In other words, the swimmer should perform both the strength and swim training programs at speeds that approximate or

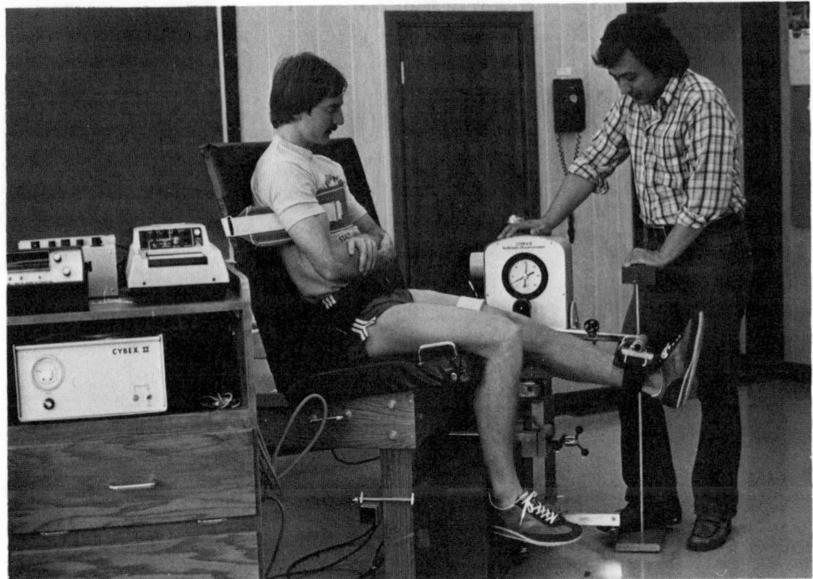


Figure 3. Subject prepared to perform isokinetic exercise.

exceed those used in competition. These observations are supported by the recent findings of Pipes and Wilmore (1975).

Muscle biopsy specimens obtained from the vastus lateralis muscles before and after training were used for enzyme and histochemical analyses. The enzymes of the ATP-CP and ADP-ATP systems (Figure 2), namely CPK and MK, showed significant increases in activity as a result of the 30-sec training bouts, but were unchanged in the leg trained with 6-sec maximal efforts (Figure 4). These findings fail to support the data of Thorstensson, Sjödin, and Karlsson (1975), who observed increases in MK and CPK activities with repeated 5-sec sprint bouts on an inclined treadmill. One obvious difference between their investigation and these findings was the shorter rest interval permitted between bouts on the treadmill (25–55 sec) as compared with this study's maximal isokinetic work (114 sec). In any event, these studies demonstrate that the enzyme mechanisms responsible for resynthesising ATP from secondary phosphogen bonds are adaptable with maximal strength sprint training. Whether these changes enable the muscle to perform more work anaerobically remains unanswered.

The effects of the 6- and 30-sec type training on the enzymes of glycolysis and glycogenolysis seem to be related to the duration of training bouts. Total muscle phosphorylase and phosphofructokinase, for example, both increased significantly more in the leg trained with repeated 30-sec work bouts than they did in the "6-sec leg" (Figure 5).

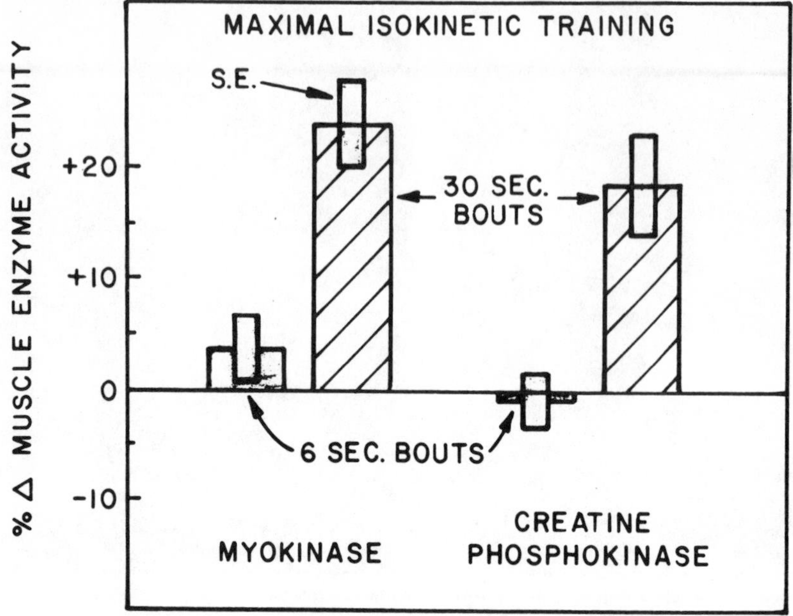


Figure 4. Changes in muscle myokinase (MK) and creatine phosphokinase (CPK) activities as a result of 6-sec and 30-sec bouts of maximal isokinetic training.

This difference in response to training is apparently the result of the greater glycolytic demands imposed during the longer maximal efforts. Because both of these enzymes serve as rate-limiting steps in the anaerobic yield of ATP, it seems that short-term, high intensity training will enhance the glycolytic capacity and should, theoretically, enable the muscle to develop maximal isotonic tension for longer periods.

This theory was not supported by the results of a 1-min performance test of maximal isokinetic knee extension (Figure 6). As would be expected, the maximal power generated during the early seconds (0–25 sec) of the test was significantly greater ($P < 0.05$) after training. Each leg increased its anaerobic power yield with training, but no differences were found between the 6- and 30-sec legs. Thus, this enhanced power output was probably a function of improved contractile force (i.e., strength), and was not paralleled by a similar increase in anaerobic energy production. To the contrary, the rapid fatigue experienced in the initial 30 sec of the test suggests that although the knee extensor muscles had increased in maximal tension capability with training, they did not experience a proportional gain in their resistance to fatigue (Figure 6). Despite the 26% improvement in maximal power output with training shown in the early seconds of the fatigue test, the

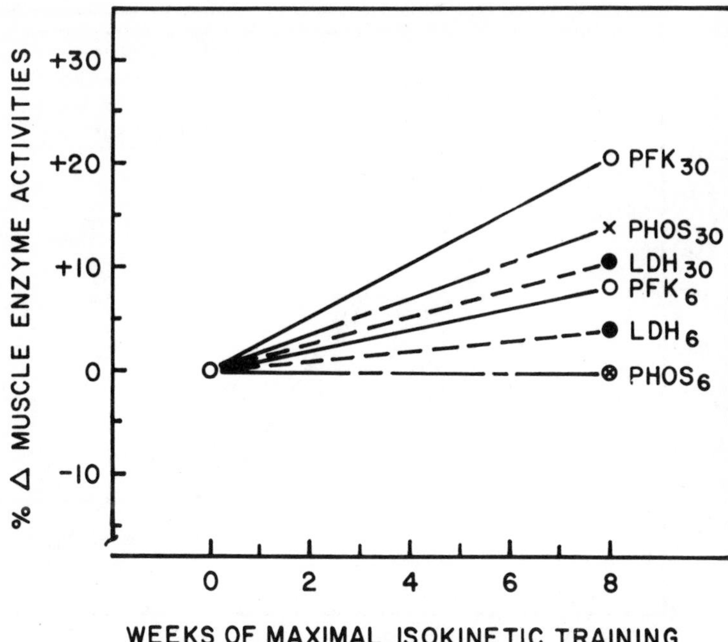


Figure 5. Changes in muscle glycolytic enzyme activities as a result of 6- and 30-sec bouts of maximal isokinetic training are illustrated here.

men could generate only 30% of their maximal power at the end of the 1-min test, which was relatively less than the power output in the untrained state (38% of value at 5 sec of the test).

Thus, it has been shown that high intensity anaerobic training will increase muscular power but does little to improve the fatigability of the muscle during maximal efforts lasting more than a few seconds, despite an apparent increase in the mechanisms of anaerobic energy production (e.g., glycolytic enzyme activities). One might ask the obvious question: Is it possible to improve the swimmer's anaerobic capacity? Before offering an answer to this question, the possible causes for fatigue and ultimate exhaustion during sprint swimming events (100- and 200-m events) should be considered.

Available data suggest that neither the depletion of the phosphogen pool nor the depletion of muscle glycogen stores is responsible for exhaustion in maximal sprint exercise (Karlsson, 1971). The accumulation of lactic acid in skeletal muscle has been proposed as the limiting factor during maximal work of short duration (Gollnick and Hermansen, 1973; Karlsson, 1971). However, it is probably not the lactate per se that causes fatigue, but the lowering of tissue pH that accompanies lactate accumulation. Previous studies have reported pH values of 6.40

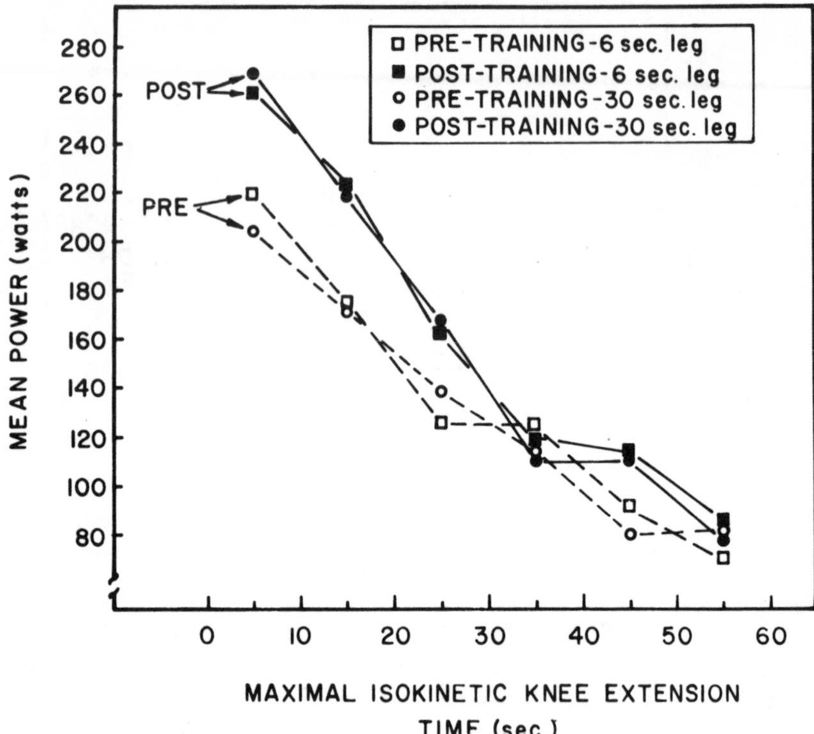


Figure 6. Effects of maximal isokinetic training on power development during a maximal 60-sec work bout.

in the skeletal muscle of men immediately after 40–60 sec of exhaustive exercise. Hill (1955-56) (Bergström, 1962; Hermansen and Osnes, 1972) has shown that formation of lactic acid in response to stimulation stopped when the internal pH dropped to about 6.30, suggesting an inhibition of glycolysis and a concomitant decline in available ATP.

What, then, does the sprint swimmer gain from the anaerobic power type of training? As mentioned earlier, the predominant adaptation to this type of training is greater muscular power. The mechanisms underlying this change can, in part, be explained from the histological observation made before and after the 6- and 30-sec isokinetic training study. As is shown in Table 1, this training increased the percentage of the area occupied by the Type II-A (fast twitch, oxidative) fibers. At the same time, there was a decrease in the percentage of area occupied by the Type I fibers. In view of the few subjects studied and possible error in these histological measurements, some caution should be taken in the interpretation of these findings. If, in fact, the muscle fiber composition does change as a result of maximal isokinetic training,

Table 1. Effects of maximal isokinetic training on the fiber composition of the vastus lateralis muscle

| | Histochemical data 7 weeks of maximal isokinetic training | |
|---|---|---|
| % Fiber composition | Pretraining | Posttraining |
| I | 46.5 (±3) | 38.8 (±5) |
| II-A | 29.2 (±3) | 33.0 (±2) |
| II-B | 24.3 (±2) | 23.5 (±2) |
| Fiber areas ($\mu^2$) | | |
| I | 5485 (±374) | 5432 (±321) |
| II-A | 6801 (±511) | 7455 (±451) |
| II-B | 6262 (±391) | 6372 (±318) |
| % Fiber area | | |
| I | 42.1 (±4) | 35.7 (±3)[a] |
| II-A | 32.7 (±4) | 40.9 (±3)[a] |
| II-B | 25.2 (±2) | 23.1 (±2) |

[a] Significance between pre- and posttraining values ($p < 0.05$).

then there are at least two possible explanations for this change. First, it may be argued that some of the Type I fibers are converted to Type II fibers. Such a change would require marked modifications in the neurological input to these fibers. Because this has only been demonstrated in surgical cross-enervation and electrical stimulation, it is an unlikely explanation for these changes to occur in the intact man.

A second alternative is that some muscle fibers may split, thereby producing an increase in the fractional composition of that fiber type. Recent research by Gonyea, Ericson, and Bonde-Petersen (1977) has demonstrated this phenomenon during strength training in cats. These studies reveal an increase in fiber numbers and cross-sectional areas of both slow twitch (Type I) and fast twitch (Type II) fibers. In light of the volume of information that describes skeletal muscle regeneration in humans, muscle fiber splitting seems to be a reasonable explanation for the increased area occupied by the Type II-A fibers observed in the anaerobic power training study.

The next logical questions seem to be: Why does the alteration in fiber composition favor the production of Type II-A fibers? Is it because these fibers play a larger role in maximal tension development? An examination of muscle glycogen depletion patterns in maximal isokinetic exercies (knee extension) reveals that all muscle fibers are metabolically active. As illustrated in Figure 7, however, the Type II fibers are nearly all depleted of glycogen after 1.5–2 hr of intermittent, maximal isokinetic work (30 sec bouts). Quantitative measurements of glycogen in single muscle fibers following maximal isokinetic exercise

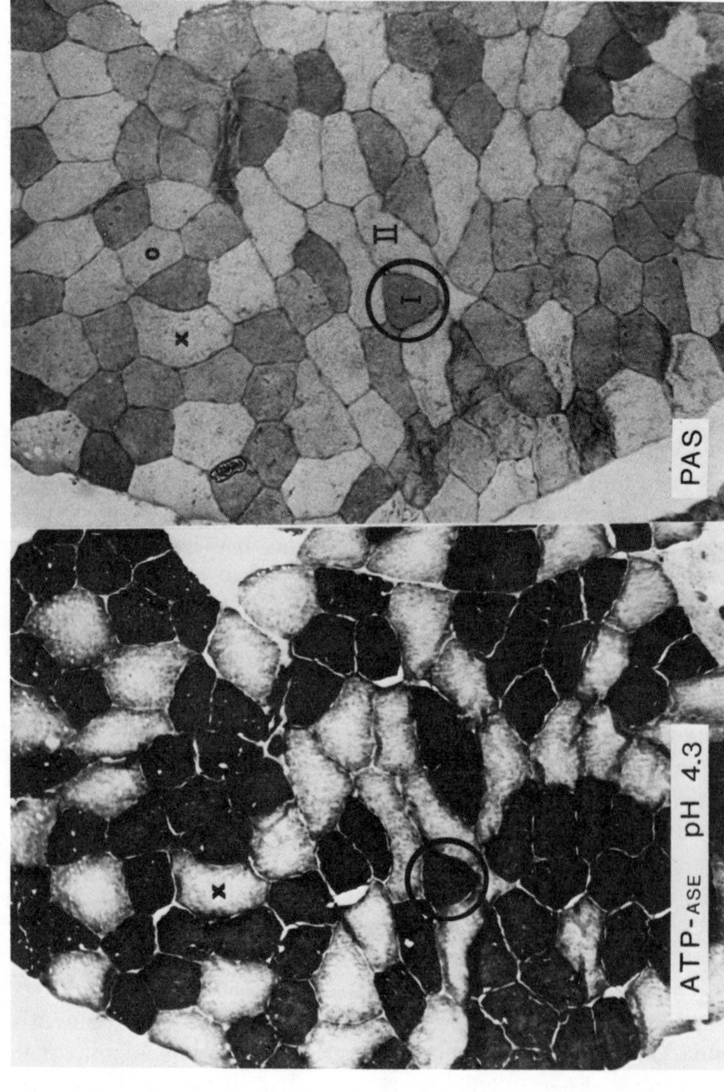


Figure 7. Glycogen depletion patterns in vastus lateralis muscle following repeated bouts of maximal isokinetic knee extension. The circled fiber (Type I) is only partly depleted of glycogen. The Type II fibers (noted with an X) are almost completely empty of glycogen. The fiber marked with an "O" identifies a Type I fiber that is also depleted of glycogen.

reveal a sizeable decrease in both fiber types (Type I, −233 and Type II, −273 mmoles/kg dry tissue). In nearly all subjects, however, greater demands seem to be placed on the Type II fibers with little distinction between the II-A and II-B fibers. These findings lead to the conclusion that maximal isokinetic effort involves all fiber types with a somewhat greater stress on the Type II fibers. This latter point may account for the changes seen in the population and cross-section areas of the II-B fibers. The actual mechanisms underlying any change in muscle fiber composition remain to be detailed.

Studies have observed a close relationship between muscle glycolytic enzyme activities and fiber composition (Costill et al., 1976). Because the Type II fibers are characterized as highly glycolytic, at least part of the increase in muscle LDH, phosphorylase, and PFK activities may be accounted for by the observed increase in the area occupied by the Type II-A fibers during power training. Thus, the glycolytic capacity of each muscle fiber may change little with this type of training.

## ENDURANCE TRAINING

As pointed out earlier (Figure 1), today's swimmers seem to have greater maximal power, but large volumes of training have not improved their ability to resist fatigue in the highly anaerobic sprint events (45–200-m). It is only in events lasting more than a few minutes that the endurance gains that result from current training methods become evident. This finding is not too surprising, because it is in these events (400–1500-m) that the aerobic mechanisms for energy production play a greater role in maximal muscular effort. Unlike glycolysis, endurance in such events as the 1500-m is determined for the most part by the rate of aerobic ATP production. This must not be interpreted to mean that all of the energy needed for these intermediate distance events can be derived via oxidative phosphorylation. To the contrary, the muscle fibers place considerable demand on glycolysis; this results in a large accumulation of blood lactic acid (>16 mM after 400-m freestyle).

As has been pointed out, fatigue in events up to and including 200-m is probably the result of a decrease in muscle pH and a subsequent decline in the speed of many biochemical reactions, thereby limiting the availability of ATP. In the more endurance oriented events (400–1500-m), fatigue is generally associated with diminished oxygen supply and/or available substrate (i.e., muscle glycogen). Nevertheless, changes in intracellular pH may also serve as the ultimate deterrent to success in these longer events. Only with the support of a capable oxygen transport system can the swimmer minimize his /her use of glycolysis and the effects of altering the tissue pH.

As can be seen in Figure 8, the enzymatic reactions that occur in the mitochondria provide a rich source of ATP for sustained muscular effort. Because none of these enzymatic steps are deemed limiting to the rate of oxidative metabolism, changes in mitochondrial enzyme activities are considered to reflect alterations in the aerobic potential of muscle.

Endurance training is known to increase the activity of numerous oxidative enzymes. Succinic acid dehydrogenase (SDH), a Krebs Cycle marker has been shown to increase 30–95% with 4 weeks to 4 months of endurance training (Eriksson, Gollnick, and Saltin, 1973; Gollnick et al., 1973; Saltin et al., 1976). A 38% increase in SDH activity was recently observed in the gastrocnemius muscles of men following 8 weeks of endurance running (30 min/day) (Costill et al., 1978). A similar increase was noted for malic acid dehydrogenase (MDH). Although hexokinase is an extramitochondrial enzyme, its activity seems to parallel the changes seen in most Krebs Cycle enzymes with endurance training. Most glycolytic enzymes, however, fail to show any change in activity following chronic endurance work. Thus, changes in muscle enzyme activities with training are specific to training intensity. That is to say, if the swimmer concentrates on short-burst, maximal efforts (25–100 m) during training, an increase in the activities of the muscle glycolytic enzymes (e.g., phosphorylase, PFK, and LDH) can be anticipated. If, on the other hand, training is principally aerobic, only increases in the Krebs Cycle enzymes will occur.

Current training methods, however, encompass a large volume of work (10,000–15,000 m per day), requiring several hours to complete. Much of this swimming is performed at relatively high velocities, and in repeated bouts. The current world record holder for the 100-m freestyle, for example, swims about 10,000 m per day, with most of the work performed in intermittent bouts of 50- and 100-m sprints (~26- and 56-sec bouts, respectively). Muscle biopsies obtained from the posterior deltoid reveal that both the glycolytic and Krebs Cycle enzyme levels are elevated above those generally observed in the deltoids of untrained men and women. In sprint swimmers the composition of this muscle is roughly 60–65% Type II fibers; this could explain their high glycolytic enzyme activites. SDH activity in the sprinter's deltoid muscle was found to be 50% higher than in the untrained muscle. Thus, current sprint training methods appear to place considerable demands on the oxidative capacity of the swimming musculature.

Histological observations of muscle (deltoid) glycogen depletion during swim training (60 repeats of 100-yard freestyle with 1 min rest between bouts) reveals a pattern quite like that seen during maximal

AEROBIC METABOLISM
ENERGY FOR MUSCLE METABOLISM

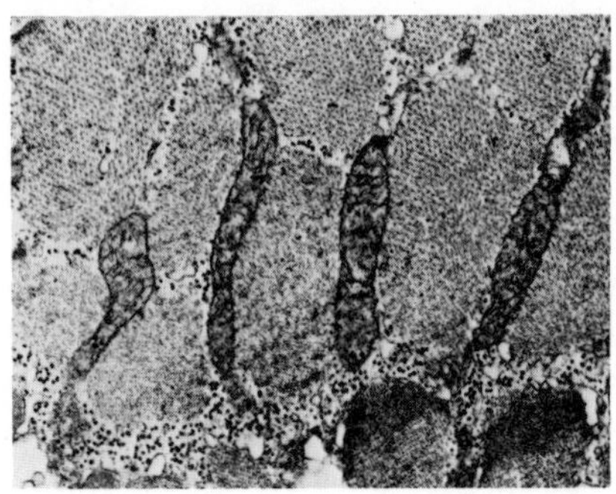

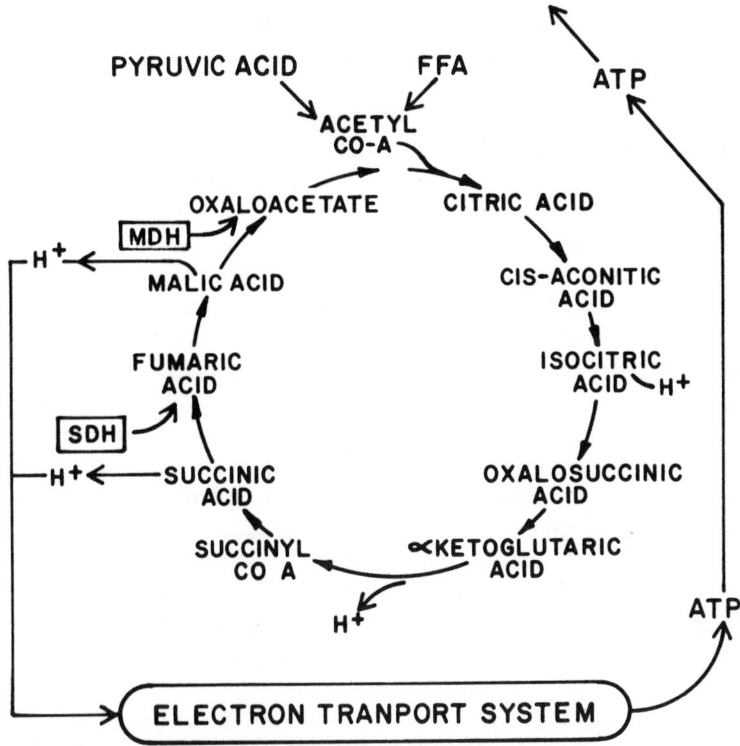


Figure 8. Schematic illustration of the Krebs Cycle and the electron transport system. Enzymes examined during endurance training have been denoted by the rectangular enclosures.

isokinetic exercise. That is, both Type I and Type II fibers have diminished glycogen stores throughout the swimming bouts, with the Type II fibers depleting first. At the completion of the 60, 100-yard sprints, all of the fibers were completely empty of glycogen as indicated by the PAS stain. A somewhat different pattern was observed during training for the intermediate distance freestyle events (400–1500-meter). During repeated 400-m training bouts, the Type I fibers were seen to glycogen deplete more rapidly than the Type II-A and II-B fibers. Still, all fibers diminished their glycogen storage and were depleted at the end of the training session.

Muscle SDH activities measured in the posterior deltoid of these swimmers were somewhat higher (+28%) than in the trained sprinters, and 92% greater than values obtained for untrained men. Muscle PFK, phosphorylase, and LDH values were not significantly different from untrained and endurance trained men (Costill et al., 1976). Venous blood samples taken during repeated 400-m training bouts show only a modest accumulation of lactic acid (3.9–5.9 mM). Thus, such training stresses principally the oxidative metabolism in skeletal muscle. The oxidative enzyme changes seen probably reflect an increase in mitochondrial number and size, thereby enhancing each muscle fiber's capacity to generate ATP during the longer competitive events. This reduces the fibers' dependence on anaerobic energy sources and minimizes the drop in intracellular pH.

Another major metabolic change that occurs with endurance training is the enhanced capacity of muscle to oxidize lipids, thereby reducing the demands on muscle glycogen stores during training and competition. The free fatty acids (FFA) derived from the fat cells and/or the breakdown of plasma triglyceride (TG) are transported across the mitochondrial membrane under the direct action of carnitine palmitoyl transferase (CPT). Since FFA have only a limited ability to cross the inner mitochondrial membrane as Co A esters, their entry is greatly stimulated by CPT. Fritz (1963) has shown this enzyme has a regulatory influence on the rate of FFA oxidation.

Thus, it is of considerable significance to find that the activity of CPT in skeletal muscle increases approximately 30% as a result of endurance training (Costill et al., 1978). This increased capacity for FFA entry into the mitochondria complements the enhanced oxidative capacity observed in endurance trained skeletal muscle. The resultant benefits for the swimmer are a partial shift in carbon source from carbohydrates to lipids and a subsequent sparing of muscle glycogen.

## CONCLUSION

Based on the preceding discussion, it is apparent that the rapid improvements in swimming performances seen in the past 20 years are the result of training programs that meet the physiological demands of competition. Maximal anaerobic training has enabled the swimmer to develop the muscular power essential for sprint events. Although these strength gains are frequently accompanied by increased glycolytic enzymes (phosphorylase, PFK, LDH, and hexokinase) and anaerobically related enzyme activities (CPK and MK), it is difficult to speculate on their role in events lasting only 20–120 sec. Endurance training, on the other hand, results in skeletal muscle adaptations that are specific to oxidative metabolism. Increased activities of Krebs Cycle enzymes (SDH and MDH) reflect an enhanced capacity for oxidation of carbohydrates and fats. As the muscle increases its ability to oxidize fats, it is able to reduce the demands placed on muscle glycogen, thereby minimizing the threat of chronic exhaustion during repeated days of heavy training. Future improvements in swimming performance will depend on efforts to match the training regimen to the physiological demands of the event and the physiological adaptability of the athlete.

## ACKNOWLEDGMENTS

The author wishes to express his appreciation to all those who were instrumental in the collection and analysis of the data presented in this paper: W. Fink, C. Foster, G. Lesmes, E. Coyle, G. Dalsky, F. Witzmann, and D. Benham.

## REFERENCES

Bergström, J. 1962. Muscle electrolytes in man. Scand. J. Clin. Lab. Invest. Suppl. 68.

Carlson, B. M. 1973. The regeneration of skeletal muscle: A review. Am. J. Anat. 137:119–150.

Costill, D. L., Daniels, J., Evans, W., Fink, W., Krahenbuhl, G., and Saltin, B. 1976. Skeletal muscle enzymes and fiber composition in male and female track athletes. J. Appl. Physiol. 40:149–154.

Costill, D. L., Benham, D., and Lesmes, G. 1977. Muscle lactate and glycogen depletion patterns during isokinetic exercise. In preparation.

Costill, D. L., Fink, W. J., Foster, C., and Ivy, J. 1978. Adaptations in skeletal muscle of juvenile diabetics during physical training. In preparation.

Eriksson, B. O., Gollnick, P. D., and Saltin, B. 1973. Muscle metabolism and enzyme activities after training in boys 11–13 years old. Acta Physiol. Scand. 87:485–497.

Fritz, I. B. 1963. Carnitine and its role in fatty acid metabolism. Adv. Lipid Res. 1:285–334.

Gollnick, P. D., Armstrong, R. B., Saltin, B., Saubert, C. W., IV, Sembrowich, W. L., and Shephard, R. E., 1973. Effect of training on enzyme activities and fiber composition of human skeletal muscle. J. Appl. Physiol. 34:107–111.

Gollnick, P. D., Armstrong, R. B., Saubert, C. W., IV, Piehl, K., and Saltin, B. 1972. Enzyme activity and fiber composition in skeletal muscle of untrained and trained men. J. Appl. Physiol. 33:312–319.

Gollnick, P. D., and Hermansen, L. 1973. Biochemical adaptations to exercise: Anaerobic metabolism. In: Exercise and Sports Science Reviews, J. Wilmore (ed.). pp. 1–43. Academic Press, New York.

Gonyea, W., Ericson, G. C., and Bonde-Petersen, F. 1977. Skeletal muscle fiber splitting induced by weight lifting exercise in cats. Acta Physiol. Scand. 99(1):105–109.

Hermansen, L., and Osnes, J.-B. 1972. Blood and muscle pH after maximal exercise in man. J. Appl. Physiol. 32:304–308.

Hill, A. V. 1955-1956. The influence of the external medium on the internal pH of muscle. Proc. Roy. Soc., London, Ser. B. 144:1–22.

Karlsson, J. 1971. Lactate and phosphagen concentrations in working muscles of man. Acta Physiol. Scand. 82(Suppl. 358).

Pipes, T. V., and Wilmore, J. H. 1975. Isokinetic versus isotonic strength training in adult men. Med. Sci. Sports 7:262–274.

Saltin, B. 1973. Metabolic fundamentals in exercise. Med. Sci. Sports 5:137–146.

Saltin, B., Nazar, K., Costill, D. L., Stein, E., Jansson, E., Essén, B., and Gollnick, P. D. 1976. The nature of the training response: Peripheral and central adaptations to one-legged exercise. Acta Physiol. Scand. 96:289–305.

Thorstensson, A., Larsson, L., Tesch, P., and Karlsson, J. 1977. Muscle strength and fiber composition in athletes and sedentary men. Med. Sci. Sports 9:26–30.

Thorstensson, A., Sjödin, B., and Karlsson, J. 1975. Enzyme activities and muscular strength after "spring training" in man. Acta Physiol. Scand. 94:313–318.

# Blood Lactic Acid Concentrations in High Velocity Swimming

**P. E. di Prampero, D. R. Pendergast, D. W. Wilson, and D. W. Rennie**

The majority of well trained swimmers reach their maximal $O_2$ consumption at speeds between 0.9 and 1.2 m/sec. Hence, higher swimming speeds are necessarily accompanied by an appreciable anaerobic contribution to the overall energy requirement.

The purpose of this study was to investigate the anaerobic contribution to energy expenditure in swimming from measurements of lactic acid in the blood, following the same approach applied by Margaria et al. (1963) to running.

## EXPERIMENTAL PROCEDURE AND METHODS

The experiments were performed on nine well trained men (Table 1) swimming the front crawl at 0.6–1.8 m/sec in an annular swimming pool of 60 m circumference, at water temperatures of 28–30°C. The subjects swam at constant velocity, paced by a platform moving over the water surface. The overall energy requirement ($\dot{E}$) to swim at any given speed for each subject was known from a previous series of experiments (di Prampero et al., in press).

Each subject swam for a timed period at a predetermined speed for which his $\dot{E}$ was known. The speeds were selected for individual subjects to produce exhaustion between 30 sec and 5 min. This assured that there was an appreciable anaerobic contribution to total energy expenditure.

To avoid an acceleration phase, the subjects were towed by the monitoring platform until a steady speed was attained and were cast off at time zero. They were instructed to maintain an exact position with

Table 1. $O_2$ consumption and blood La in swimming[a]

| W (kg) | v (m/sec) | $\dot{E}$ (ml/kg/min) | $t_{ex}$ (min) | $\dot{La}_b$ (mM/min) | $\dot{V}_{O_2}$ (ml/kg/min) | $V_{O_2}$ (ml/kg)[c] | $V_{O_2}$ (ml/kg)[d] | $\hat{La}_b$ (mM) |
|---|---|---|---|---|---|---|---|---|
| 72 | 1.20 | 55.5 | 4.91 | 2.0 | 55.0 | 237.0 | | 8.6 |
| | 1.30 | 63.9 | 0.54[b] | | 40.0 | 11.6 | 10.7 | 1.4 |
| | 1.30 | 63.9 | 1.52[b] | | 59.0 | 62.5 | 64.0 | 8.2 |
| | 1.30 | 63.9 | 2.11 | 6.4 | 63.0 | 96.6 | 79.0 | 11.4 |
| | 1.40 | 71.8 | 1.47 | 9.4 | 63.0 | 58.2 | | 12.1 |
| | 1.50 | 84.7 | 0.77[b] | | 63.0 | 28.8 | 28.1 | 5.6 |
| | 1.50 | 84.7 | 0.97 | 15.1 | 63.0 | 42.0 | 40.3 | 10.4 |
| 68 | 1.40 | 77.7 | 1.62 | 9.8 | 53.0 | 74.4 | | 12.2 |
| | 1.50 | 84.0 | 0.73 | 15.7 | 53.0 | 25.3 | | 10.3 |
| 73 | 1.00 | 42.5 | 2.65 | 5.7 | 30.5 | 73.0 | | 14.4 |
| | 1.20 | 56.2 | 1.44 | 11.6 | 30.5 | 37.4 | | 14.6 |
| 71 | 0.87 | 41.3 | 5.09 | 1.7 | 36.2 | 163.0 | | 6.9 |
| | 0.93 | 36.6 | 2.13 | 3.3 | 34.3 | 53.2 | | 5.2 |
| | 1.04 | 48.7 | 1.82 | 5.1 | 34.6 | 53.6 | 46.3 | 6.8 |
| 76 | 0.93 | 34.9 | 5.42 | 0.6 | 31.0 | 145.0 | | 1.7 |
| | 1.10 | 42.0 | 1.62 | 6.4 | 31.2 | 39.0 | | 7.4 |
| 100 | 0.75 | 19.7 | 5.01 | 1.7 | 22.0 | 97.3 | | 6.9 |
| | 0.87 | 22.5 | 5.94 | 1.4 | 22.4 | 120.1 | | 7.3 |
| 89 | 0.64 | 22.3 | 4.08 | 0.9 | 22.0 | 77.5 | | 2.4 |
| | 0.75 | 40.1 | 1.72 | 5.8 | 24.1 | 31.0 | 34.3 | 7.8 |
| 87 | 0.70 | 30.1 | 6.00 | 0.9 | 29.0 | 137.3 | 145.0 | 4.3 |
| | 0.75 | 32.2 | 2.63 | 2.2 | 26.8 | 55.0 | | 4.4 |
| 84 | 1.40 | 71.7 | 0.77 | 10.8 | 54.0 | 23.0 | | 5.0 |

[a] Rate of energy expenditure ($\dot{E}$), exhaustion time ($t_{ex}$), rate of La accumulation in blood ($\dot{La}_b$), $O_2$ uptake in the last 15–30 sec ($\dot{V}_{O_2}$), overall $O_2$ consumed during the swim ($V_{O_2}$) and peak blood La concentration in recovery after the swim ($\hat{La}_b$), are indicated for all subjects at all investigated speeds. Subjects' body weight is also indicated.

[b] Interrupted before exhaustion

[c] Calculated (see text)

[d] Measured

respect to a towed underwater marker. Exhaustion time was defined as the time at which the subjects could no longer maintain the pace. After having determined the total swimming time to exhaustion for a given subject at a given speed, subsequent swims were performed, the durations of which were approximately 0.8, 0.5, and 0.3 of the exhaustion time. The subjects recovered for 24–48 hr between successive swims.

Expired gas was collected for the final 15–30 sec of the swim in order to determine $O_2$ consumption ($\dot{V}_{O_2}$). In addition, $\dot{V}_{O_2}$ was measured by continuous collection and analysis of expired gas from the time of onset of swimming until exhaustion occurred in eight trials in four subjects in order to determine: the kinetics of $\dot{V}_{O_2}$ at the onset of exercise, and the total amount of $O_2$ consumed ($\dot{V}_{O_2}$) for the duration of the swim.

After each trial, venous blood samples were drawn at 1 or 2 min intervals during the first 10 min of recovery and at 5 or 10 min intervals from 10 to 40–60 min after the end of the exercise. The blood samples were subsequently analyzed for lactate (La) concentration according to standard enzymatic techniques.

## RESULTS

The time course of blood La concentration ($La_b$) following the termination of swimming is indicated in Figure 1. For the first minutes of recovery, $La_b$ in peripheral venous blood increased until a peak concentration was reached between 5 and 8 min into recovery. Within 40 min of recovery, the decrease of $La_b$ following the peak could be approximated by a simple exponential with a $t_{1/2}$ of ~ 20 min, independent of the absolute peak concentration. The peak concentration above resting following exercise will be designed as $L\hat{a}_b$.

The early shape of the $La_b$ curve in recovery is presumably the net result of diffusion of La from the muscles, mixing by the circulation, and removal of La by different organs. However, at the time when $L\hat{a}_b$ is reached it will be assumed that equilibrium of La has occurred in the water compartments of highly perfused tissues of the body.

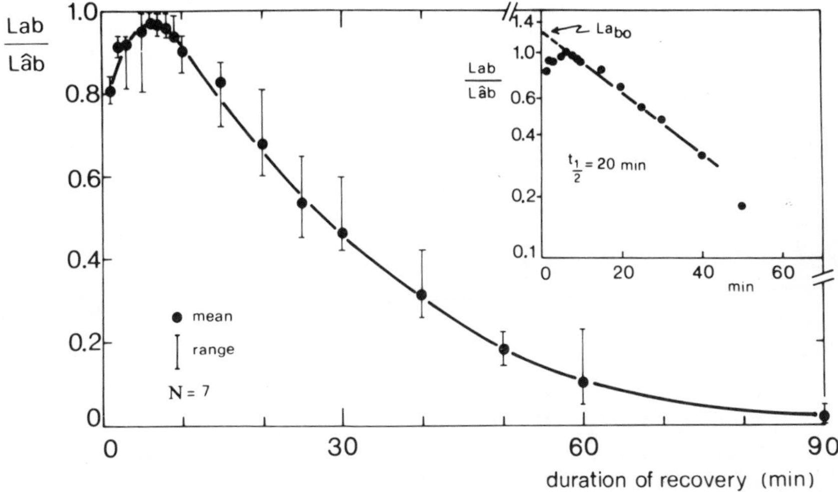


Figure 1. Average La concentration in blood ($La_b$) is shown as a function of the time of recovery after swimming in seven subjects. $La_b$ is given as a fraction of the peak blood La concentration attained in recovery ($L\hat{a}_b$). Range is indicated. Highest and lowest $L\hat{a}_b$s amounted to 15.5 and 10.5 mM, respectively. Insert shows mean values on semilog plot. Half time of the simple exponential drawn through the data from 6 to 40 min is ~ 20 min.

$L\hat{a}_b$ after exercise is plotted as a function of the swimming time for one subject in Figure 2. Data for each line were obtained at a predetermined speed as indicated. After the first 20–40 sec of exercise, $L\hat{a}_b$ approximated as a linear function of the swimming duration and, for any given duration of exercise, was greater with greater velocity.

The rate at which $L\hat{a}_b$ increased ($\dot{L\hat{a}}_b$) is represented by the slopes of the straight lines of Figure 2. $\dot{L\hat{a}}_b$ is an increasing function of exercise intensity, i.e., swimming velocity. This is noted for all subjects, at all investigated speeds, in Table 1, as are the energy requirements of the exercise ($\dot{E}$), and the $O_2$ consumption measurements.

The swimming speed at which $\dot{L\hat{a}}_b$ became appreciably greater than zero is related to the subject's $\dot{V}_{O_2}$ max. As seen in Table 1, this speed was about 0.75 m/sec in the subjects with the lowest $\dot{V}_{O_2}$ max (26–30 ml/kg/min) and was about 1.2 m/sec in the most fit subject ($\dot{V}_{O_2}$ max = 63 ml/kg/min).

The relationship between the rate of La accumulation in blood ($\dot{L\hat{a}}_b$) (as calculated from graphs such as Figure 2, and neglecting the first 30 sec of exercise) and the energy requirement of swimming ($\dot{E}$), measured independently on the same subjects (Table 1), is indicated in

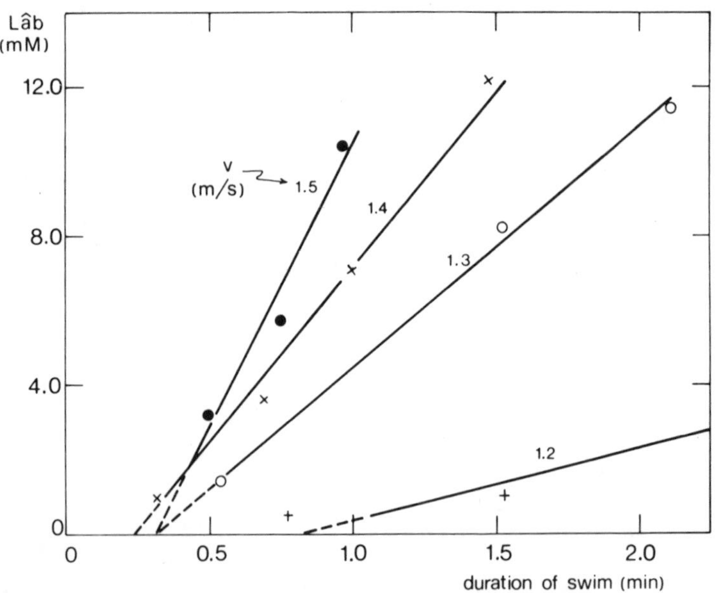


Figure 2. Peak blood La concentration attained after swimming ($L\hat{a}_b$, mM) is shown as a function of the duration of the preceding swim. The four sets of symbols designate four different velocities, as marked. The slope of the straight lines is a measure of the rate at which La accumulates in blood ($\dot{L\hat{a}}_b$). The line for the 1.2 m/sec velocity was obtained from four points, two of which were for t > 2.5 min.

Figure 3. The three subjects with the highest $\dot{V}_{O_2}$ max (53–63 ml/kg/min) have been separated from the five subjects with the lowest $\dot{V}_{O_2}$ max (24–30 ml/kg/min). In both groups, $\dot{La}_b$ and $\dot{E}$ are approximately linearly related.

The intercepts on the $\dot{E}$ axis of the two functions of Figure 3 indicate the intensity of swimming that can be sustained without any appreciable La accumulation in the blood. This amounts to 24 and 51 ml/kg/min in the low and high $\dot{V}_{O_2}$ max groups, respectively, corresponding to velocities of 0.75 and 1.2 m/sec. Thus, $\dot{La}_b$ becomes appreciable when the velocity of swimming requires about 85–90% of the subjects' $\dot{V}_{O_2}$ max, without regard to its absolute magnitude.

## DISCUSSION

When the energy requirement of swimming is such that a significant accumulation of La in blood takes place, the energy for work performance is derived from three sources: oxidative phosphorylations ($\dot{V}_{O_2}$); anaerobic glycolysis, leading to a net accumulation of lactic acid in the body ($\dot{La}_m$); and net depletion of alactic energy stores ($\dot{Al}$), i.e.,

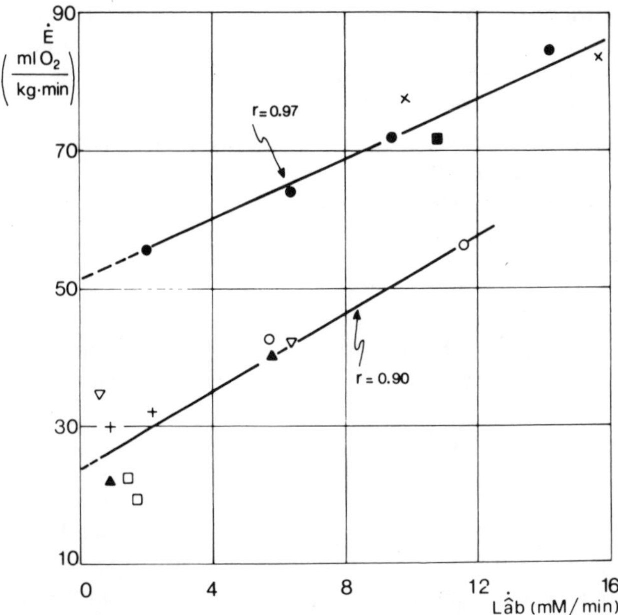


Figure 3. Energy requirement of swimming ($\dot{E}$, ml/kg/min) is shown as a function of the rate of La accumulation in blood ($\dot{La}_b$, mM/min) in the three subjects with highest and the five with lowest $\dot{V}_{O_2}$ max. The upper and lower functions are described by the equations $y = 51.5 + 2.15 \times$ (r = 0.97) and $y = 23.7 + 2.83 \times$ (r = 0.90), respectively. See Table 1 for explanation of symbols.

$O_2$ stores and high energy phosphates. Hence, the overall rate of energy expenditure ($\dot{E}$, in $O_2$ equivalents) can be described as:

$$\dot{E} = \dot{V}_{O_2} + a \, \dot{La}_m + \dot{Al} \quad (1)$$

where all terms are referenced to 1 kg of body weight, $a$ is the energy released (in $O_2$ units) per unit La formed, and $\dot{Al}$ is expressed in $O_2$ equivalents.

$\dot{La}_m$ indicates the net amount of La produced, per unit of time and per unit of body weight, by the working muscles, a measure of the anaerobic glycolytic contribution to the whole body energy expenditure. This is so despite the fact that a constant $La_b$ may be the result of a balance between La production and removal (Hermansen and Stensvold, 1972). In fact, as the excretion of La through the kidney is negligible, La can be removed in substantial amounts only via oxidations at the muscle level (Hermansen and Stensvold, 1972; Jorfeldt, 1970). To a minor extent, it can also be resynthesized to glycogen, a process requiring an oxidative energy input at least equal to the free energy change of the reverse transformation glycogen → lactate. Hence, any La production accompanied by simultaneous removal will be reflected in the $O_2$ consumption of the whole body ($\dot{V}_{O_2}$ in Equation 1). It can therefore be concluded that, when no net La accumulation takes place in the body, the whole body can be considered in aerobic conditions even while some muscles are actually producing La, and others (or other organs) are removing it.

$\dot{La}_m$ cannot be easily measured. However, as a first approximation it can be assumed that the peak La concentration in blood, after exercise ($\hat{La}_b$) is proportional to the total amount of La accumulated in the body (Margaria and Edwards, 1934):

$$\hat{La}_b = \alpha \, La_m \quad (2)$$

where $\alpha = (\hat{La}_b/La_m)$ is a proportionality constant that depends on the La distribution within the body fluids and on the amount of La that may disappear within the 5–8 min required to reach $\hat{La}_b$ after the end of the exercise.

From Equations 1 and 2:

$$\dot{E} = \dot{V}_{O_2} + (a/\alpha) \, \dot{La}_b + \dot{Al} \quad (3)$$

In these experimental conditions, $\dot{La}_b$ was obtained from the slope of the straight line in Figure 2. These lines, when extrapolated to $\hat{La}_b = O$, indicate that a delay of approximately 15–30 sec occurred from the sudden onset of exercise before net accumulation of La in blood could be detected. This has been observed in other forms of exercise (Margaria, Cerretelli, and Mangili, 1964), and has been interpreted as the time during which the alactic energy stores are utilized. After this time, during supramaximal exercise: the alactic energy sources presumably do not contribute appreciably to the energy requirement of the exercise (Margaria, Cerretelli, and Mangili, 1964); and $\dot{V}_{O_2}$ has reached an approximately constant and maximal value (Margaria et al., 1965). Therefore, in Equation 3, $\dot{A}l = O$, and $\dot{V}_{O_2}$ = constant = $\dot{V}_{O_2}$ max. Equation 3 is therefore reduced to:

$$\dot{E} = \dot{V}_{O_2}\ \text{max} + (a/\alpha)\dot{La}_b \tag{4}$$

Hence, the relationship between $\dot{E}$ and $\dot{La}_b$ in each subject should be a straight line displaced to a higher level the higher the subject's $\dot{V}_{O_2}$ max is, as experimentally found (Figure 3). Furthermore, from Equation 4, the slope of the lines in Figure 3 should be equal to $a/\alpha$ and independent of the subject's $\dot{V}_{O_2}$ max. The slopes of the two straight lines in Figure 3 were indeed fairly close, amounting to 2.2 and 2.8 ml $O_2$/kg)/mM, respectively.

To calculate $a/\alpha$ on a larger number of data, whatever the subjects' $\dot{V}_{O_2}$ max, the ratio $E/\dot{V}_{O_2}$ max has been plotted in Figure 4 as a function of the ratio $\dot{La}_b/\dot{V}_{O_2}$ max for all subjects. In fact, rearranging Equation 4:

$$\frac{\dot{E}}{\dot{V}_{O_2}\ \text{max}} = 1 + \frac{a}{\alpha}\frac{\dot{La}_b}{\dot{V}_{O_2}\ \text{max}} \tag{4a}$$

it is apparent that this plot should yield a straight line with a slope equal to $a/\alpha$.

Figure 4 shows that the relationship between these two variables can indeed be approximated by a straight line described by:

$$y = 0.86\ (\pm 0.046) + 2.71\ (\pm 0.24)\ x\ (r = 0.91) \tag{4b}$$

It can therefore be concluded that: the accumulation of La in blood becomes appreciable when the energy requirement of the exercise is about 86% of the subject's $\dot{V}_{O_2}$ max; and the ratio $a/\alpha$, as calculated on all subjects, amounts to about 2.7 ml $O_2$/kg/mM. This represents the amount of energy (in $O_2$ equivalents) set free per kg of body weight when the amount of La produced by the muscles is such that $\dot{La}_b$ increases by 1 mM.

The value of $a/\alpha$ in running was calculated by Margaria, Aghemo, and Sassi (1971) and Margaria et al. (1963) and found to be of the order of 3.0–3.3 (ml/kg)/mM, a value about 20% higher than the present one. This difference can presumably be attributed to the slower decline of $La_b$ after swimming ($t_{1/2} \cong 20$ min, (Figure 1)) than after running ($t_{1/2} \cong$ 15 min (Margaria, Edwards, and Dill, 1933)).

The values of $a/\alpha$ in this study, as well as in the experiments of Margaria, Aghemo, and Sassi (1971) and Margaria et al. (1963) were calculated on the assumption that, after about 20 sec of exercise, Al is

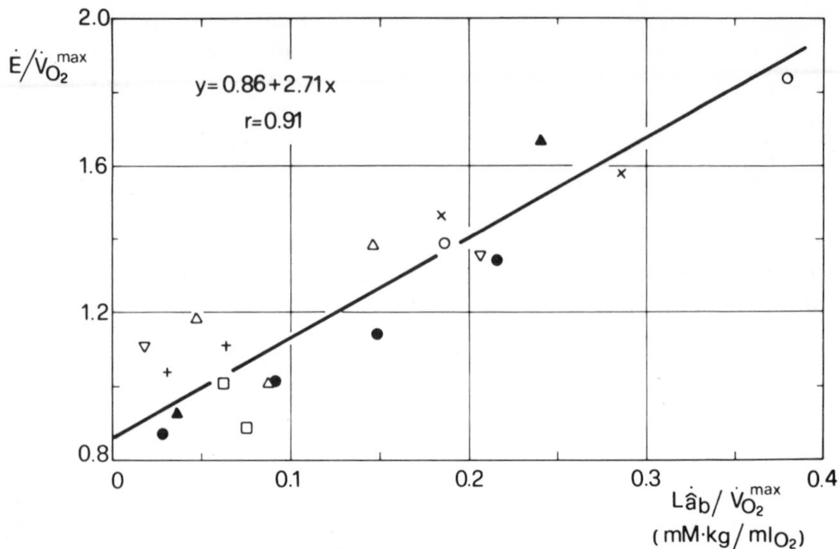


Figure 4. Energy requirement of swimming ($\dot{E}$) is shown as a function of the rate of La accumulation in blood ($\dot{La}_b$), each expressed as a ratio of the individual $\dot{V}_{O_2}$ max of the subject. The ordinate is therefore dimensionless, both $\dot{E}$ and $\dot{V}_{O_2}$ max being given in ml $O_2$/kg/min. The dimensions of the abscissa are mM/kg/ml $O_2^{-1}$. The straight line regression is described by: y = 0.86 (± 0.046) + 2.71 (±0.24) x, r = 0.91, N = 19. See Table 1 for explanation of symbols.

negligible and $\dot{V}_{O_2}$ is constant and maximal, independent of the exercise intensity.

To circumvent these assumptions, a different approach can be utilized. In an exercise of duration, t, and intensity, $\dot{E}$, the overall energy consumed ($\dot{E} \cdot t$) must be derived from the three energy sources described in Equation 1. Hence, by analogy with Equation 3, and by rearranging, it is found that:

$$\dot{E} \cdot t - V_{O_2} = (a/\alpha)\, L\hat{a}_b + Al \qquad (5)$$

where $\dot{V}_{O_2}$ indicates the overall $O_2$ consumed during time t. $\dot{V}_{O_2}$ was either directly measured or calculated from the $O_2$ uptake observed in the last 15–30 sec of swimming (Table 1) and the kinetics of $\dot{V}_{O_2}$ at the onset of the exercise (Margaria et al., 1965). The latter was determined in eight trials on four subjects and found to be a simple exponential with a $t_{1/2}$ of 0.4 min. In the cases where the total amount of $O_2$ consumed during the swim was directly measured, it was found to be within a few percent of that calculated from $t_{1/2}$ (Table 1).

$\dot{E} \cdot t - V_{O_2}$ was found to be a linear function of $L\hat{a}_b$ (Figure 5). The slope of this function yields another measure of $a/\alpha$ (Equation 5). This amounts to about 2.5 (ml/kg)/mM, a value of the same order as that obtained from Figure 4. In this graph, the vertical scatter of the data is

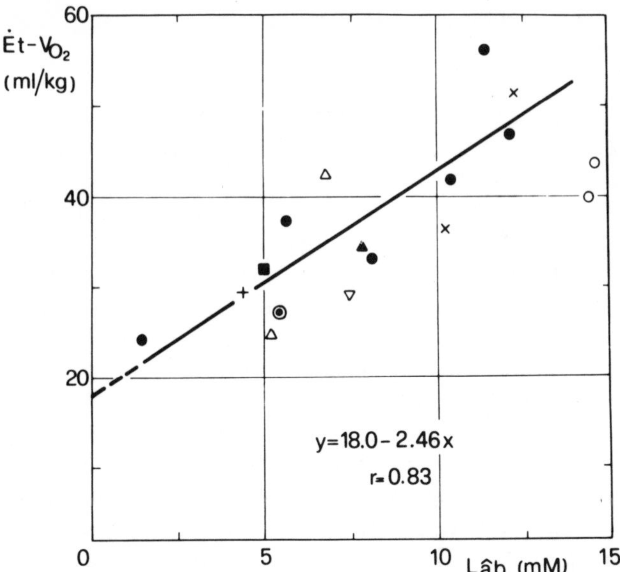


Figure 5. This graph illustrates total amount of energy derived from anaerobic sources during swimming for time t ($\dot{E}t - \dot{V}_{O_2}$) as a function of peak La concentration attained in blood after the swim ($L\hat{a}_b$). The circled dot (⊙) is the average of all data for $t > 3$ min. The $\dot{V}_{O_2}$ value used in the calculation of the ordinate was directly measured in eight instances. In the other cases, $\dot{V}_{O_2}$ was calculated from the kinetics of $\dot{V}_{O_2}$ at the onset of the swim (see text and Table 1). The straight line regression, described by: $y = 18.0\,(\pm 2.15) + 2.46\,(\pm 0.48)\,x$ ($r = 0.83$; N = 14) was calculated on the data for $t < 3$ min, neglecting subject B.R.

somewhat larger than in the previous ones (Figures 3 and 4) because any error in the estimate of $\dot{E}$ is multiplied by t. Therefore, the value of $a/\alpha$ was calculated only from the data for $t < 3$ min.

The intercept on the $\dot{E} \cdot + - \dot{V}_{O_2}$ axis of Figure 5 (≅ 18 ml/kg) is a measure of the amount of energy (in $O_2$ equivalents) that was derived from depletion of alactic stores during high velocity swimming. This on the average is about half the maximal value observed in running, which is ~ ml/kg in well trained subjects during exercises leading to exhaustion in 30–50 sec (di Prampero, Peeters, and Margaria, 1973). This finding may be attributed to a smaller amount of muscle being exhausted during high velocity swimming than in running.

## GENERAL DISCUSSION

The results obtained in this study indicate that $a/\alpha$ is constant and amounts to 2.7 ml $O_2$/kg/mM (Figure 4). Hence, if the value of $\alpha$ were known, $a$ could be calculated. This would then be a measure of the amount of energy released per unit La formed from glycogen under physiological conditions of pH, temperature, and buffer composition of body fluids.

To assign a numerical value to *a*, Margaria, Edwards, and Dill (1933) assumed that: La is uniformly distributed throughout the water phase of the body at the time when $\hat{La}_b$ is reached; and the amount of La metabolized is negligible during the 5–8 min of recovery to reach $\hat{La}_b$. Because the water phase of the blood is about 0.8, and that of the whole body 0.6, $\alpha = \hat{La}_b/La_m$ was estimated as 0.8/0.6 = 1.33. From the observed value of $a/\alpha$ (= 3.0 ml/kg$^{-1}$/mM$^{-1}$), they therefore calculated $a = 3.0 \times 1.33 = 3.99$ liters $O_2$/mole La, i.e., about 20 kcal/mole (Margaria et al., 1963).

Both the above assumptions are incorrect because the La distribution across the cell membrane is not homogeneous (Roos, 1975) and because a certain amount of La is inevitably metabolized in the time of recovery necessary to reach $\hat{La}_b$. Thus, although the above two assumptions tend to compensate for each other so that the numerical value of *a* arrived at by Margaria, Aghemo, and Sassi (1971); Margaria et al. (1963), as well as by others along similar lines (Cerretelli et al., 1964), is reasonable, a rediscussion of this whole problem is needed.

In Equation 3, $\hat{La}_b$ denotes the peak La concentration attained 5–8 min after the end of the exercise. During this time, diffusion and mixing of La take place, along with La removal from the body. Therefore, $\hat{La}_b$ is lower than the hypothetical blood La concentration that would be attained at time zero of recovery ($La_{b_0}$), if the La diffusion and mixing were instantaneous. Furthermore, $La_m$ in Equation 3 is the mean La concentration per kg of body weight at the end of the exercise, i.e., at time zero of recovery. It follows that the ratio between these two hypothetical blood and whole body concentrations ($La_{b_0}/La_m$) depends only on the La distribution in the body, because no net removal of La has yet occurred at time zero of recovery.

It is the purpose of what follows to show that it is possible: to estimate $La_{b_0}$, i.e., the hypothetical equilibrium concentration of La at time zero of recovery; to evaluate the La distribution throughout the body; and, hence, to calculate a tentative numerical value of $\alpha$.

$La_{b_0}$ can be calculated on the assumption that La has reached an equilibrium in the water phase of the highly perfused tissues of the body at the time when $\hat{La}_b$ is reached. The decline of $La_b$ after 8 min of recovery (Figure 1) can then be attributed mainly to La removal from the body rather than to further distribution. Hence, $La_{b_0}$ can be obtained by extrapolating to t = O, the linear relationship observed from 8–40 min of recovery between log $La_b$ and time (Figure 1, insert). The following relationship is then empirically obtained:

$$\hat{La}_b = 0.80\ (\pm 0.02\ \text{SD})\ La_{b_0} \qquad (6)$$

independently of the absolute $\hat{La}_b$ level. Because $\alpha = \hat{La}_b/La_m$ (Equation 2), the following is obtained by substituting into Equation 6:

$$\alpha = 0.80\ La_{b_o}/La_m \tag{7}$$

As previously pointed out, $La_{b_o}/La_m$ depends only on the La distribution within the body. Its value could therefore be calculated, provided the following were known: the amount of body water in which La is distributed; the partition of body water into intra- and extracellular compartments; and the La distribution across cell membranes.

The water content of the highly perfused tissues of the body, in which La was assumed to have reached an equilibrium, constitutes about 85% of the total body water (Cizek, 1968), or about 50% of the body weight. It will further be assumed that the body water in which La is distributed is 45% extracellular and 55% intracellular, i.e., the same as for the body as a whole (Altman and Dittmer, 1974).

The La concentration ratio of intracellular to extracellular compartments ($La_i/La_e$) was shown by Roos (1975) to be ~ 0.4 in the rat diaphragm at equilibrium at normal intra- and extracellular pH (7.0 and 7.4, respectively). Roos further observed that $La_i/La_e$ is constant over a range of $La_e$ between 2 and 119 mM, and that it depends only on the $H^+_e/H^+_i$ ratio and not on membrane potential. If it is assumed that the intra- and extracellular pH are not substantially altered at the time $\hat{La}_b$ is attained, the La concentration in blood and in the body as a whole can be calculated from the above. Setting the La concentration in extracellular water as 1.0 arbitrary units (corresponding to an intracellular water concentration of 0.4), at equilibrium the mean La concentration in whole blood of 44% hematocrit will be $La_{b_o} = 0.94 \times (0.56 \times 1.0 + 0.73 \times 0.44 \times 0.40) = 0.65$ where 0.94 and 0.73 are the water fractions of plasma and red blood cells, respectively (Altman and Dittmer).

The concentration in the body as a whole will be $La_m = 0.50 \times (0.45 \times 1.0 + 0.55 \times 0.40) = 0.34$ where 0.50 is the fraction of the body in which La is at equilibrium, i.e., 85% of the total body water, and 0.45 and 0.55 are the corresponding extra- and intracellular fractions (Altman and Dittmer, 1974).

Hence:

$$La_{b_o}/La_m = 0.65/0.34 = 1.91 \tag{8}$$

It must be pointed out that this ratio applies to any equilibrium condition, of which $La_{b_o}/La_m$ is one particular instance.

Substituting Equation 8 into Equation 7 yields this result:

$$\alpha = 0.80 \times 1.91 = 1.53 \tag{9}$$

Thus, $a = 2.7 \times 1.53 = 4.13$ liters $O_2$/mole, i.e., about 20.5 kcal/mole. This value is of the same order as that calculated by Margaria,

Aghemo, and Sassi, 1971; Margaria et al. (1963) in man and by Cerretelli, di Prampero, and Piiper (1969) on the isolated perfused dog gastrocnemius (22.8 kcal/mole). This last observation is particularly interesting because, in these latter experiments, no assumptions on La distribution within the body fluids were needed.

The above assumption may be modified by further studies of La distribution in the body thus leading to a different estimate of $a$. However, the preceding discussion shows that, within certain limits and approximations, it is legitimate to evaluate the amount of energy derived from anaerobic glycolysis during exercise from measurements of net La accumulation in the blood. The proportionality constant between La accumulated in blood and energy released by anaerobic glycolysis ($a/\alpha$) is known with reasonable accuracy from this, as well as from previous studies (Margaria, Aghemo, and Sassi, 1971; Margaria et al., 1963). It amounts to about 2.7 and 3.3 ml $O_2$/kg/mM in swimming and running, respectively.

From the practical point of view, this allows the researcher to determine the overall energy expenditure of swimming, as well as of other forms of exercise, from measurements of $O_2$ consumption and of La accumulation in blood, without regard to the relative contribution of these two energy sources.

## REFERENCES

Altman, P. L., and Dittmer, D. S. (eds.). 1974. Biology Data Book 2nd Ed. 3:1833 and 2041. FASEB, Bethesda, Md.

Cerretelli, P., di Prampero, P. E., and Piiper, J. 1969. Energy balance of anaerobic work in the dog gastrocnemius muscle. Am. J. Physiol. 217:581–585.

Cerretelli, P., Piiper, J., Mangili, F., and Ricci. B. 1964. Aerobic and anaerobic metabolism in exercising dogs. J. Appl. Physiol. 19:29–32.

Cizek, L. J. 1968. Total body water and the fluid compartments. In: V. B. Mountcastle, (ed.), Medical Physiology. pp. 287–306. C. V. Mosby Company, St. Louis.

di Prampero, P. E., Peeters, L., and Margaria, R. 1973. Alactic $O_2$ debt and lactic acid production after exhausting exercise in man. J. Appl. Physiol. 34:628–633.

di Prampero, P. E., Pendergast, D. R., Wilson, D. W., and Rennie, D. W. In press.

Hermansen, L., and Stensvold, I. 1972. Production and removal of lactate during exercise in man. Acta Physiol. Scand. 86:191–201.

Jorfeldt, L. 1970. Metabolism of (L+)-lactate in human skeletal muscle during exercise. Acta Physiol. Scand. (suppl. 338).

Margaria, R., Aghemo, P., and Sassi, G. 1971. Lactic acid production in supramaximal exercise. Pflügers Arch. 326:152–161.

Margaria, R., Cerretelli, P., di Prampero, P. E., Massari, C., and Torelli, G. 1963. Kinetics and mechanism of oxygen debt contraction in man. J. Appl. Physiol. 18:371–377.

Margaria, R., Cerretelli, P., and Mangili, F. 1964. Balance and kinetics of anaerobic energy release during strenuous exercise in man. J. Appl. Physiol. 19:623–628.

Margaria, R., and Edwards, H. T. 1934. The removal of lactic acid from the body during recovery from muscular exercise. Am. J. Physiol. 107:681–686.

Margaria, R., Edwards, H. T., and Dill, D. B. 1933. The possible mechanism of contracting and paying the oxygen debt and the role of lactic acid in muscular contraction. Am. J. Physiol. 106:689–714.

Margaria, R., Mangili, F., Cuttica, F., and Cerretelli, P. 1965. The kinetics of the oxygen consumption at the onset of muscular exercise in man. Ergonomics 8:49–54.

Roos, A. 1975. Intracellular pH and distribution of weak acids across cell membranes. A study of D- and L-lactate and of DMO in rat diaphragm. J. Physiol. (London) 249:1–25.

# Metabolic Prediction of Swimming Performance

**V. Klissouras and W. S. Sinning**

The prediction of potential physical performance capacity has long been of interest to physiologists and others who are concerned with the attainment of maximum human performance. Over 40 years ago, Sargent (1926) estimated the potential speed of a runner over different distances on the basis of his maximal oxygen uptake, maximal oxygen debt, and oxygen requirements while running at different speeds. A similar approach to studying swimming was later used by Greene (1930) with the crawl stroke, and by Karpovich and LeMaistre (1940) with the back stroke. They showed in swimming, as Sargent had shown in running, that the rate of energy expenditure is the primary limitation to maximal performance.

The purpose of this investigation was to present further evidence of the dependence of maximum swimming performance on the ability of the body to provide oxygen to the tissues.

## METHODS

### Subjects

Five college students who routinely used the dolphin-butterfly stroke in competition served as subjects. Testing was completed immediately after the competitive season; therefore, it could be assumed that subjects were at or near their peak physical condition. The physical characteristics of the subjects and their best competitive swimming performances are shown in Table 1. Data obtained from a sixth subject, who had a much lower maximal aerobic power and inferior swimming performance times, were not considered in the present study in order to maintain the homogeneity of the group.

Table 1. Physical characteristics and best competitive swimming performances of subjects

| Subject | Age (years) | Height (cm) | Weight (kg) | Swimming times: Dolphin-Butterfly 100 yards | Dolphin-Butterfly 200 yards | Freestyle Stroke 400 yards | Freestyle Stroke 500 yards |
|---|---|---|---|---|---|---|---|
| RF | 20 | 185 | 76 | 0:54.4 | 2:09.0 | 4:03 | 5:07 |
| DH | 20 | 181 | 75 | 0:55.6 | 2:04.7 | 4:03 | 5:07 |
| SO | 20 | 185 | 73 | 0:54.7 | 2:12.5 | 4:08 | 5:12 |
| JS | 20 | 175 | 72 | 0:57.6 | 2:12.8 | 4:13 | 5:25 |
| DS | 19 | 167 | 64 | 0:56.0 | 2:06.3 | 4:18 | 5:40 |
| Mean | 19.8 | 178.6 | 72.0 | 0:55.6 | 2:09.6 | 4:09 | 5:18 |
| SD | ±0.447 | ±7.668 | ±4.743 | ±1.264 | ±0:03.6 | ±0:065 | ±0:142 |

## Measurements

Four measurements were taken to provide data for the computations of predicted times for swimming the various distances with the dolphin-butterfly stroke. These were: the oxygen requirements while swimming the dolphin-butterfly at various speeds; oxygen requirements and elapsed time for making the swimming turns used while swimming the dolphin-butterfly in competition; maximal oxygen uptake; and maximal oxygen debt.

The methods used to measure the oxygen requirements while swimming and performing open butterfly turns were described elsewhere (Klissouras, 1968). Briefly, during maximal speeds and swimming turns, the swimmer held his breath throughout the effort and the expired gases were collected during recovery. This technique, the oxygen debt technique, was previously reported and used (Sargent, 1926; Greene, 1930; Karpovich and LeMaistre, 1940; Adrian, Singh, and Karpovich, 1966; Klissouras, 1968). During submaximal speeds, the expired gases were collected while the subjects swam one length of the pool after swimming continuously for not less than 5 nor more than 6 min. In all tests, the open circuit method was used for the collection of expired air. Air samples were taken from Douglas bags into small butyl rubber bags and later analyzed for concentrations of oxygen and carbon dioxide by use of a Beckman Model LB-1 carbon dioxide analyzer and a Beckman Model E2 oxygen analyzer.

A tethered swimming test was used to measure the maximal oxygen uptake of the subjects. Each subject was allowed to warm-up in his usual manner. After being attached to the gas collection assembly by means of a low resistance one-way valve, the subject was tethered to a weight resistance device. In this device, a weight was suspended from a wire that passed through a pulley system and was attached to the waist of the subject. The subject first swam against the pull of a 10-pound weight at a rate that enabled him to maintain a constant position in the pool. Two min later a 2.5-pound weight was added. A similar weight was added every min thereafter until the subject was exhausted. This procedure is a modification of the one described by Magel and Faulkner (1967).

Expired air was collected throughout the test and analyzed to determine each subject's maximal oxygen uptake. The criteria used to evaluate whether subjects attained their maximal oxygen uptakes were that: oxygen uptake did not increase despite an increase in work load; the respiratory exchange ratio was higher than 1.15 (i.e., an R of about 0.40 from resting value) and there was evidence of hyperventilation. Heart rate immediately after maximal exercise was also used as an indication of the intensity of the effort. The heart beat was counted by palpating the carotid artery for the first 15 sec after the cessation of swimming. The oxygen debt was measured by having subjects swim to exhaustion. Expired gases were collected for 1 hr in a series of Douglas bags while the subject was seated, well covered, beside the pool. Oxygen consumption was measured prior to exercise for 10 min following a rest period of 30–40 min in order to establish a reference baseline value for computing the oxygen debt.

The prediction of performance time for swimming the dolphin-butterfly stroke consisted of several steps. The mean values obtained from the five subjects were used to make the computations. The steps are described in the following paragraphs. All predictions were made for swimming in a 25-yard (23-m) pool.

The quantity of oxygen required for swimming each of the distances studied over given periods of time was determined first. It was assumed that the total amount of oxygen subjects could consume in a race would be equal to the sum of the oxygen uptake (aerobic) and oxygen debt (anaerobic) processes. It was also assumed that the maximal oxygen debt would be the same after each swimming effort if a subject were completely exhausted at the end of the swim.

Because the maximal $\dot{V}_{O_2}$ can neither be reached instantly at the onset of work nor maintained indefinitely, the oxygen uptake of the subjects during a race must always be a proportion of their maximal $\dot{V}_{O_2}$. The average proportion of the maximal $\dot{V}_{O_2}$ (% $\dot{V}_{O_2}$ max) that subjects could use when swimming for periods of time (t min) was obtained from the following equation (see Appendix for the method used for its derivation):

$$\% \dot{V}_{O_2} \max = 87.74 + 20.65 \log t - 16.19 (\log t)^2 \qquad (1)$$

The total volume of oxygen that was available for a given time period (aerobic and anaerobic processes) was thereafter computed according to the equation:

$$\text{Available } V_{O_2} = (\% \ \dot{V}_{O_2} \text{ max} \times \dot{V}_{O_2} \text{ max} \times t) + V_{O_2} \text{ debt} \quad (2)$$

The amount of oxygen necessary for performing the swimming turns during each event was subtracted from the available $V_{O_2}$ as calculated from Equation 2. The total requirement for the turns depended upon the number of turns completed rather than the velocity of the swim. For example, when swimming the 200-yard distance in the 25-yard pool, the calculated mean oxygen requirement for the subjects for performing seven swimming turns was 2.24 liters and the calculated distance covered was 42 yards. The calculated elapsed time was 22.0 sec.

Once the amount of oxygen that could be made available through oxygen uptake and debt and the true swimming distances were determined, the amount of oxygen that the subjects could, on the average, make available in liters/min, and the true distance in arbitrarily selected times were computed. Regression equations were then computed by the method of least squares to show the amount of oxygen available for swimming given distances in given periods of time. This procedure was carried out for distances of 200, 400, 500, and 1650 yards. The derived regression lines are shown on Figure 1 ($a_1$, $b_1$, $c_1$, and $d_1$, respectively).

The relationship between oxygen consumption and swimming velocity for the same subjects was previously reported (Klissouras, 1968) and was used in the present study to determine the amount of oxygen necessary for swimming a specified distance at different average velocities. These velocities were used to calculate the time necessary to swim the true distances of the different races, i.e., the total distance minus the distance covered by the dive and the turns. Regression equations were again derived on the basis of these computations. The derived regression equations are also shown in Figure 1 ($a_2$, $b_2$, $c_2$, and $d_2$).

The predicted time for swimming each true distance was indicated by the point where the two regression lines crossed. The crossing of regression lines showed the point where the maximum amount of $O_2$ subjects could make available while performing a given race (lines $a_1$, $b_1$, $c_1$, and $d_1$) was equal to the amounts required for swimming that distance in a given time ($a_2$, $b_2$, $c_2$, and $d_2$). The latter was dependent upon the maximum average velocity subjects could sustain for that period of time. Finally, the predicted time for swimming each distance (including dive and turns), was derived by adding the time spent for the dive and the turns to the time value obtained by the intersection. These

$$a_1: V_{O_2} = 6.60 + 3.60\,t - 0.02\,t^2$$
$$b_1: V_{O_2} = 4.04 + 3.59\,t - 0.02\,t^2$$
$$c_1: V_{O_2} = 2.73 + 3.59\,t - 0.02\,t^2$$
$$d_1: V_{O_2} = -7.74 + 2.93\,t$$

$$a_2: \log_{10} V_{O_2} = 2.729 - 1.348\,t + 0.314\,t^2 - 0.025\,t^3$$
$$b_2: \log_{10} V_{O_2} = 3.188 - 0.748\,t + 0.089\,t^2 - 0.0036\,t^3$$
$$c_2: \log_{10} V_{O_2} = 2.683 - 0.373\,t + 0.030\,t^2 - 0.00084\,t^3$$
$$d_2: \log_{10} V_{O_2} = 3.391 - 0.128\,t + 0.003\,t^2 - 0.00003\,t^3$$

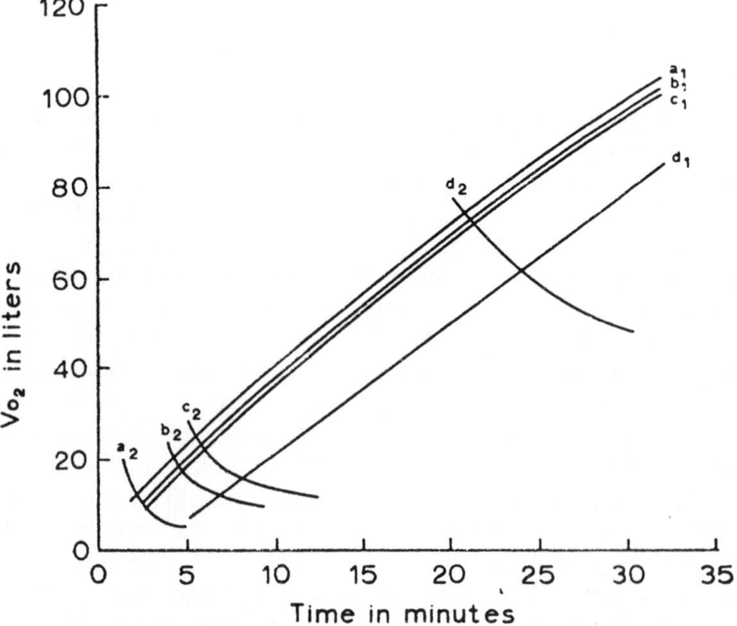


Figure 1. The intersection of regression lines shows the point at which the maximum amount of $O_2$ that subjects could make available while performing a given race is equal to the amount required for swimming that distance in a given time. The intersection of $a_1$, $a_2$ refers swimming to 200 yards; $b_1$, $b_2$ to 400 yards; $c_1$, $c_2$ to 500 yards; and $d_1$, $d_2$ to 1650 yards.

latter values were 22.9, 46.1, 57.7, and 191.1 sec for swimming 200, 400, 500, and 1650 yards, respectively.

## RESULTS

The data obtained on each subject from the maximal oxygen uptake and oxygen debt tests are shown in Table 2. The similarity of individual values for maximal $\dot{V}_{O_2}$, pulmonary ventilation ($\dot{V}_E$), respiratory ratio

Table 2. Maximal oxygen uptake values ($V_{O_2}$ max), oxygen debt ($V_{O_2}$ debt), ventilation ($\dot{V}_E$), respiratory ratio (R), and heart rate (HR)

| Subject | $\dot{V}_{O_2}$ max (liters/min) | | $\dot{V}_{O_2}$ max (ml/kg/min) | | $V_{O_2}$ debt | | $\dot{V}_E$ (liters/min) STPD | | R | | HR | |
|---|---|---|---|---|---|---|---|---|---|---|---|---|
| | $T_1$[a] | $T_2$[a] | $T_1$[a] | $T_2$[a] | $T_1$[a] | $T_2$[a] | $T_1$[a] | $T_2$[a] | $T_1$[a] | $T_2$[a] | $T_1$[a] | $T_2$[a] |
| RF | 4.01 | 3.98 | 51.8 | 52.1 | 14.00 | 13.54 | 107.1 | 103.3 | 1.25 | 1.20 | 188 | 188 |
| DH | 3.75 | 3.78 | 48.5 | 48.8 | 12.75 | 12.33 | 114.6 | 104.6 | 1.31 | 1.31 | 208 | 212 |
| SO | 3.60 | 3.65 | 49.5 | 49.9 | 6.97 | 6.93 | 103.3 | 101.5 | 1.16 | 1.27 | 192 | 180 |
| JS | 3.70 | 3.69 | 52.9 | 52.1 | 7.57 | 7.04 | 96.1 | 99.8 | 1.19 | 1.09 | 192 | 196 |
| DS | 3.25 | 3.35 | 50.7 | 52.3 | 5.51 | 5.80 | 109.5 | 95.2 | 1.27 | 1.24 | 204 | 200 |
| Mean | 3.66 | 3.69 | 50.68 | 51.04 | 9.36 | 9.13 | 106.12 | 100.88 | 1.23 | 1.22 | 196.8 | 195.20 |
| SD | ±0.28 | ±0.23 | ±1.76 | ±1.59 | ±3.77 | ±3.53 | ±6.94 | ±0.08 | ±0.08 | ±0.08 | ±8.67 | ±12.13 |
| CV | 7.5 | 6.2 | 3.5 | 3.1 | 40.2 | 38.8 | 6.5 | 6.8 | 6.8 | 6.95 | 4.4 | 6.2 |

[a] $T_1$ and $T_2$ refer to the first and second trials conducted on different days.

(R), and heart rate on the two trials and the coefficients of variation indicate that the testing techniques were reliable and that true maximal oxygen uptake values were obtained. The measured oxygen requirement values of the subjects while swimming were presented in a previous report (Klissouras, 1968), whereas data on swimming turns are in the authors' files.

Predictions of the subjects' potential performance times were made according to the computational procedures described above. On the basis of the oxygen consumption values found while subjects swam at different velocities, the following regression equations express the relationship between the amount of oxygen that subjects could make available for swimming distances of 200, 400, 500, and 1650 yards.

$$V_{O_2} = 6.60 + 3.60\ t - 0.02\ t^2 \quad (3)$$
$$V_{O_2} = 4.04 + 3.59\ t - 0.02\ t^2 \quad (4)$$
$$V_{O_2} = 2.73 + 3.59\ t - 0.02\ t^2 \quad (5)$$
$$V_{O_2} = -7.74 + 2.93\ t \quad (6)$$

The plotted regression lines are shown in Figure 1 ($a_1$, $b_1$, $c_1$, and $d_1$, respectively).

The relationship found between the different amounts of oxygen that would be required for swimming the different distances at different speeds was expressed by the following equations:

$$\log_{10} V_{O_2} = 2.729 - 1.348\ t + 0.314\ t^2 - 0.025\ t^3 \quad (7)$$
$$\log_{10} V_{O_2} = 3.188 - 0.748\ t + 0.089\ t^2 - 0.0036\ t^3 \quad (8)$$
$$\log_{10} V_{O_2} = 2.683 - 0.373\ t + 0.030\ t^2 - 0.00084\ t^3 \quad (9)$$
$$\log_{10} V_{O_2} = 3.391 - 0.128\ t + 0.003\ t^2 - 0.00003\ t^3 \quad (10)$$

These regression lines are also shown in Figure 1 ($a_2$, $b_2$, $c_2$, and $d_2$, respectively).

After the two regression equations were computed for each distance, the two equations were solved for time, which was a common unknown factor. For example, the two equations for the 200-yard distance were shown in the above two sets of equations (Equations 3 and 7). When these equations were solved simultaneously, a value of 1.80 min was obtained. This was equivalent to swimming the distance in 1 min and 48 sec. A value of 22.9 sec was added to account for the time spent during the turns and dive. Thus, the predicted performance time was 2:10.9. Predicted times for swimming the other distances were also computed. These were 5:16.6 for 400 yards, 6:45.4 for 500 yards, and 26:11.1 for 1650 yards.

## DISCUSSION

The criteria for evaluating whether subjects attained their maximal $\dot{V}_{O_2}$s were satisfied (Table 2). The mean maximal $\dot{V}_{O_2}$ of 50.86 ml/kg per min found here was comparable to a value of 51.1 ml/kg per min observed by Åstrand and Saltin (1961a) in subjects who swam the breast stroke. Magel and Faulkner (1967) found a value of 55 ml/kg/min for subjects swimming the dolphin stroke.

The mean maximal oxygen debt for the group was 9.25 liters. Individual values ranged from as low as 5.51 liters to as high as 14.00 liters. This wide interindividual variability cannot be explained on the basis of base-line values (Welch et al., 1969) or duration of recovery (Ricci, 1968), in view of the fact that all experimental conditions were the same for all subjects. Further, the high reproducibility of these observations (see Table 2) makes the possibility of error in measurement rather remote.

It is recognized, however, that the entire amount of the measured oxygen debt may not be available to the swimmer while he is performing even though it is necessary to make that assumption in the computation of performance capacity. Present theory (Margaria et al., 1963; Welch et al., 1969) assumes that the only functions of the oxygen debt are to resynthesize ATP and phosphocreatine, resaturate depleted oxygen stores, and remove and oxidize the lactic acid produced during exercise. The high values found here, as in other studies (Robinson et al., 1958), also include the oxygen cost of maintaining the elevated physiological activity of the recovery period (Keul, Doll, and Keppler, 1972; Stainsby and Barclay, 1970).

The predicted time of 2:10.9 for swimming the 200-yard distance compared favorably with the mean competitive swimming time of the group, 2:09.6. Karpovich and LeMaistre (1940) reported a predicted time of 3:00 and an observed time of 2:53 for the same distance in a breaststroke swimmer. In Sargent's (1926) observations on running, the difference between the observed and predicted times ranged from 0.7 to 2.5 sec.

A comparison can be made between the predicted time for the dolphin stroke and the best competitive swimming times of the subjects for the crawl stroke for distances greater than 200 yards by referring to Table 1. The average competitive times of the group for swimming distances using the dolphin-butterfly stroke were 5:16.6 and 6:45.4. One of the subjects (DH) had a recorded competitive time for the crawl stroke of 18:20 for the distance of 1650 yards. This is much faster than the 26.11.1 predicted for the group for this distance when using the dolphin stroke. Obviously, using the dolphin-butterfly stroke to swim any great distance would place undue physiological demands on the swimmer.

The validity of any predictive procedure depends on the acceptability of the underlying assumptions. Two crucial assumptions were made in the procedure described here. It was assumed on the one hand that the subjects always attained maximal $\dot{V}_{O_2}$ debts if they swam to exhaustion, and on the other hand that Equation 1 described the proportion of the maximal $\dot{V}_{O_2}$ that could be maintained during swimming.

The first assumption is apparently tenable. Margaria et al. (1963) and Margaria, Cerretelli, and Mangili, (1964) reported that the lactacid portion of oxygen debt contraction reaches its maximum in about 40 sec in very strenuous exercise. Margaria and his associates (1964) also reported that the alactacid portion of the debt may reach its maximum within the first 10–30 sec after strenuous exercise begins. Energy requirements in excess of maximum values for the alactacid and lactacid portions of the oxygen debt must be met through oxidative reactions. Because the shortest swimming time predicted in the present study exceeded 2 min, there is no reason to question this assumption. Unfortunately, no measurements of lactic acid concentrations were taken during the recovery period, so it is not possible to evaluate the oxygen debt measurements in terms of lactic acid formation.

Bink (1962) and Bonjer (1962) contrived an empirical equation to determine maximum working capacity in industrial tasks on the basis of the maximal $\dot{V}_{O_2}$, because it was obvious that maximal $\dot{V}_{O_2}$ cannot be maintained indefinitely. However, they based their calculations on caloric intake data and did not consider the dynamics of adjustment at the beginning of work, making the equation of limited usefulness to these predictions. Thus, it became necessary to obtain experimental data from subjects who performed to exhaustion on a cycle ergometer against different work loads (see Appendix).

Equation 1 was derived from such data and describes the period of adjustment while cycling at the beginning of exercise until a plateau

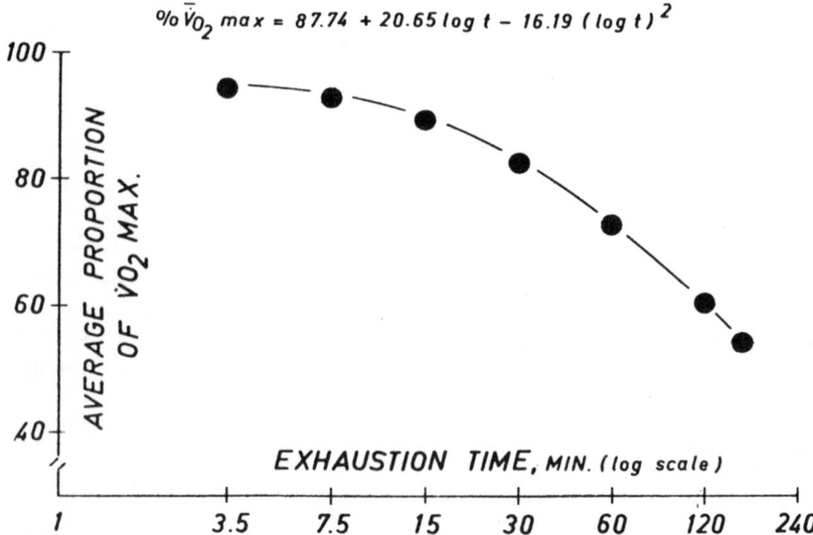


Figure 2. Average proportion of $\dot{V}_{O_2}$ max is compared with exhaustion time.

value of oxygen consumption is reached. This equation is an agreement with previous work (Åstrand and Saltin, 1961a), according to which the time it takes to establish a plateau depends on the work load: the heavier the load, the more rapid the increase. In applying Equation 1 to the prediction of swimming performance, it was assumed that the adaptational response with regard to oxygen uptake is the same for cycling and swimming. It is conceivable that the hydrostatic pressure, the prone position, and the immersion in water during swimming may affect pulmonary and cardiovascular dynamics (Magel and Faulkner, 1967) differently than does bicycle riding. Also, the maximal oxygen uptake obtained during swimming may be lower than that observed during cycling (Åstrand and Saltin, 1961b). However, there is no reason to believe that the kinetics of oxygen uptake and the metabolic pathways will be different in the two types of muscular activity.

The determination of potential performance becomes more accurate as the number of required assumptions is reduced by replacing them with quantitative data. In the present study, an attempt was made to utilize knowledge of the dynamics of oxygen uptake at the beginning of exercise to express more accurately the aerobic contribution. This investigation does, however, suffer the same limitations in regard to oxygen debt as do previous studies (Sargent, 1926; Karpovich and LeMaistre, 1940). Despite this, the predicted average best time for the group for swimming 200 yards (2:10.9) was only 1.3 seconds slower than the true average (2:09.6). The value of such procedures in predicting individual potential will become greater as other assumptions are replaced by more precise data.

## APPENDIX

Three subjects of comparable age and functional adaptability to those of the swimmers (ages: 19, 22, 20; $\dot{V}_{O_2}$ max: 61, 63, 58; heart rate max: 188, 204, 187; blood lactate max: 165, 122, 94) performed periodically on a cycloergometer at different work intensities to exhaustion while oxygen uptake was measured at frequent intervals. On the basis of data obtained, the following equations (2) were computed, which express the kinetics of oxygen uptake for the corresponding average work times (1).

| (1) Work time min | (2) $\dot{V}_{O_2}$ kinetics $y = a - b_e$ | (3) $\bar{\dot{V}}_{O_2}$ (% $\dot{V}_{O_2}$ max) = $\int_0^{t\ exh} (a - b_e{}^{-ct})\, dt \times \frac{\dot{V}_{O_2}\ max}{100 t_{exh}}$ |
|---|---|---|
| 3 | $101 - 52.82_e{}^{-2.25t}$ | 93 |
| 8 | $101 - 35.88_e{}^{-0.59t}$ | 93 |
| 30 | $90.6 - 54.72_e{}^{-0.21t}$ | 82 |
| 60 | $68.5 - 19.29_e{}^{-0.13t}$ | 71 |
| 160 | $53.2 - 19.52_e{}^{-0.02t}$ | 59 |

The $\dot{V}_{O_2}$ kinetics equation (2) and the exhaustion work time (1) were used to derive the average proportion of $\dot{V}_{O_2}$ max shown in column (3). The relationship between (1) and (3) was employed to calculate the average proportion of the maximal $\dot{V}_{O_2}$ that subjects could use when swimming for various periods of time. This relationship is plotted in Figure 2.

## ACKNOWLEDGMENTS

The authors wish to express their appreciation to the subjects who voluntarily contributed their time and effort because of their devotion to the sport of swimming: R. Fleury, D. Hart, S. Olson, J. Shea, D. Sbrega, and F. Wright.

## REFERENCES

Adrian, M., Singh, M., and Karpovich, P. V. 1966. Energy cost of leg kick, arm stroke, and whole crawl stroke. J. Appl. Physiol. 21:1763.

Åstrand, P. O., and Saltin, B. 1961a. Oxygen uptake during the first minutes of heavy muscular exercise. J. Appl. Physiol. 16:971.

Åstrand, P. O., and Saltin, B. 1961b. Maximal oxygen uptake and heart rate in various types of muscular activity. J. Appl. Physiol. 16:977.

Bink, B. 1962. The physical working capacity in relation to working time and age. Ergonomics 5:25.

Bonjer, F. H. 1962. Actual energy expenditure in relation to the physical working capacity. Ergonomics 5:29.

Greene, M. M. 1930. The energy cost of track running and swimming. Unpublished masters thesis, Springfield College, Springfield, Mass.

Karpovich, P. V., and LeMaistre, H. 1940. Prediction of time in swimming the breast stroke based on oxygen consumption. Res. Q. 11:40.

Keul, J., Doll, E., and Keppler, D. 1972. Energy Metabolism of Human Muscle. University Park Press, Baltimore.

Klissouras, V. 1968. Energy metabolism in swimming the dolphin stroke. Int. Z. Angew. Physiol. 25:142.

Magel, J. R., and Faulkner, J. R. 1967. Maximum oxygen uptakes of college swimmers. J. Appl. Physiol. 22:929.

Margaria, R., Cerretelli, P., diPrampero, P. E., Massari, C., and Torelli, G. 1963. Kinetics and mechanism of oxygen debt contraction in man. J. Appl. Physiol. 18:371–377.

Margaria, R., Cerretelli, P., and Mangili, F. 1964. Balance and kinetics of anaerobic energy release during strenuous exercise in man. J. Appl. Physiol. 19:623.

Ricci, B. 1968. Measurement of oxygen debt, and blood lactate and pryuvate, in physiological aspects of sports and physical fitness. Athletic Institute, Chicago. pp. 12–15.

Robinson, S., Robinson, D. L., Mountjoy, R. J., and Bullard, R. W. 1958. Influence of fatigue on the efficiency of men during exhausting runs. J. Appl. Physiol. 12:197.

Sargent, R. M. 1926. Relation between oxygen requirement and speed in running. Proc. Roy. Soc. B. London, 100:10.

Stainsby, W. N., and Barclay, J. K. 1970. Exercise metabolism: $O_2$ deficit, steady level $O_2$ uptake, and $O_2$ uptake for recovery. Med. Sci. Sports. 2:177–181.

Welch, H. G., and Stainsby, W. N. 1967. Oxygen debt in contracting dog skeletal muscle in situ. Resp. Physiol. 3:229.

Welch, H. G., Faulkner, J. A., Barclay, J. K., and Brooks, G. A. 1969. Some factors influencing the interpretations of $O_2$ debt. Paper presented at the 16th Annual Meeting of American College of Sport Medicine, May 1–3, Atlanta, Ga.

# Parameters of Acid-Base Equilibrium at Various Swimming Intensities and Distances

Z. D. Torma and G. Székely

## INTRODUCTION

During the last few years, considerable data have been accumulated on details of anaerobic metabolism and the oxygen debt that it represents (Dill et al., 1936; Knuttgen, 1962; Karlsson, 1971). It was found that, when the intensity of work approached or exceeded the corresponding possible oxygen uptake (supramaximal work), the level of blood lactate was increased.

In an examination of this problem (Margaria et al., 1963), the highest level of blood lactate determined perceptible using a load of this type was named *lactacid capacity*. This value depends on the muscle glycogen content, current condition, alimentary state, and age of the examined subject (Johnson and Brouha, 1943). On the basis of these findings, the measurement of lactacid capacity has been used in a few investigations as a basis for the estimation of physical fitness. The workload in these examinations was produced mainly on ergometers (Wasserman, Burton, and Van Kessel, 1965; Margaria et al., 1969; De Coster et al, 1969).

In this study, an effort has been made to examine the degree of anaerobic work of swimmers with maximal assurance of typical training schedules. The study confirms the existence of alactacid and lactacid phases of anaerobic metabolism, postulated by Margaria, Edwards, and Dill (1933), by the use of a simple workload model of short-term swimming performance.

## METHODS

Swimmers (N = 16: 8 girls and 8 boys) aged 12.9–16.2 years (mean age: 14.4 years), from one swim club in Budapest, who had been engaged in intensive training for several years were studied. The workload involved freestyle swimming for 25–200 m in two different manners: with maximal intensity for different distances (25, 50, 75, 100, 150 and 200 m), and for a constant distance with different intensities (100, 90, 80, and 70%, in relation to the intensity of the best swimming results).

Blood was drawn from an earlobe during the 3rd min of recovery. The samples were stored in a 4°C environment, in the anaerobic stage, until processing commenced. Base excess (BE) in the blood was measured by the Astrup method, and the level of blood lactate was determined enzymatically with a spectrophotofluorometer.

The measurements were repeated on 3 consecutive days; the reliability of measurement was very good (86%).

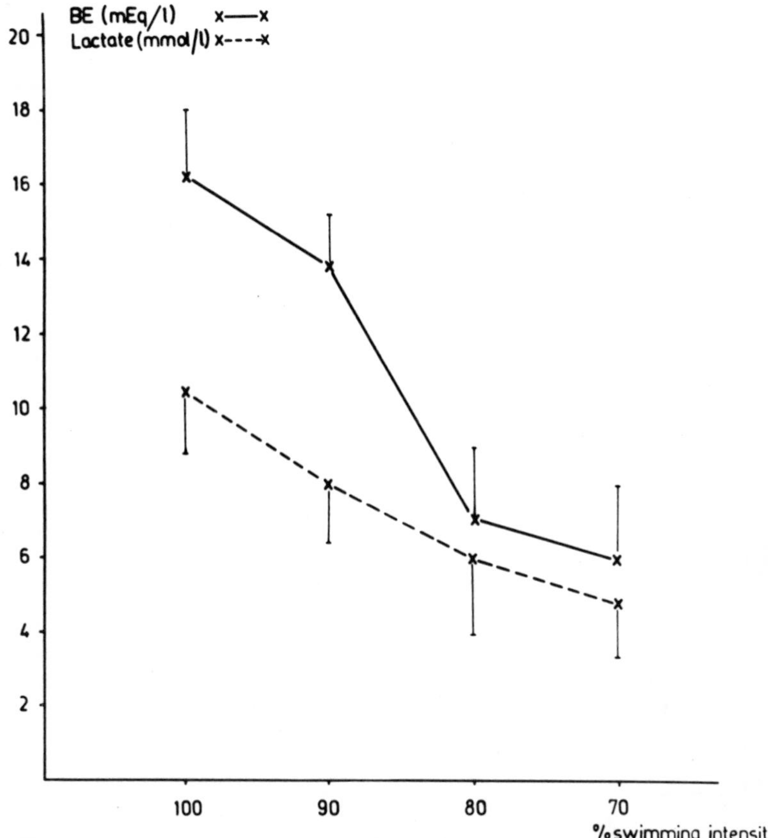


Figure 1. Relationship between blood lactate levels and BE during swimming for 200 m with different intensities.

## RESULTS

The relationships between the intensity of swimming, the level of blood lactate, and BE, respectively, is shown in Figure 1. This curve suggests a linear relationship between the intensity of freestyle swimming for 200 m and the level of lactate production. In further experiments, changes in lactate level and BE resulting from swimming with maximal intensity for different distances were studied. It seems, as Figure 2 demonstrates, that minimal increase of blood lactate occurs in the 25-m distance. The highest lactate levels followed the swimming of 100–200 m.

Figure 3 presents the distribution of lactate levels in relation to swimming rates for different distances. It can be seen from the observed lactate values that the higher lactate levels were associated with the higher swimming velocities, except for the 25-m distance, where despite the very high velocity the swimmers' lactate levels were nearly as low as those of the controls.

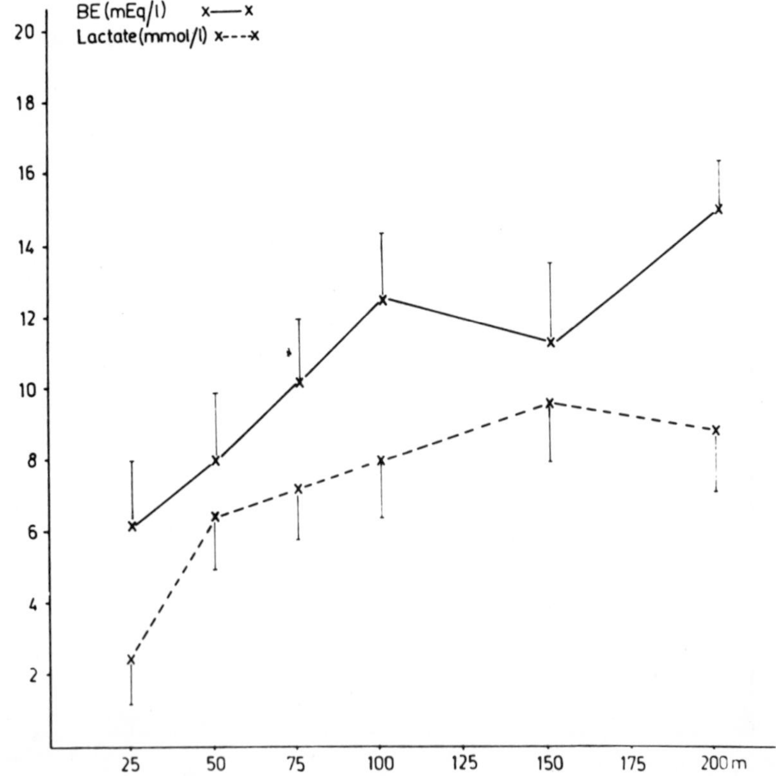


Figure 2. Relationship between blood lactate levels and BE during swimming for different distances with maximal intensity.

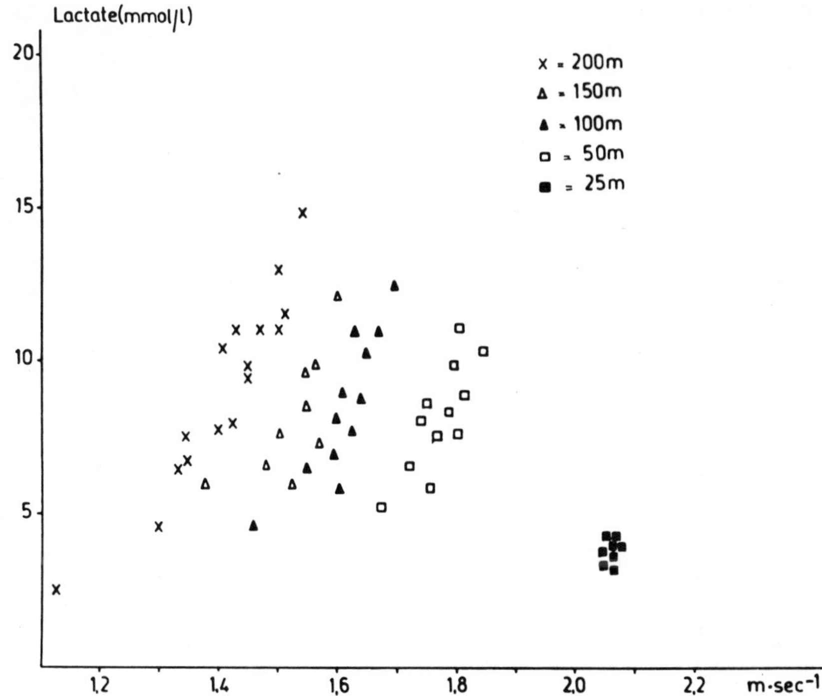


Figure 3. Values of blood lactate are shown in relation to swimming velocities over different distances (25–200 m).

Figure 4 shows the regression lines that were calculated from the data in Figure 3. Use of the equations of the lines can establish that, for individual distances (except 25 m), the relationship between lactate values and swimming velocity (i.e., intensity) is highly significant.

The relationship between lactate production and the velocity achieved at various distances (50–200 m) is shown in Figure 5. The lactacid phase reached maximal level in 40–65 sec.

## DISCUSSION

The concentration of lactate in arterial blood is generally regarded as an indicator of an anaerobic condition in the working muscles (Lundin and Ström, 1947; Williams et al., 1962; Asmussen et al., 1974). It is therefore possible to answer the question: How can the organism adapt to the work and satisfy the energy requirements immediately while the aerobic processes are striving to establish equilibrium at the increased level of work?

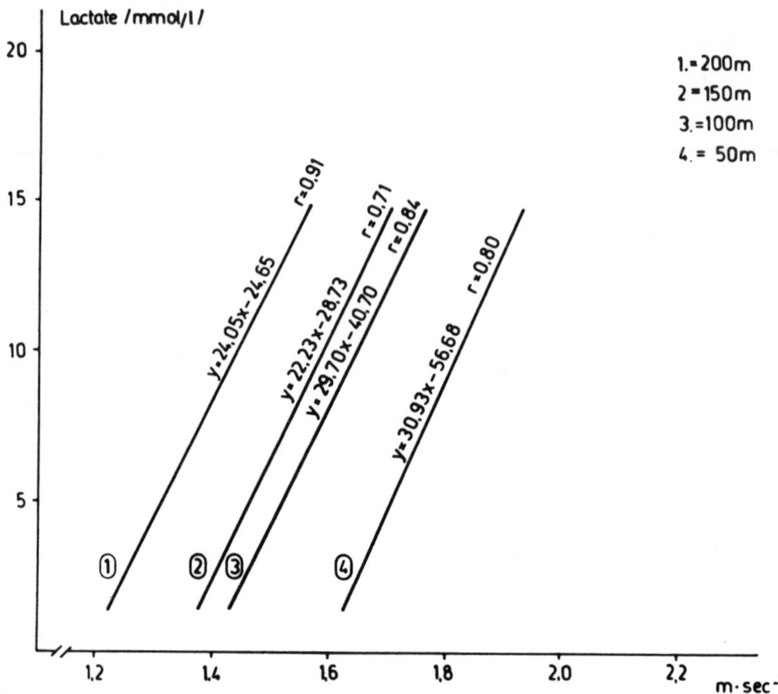


Figure 4. The relationship of blood lactate levels to swimming distances of 50–200 m is illustrated.

Some studies have shown that there is a relationship between the intensity of short-term work and the level of blood lactate (Saltin and Essén, 1971). In this study, the results agreed with previous investigations where this relationship was shown to be linear in the case of short-term (200-m) swimming loads.

In an examination of the dependence of lactate formation on distance, it was discovered that, in swimming with maximal intensity for 25 m, it is difficult to perceive any additional formation of lactate. This fact is in agreement with other data (Margaria et al., 1969; di Prampero, 1971; Saltin and Karlsson, 1971) that has shown an increase in lactate level to be impossible when the duration of work does not exceed 10–15 sec, even if the intensity of work is maximal.

Under short-term conditions, the energy required by the load is supplied by alactacid-anaerobic processes. Swimming for 50 m represents the transitional range between alactacid- and lactacid-anaerobic energy supply. The lactacid-anaerobic capacity is not fully exhausted by a single swimming bout of 50 m. According to some estimates, the prompt chemical reactions of disposable macroergophosphates enable

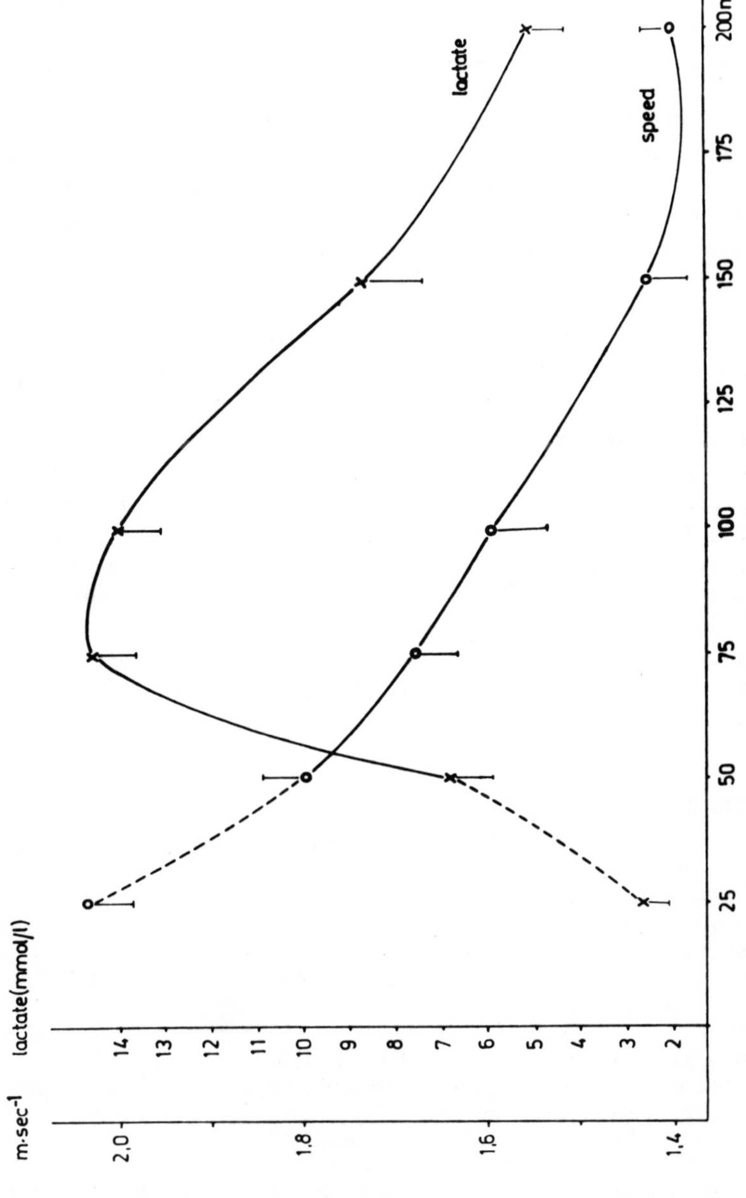


Figure 5. The relationships of lactate level and swimming velocity to swimming distances of 50–200 m are shown.

the work to be continued for as much as 20 sec (Piiper, di Prampero, and Cerretelli, 1968).

In this experiment, the highest blood lactate levels were found for swimming distances of 100–200 m. The energy requirement of these loads are supplied mainly by lactacid-anaerobic energy supply; thus, the measurement of lactacid capacity in swimming is practical when these distances are involved.

A significant relationship between the lactate levels and swimming rates was found by examining instances of different swimming distances. The regression lines calculated for individual distances were parallel to each other. This fact supports the concept that the degree of lactacid capacity is influenced by the quality of individual tolerance to lactate (Johnson and Brouha, 1943; Hermansen, 1969). The parallel regression lines also reinforce the finding that the energy needed to swim 25–200 m is satisfied by the lactacid-anaerobic energy supply.

Observing the occurrence of the highest lactate levels at distances from 100–200 m confirms the theoretical concept that the lactacid phase reaches the maximal intensity in 40–65 sec. Hence, if a measure of the anaerobic capacity is desired, a load that will result in exhaustion at the cessation of the exercise period must be chosen (Hermansen, 1969; Hultman, 1967). These results, then, support the concept proposed by Margaria, Edwards, and Dill (1933) concerning alactacid and lactacid phases of anaerobic metabolism in instances of short-term swimming with maximal intensity. Similar loads may also be valuable for quick assessments of the physical conditions of sprinters, because the degree of lactacid capacity is considered useful additional data over and above the aerobic indices of physical fitness.

## REFERENCES

Asmussen, E., Klausen, K., Nielsen, L. E., Techow, O. S. A., and Tønder, P. J. 1974. Lactate production and anaerobic work capacity after prolonged exercise. Acta Physiol. Scand. 90:731–742.

De Coster, A., Denolin, H., Messin, R., Degre, S., and Vandermoten, P. 1969. Role of the metabolites in the acid-base balance during exercise. In: J. R. Poortmans (ed.), Biochemistry of Exercise. Medicine and Sport, Vol. 3, pp. 15–34. Karger, Basel.

Dill, D. B., Edwards, H. T., Newman, E. V., and Margaria, R. 1936. Analysis of recovery from anaerobic work. Arbeitsphysiologie. 9:299–307.

di Prampero, P. E. 1971. Anaerobic capacity and power.In: R. J. Shephard (ed.), Frontiers of Fitness, pp. 172–178. Charles C. Thomas, Springfield, Ill.

Hermansen, L. 1969. Anaerobic energy release. Med. Sci. Sport 1:32–41.

Hultman, E. 1967. Studies on muscle metabolism of glycogen and active phosphate in man with special reference to exercise and diet. Scand. J. Clin. Lab. Invest. 19:(suppl. 94).

Johnson, R. E., and Brouha, L. 1943. Pulse rate, blood lactate, and duration of effort in relation to ability to perform strenuous exercise. Rev. Can. Biol. 1:171–178.

Karlsson, J. 1971. Pyruvate and lactate ratios in muscle tissue and blood during exercise in man. Acta Physiol. Scand. 81:455–458.

Knuttgen, H. G. 1962. Oxygen debt, lactate, pyruvate, and "excess lactate" after muscular work. Am. J. Physiol. 17:639–664.

Lundin, G., and Ström, G. 1947. The concentration of blood lactic acid in man during muscular work in relation to the partial pressure of oxygen of the inspired air. Acta Physiol. Scand. 13:253–266.

Margaria, R., Edwards, H. T., and Dill, D. B. 1933. The possible mechanism of contracting and paying the oxygen debt and the role of lactic acid in muscular contraction. Am. J. Physiol. 106:689–715.

Margaria, R., Cerretelli, P., di Prampero, P. E., Massari, C., and Torelli, G. 1963. Kinetics and mechanism of oxygen debt contraction in man. J. Appl. Physiol. 18:371–377.

Margaria, R., Oliva, R. D., di Prampero, P. E., and Cerretelli, P. 1969. Energy utilization in intermittent exercise of supramaximal intensity. J. Appl. Physiol. 26:752–756.

Piiper, J. P., di Prampero, P. E., and Cerretelli, P. 1968. Oxygen debt and high-energy phosphates in gastrocnemius muscle of the dog. Am. J. Physiol. 215:523–527.

Saltin, B., and Essén, B. 1971. Muscle glycogen, lactate, ATP, and CP in intermittent exercise. In: B. Pernow and B. Saltin (eds.), Muscle Metabolism During Exercise, pp. 419–423. Plenum Publisher, New York.

Saltin, B., and Karlsson, J. 1971. Muscle ATP, CP, and lactate during exercise after physical conditioning. In: B. Pernow and B. Saltin (eds.), Muscle Metabolism During Exercise, pp. 395–399. Plenum Publisher, New York.

Wasserman, K., Burton, G. G., and Van Kessel, A. L. 1965. Excess lactate concept and $O_2$ debt of exercise. J. Appl. Physiol. 20:1299–1304.

Williams, C. G., Bedell, G. A. G., Wyndham, C. H., Strydom, N. B., Marrison, J. F., Peter, J., Fleming, P. W., and Ward, J. S. 1962. Circulatory and metabolic reactions to work in heat. J. Appl. Physiol. 17:625–638.

# Skeletal Muscle Fiber Capillarization with Extreme Endurance Training in Man

**E. Nygaard and E. Nielsen**

Studies on man's maximal aerobic performance capacity have for many years involved measures of the central circulatory and respiratory functions. Accordingly, adaptations taking place with heavy endurance training have been studied in terms of changes in cardiovascular and respiratory dimensions, as well as in maximal oxygen uptake.

In recent years, new techniques have made it possible to investigate the characteristics of the skeletal muscle of man in detail. Different fiber types have been identified by histochemical techniques on the basis of stains for structural components, enzyme activities, and substrate contents. Biochemical analyses have contributed information on the metabolic profile of the fibers; and measurements on contractility, tension development, and fatiguability have provided some clarification on the functional capacity of the fibers (Saltin et al., 1977).

Also, data are available on changes in skeletal muscle of man in response to increased levels of physical activity. Reports have been given on increased activities of enzymes in the Krebs Cycle (Henriksson and Reitman, 1977), of increased capacity of fat oxidation (Bass et al., 1976), and of conversion between the subgroups of the fast twitching fibers (Andersen and Henriksson, 1977). Studies on capillary supply are somewhat conflicting. One study reports that no difference exists in capillary supply of untrained and endurance trained individuals (Hermansen and Wachtlova, 1971). Recent studies, however, have shown a higher capillary density in trained compared with untrained

This study was supported by grants from the Danish National Science Research Council and from the Research Council of the Danish Sports Federations.

subjects, and an increase in capillary density with endurance training (Andersen, 1975; Brodal, Ingjer, and Hermansen, 1976; Andersen and Henriksson).

The present study was undertaken in an attempt to determine the optimal adaptability to endurance training in terms of fiber distribution, fiber areas, and capillary density in the skeletal muscle of man.

## SUBJECTS AND METHODS

Twenty-five young competitive swimmers, 14 boys and 11 girls, participated in the study. They were all fully informed of the risks and discomfort associated with the procedure before they volunteered to participate. Mean values of age, weight, periods of intense training, and points obtained according to Schwimmsportliche Leistungstabelle 1973–1976 are presented in Table 1. Swimming maximal oxygen uptake averaged 4.1 liters/min for the boys, and 3.3 liters/min for the girls. Table 1 also gives the time for the best performance for the best swimmer in each group. Because upper body muscles are used more in swimming than are lower extremity muscles, the individuals, besides having trained heavily over an average of 5 years, constitute examples of graded adaptability among the muscles examined.

Muscle biopsies were obtained with the Bergström technique (Bergström, 1962) from the rectus femoris of the quadriceps muscle group, from the middle portion of the deltoid muscle, and from the latissimus dorsi muscle.

Using histochemical stains for myofibrillar ATPase at various pH values, muscle fibers were identified as ST fibers (slow twitch, high

Table 1. Characteristics of swimmers

| | | | Age (years) | Weight (kg) | Intensive training (years) | SL[a] 1973-1976 (points) | Best performance |
|---|---|---|---|---|---|---|---|
| Males | (N=14) | Mean | 17.8 | 67 | 4.8 | 796 | |
| | | Range | (13–25) | (56–81) | (3–8) | (617–938) | |
| | | JB[b] | 17 | 62 | 5 | 938 | 400-m freestyle 4:05.3 |
| Females | (N=11) | Mean | 15.9 | 54 | 4.6 | 860 | |
| | | Range | (14–20) | (45–63) | (3–8) | (661–1061) | |
| | | SN[b] | 16 | 59 | 3 | 1061 | 200-m breast stroke 2:35.4 |

[a] Schwimmsportliche Leistungstabelle 1973–1976
[b] Best male and female swimmer of the group

oxidative), FTa fibers (fast twitch, oxidative-glycolytic) and FTb fibers (fast twitch, high glycolytic) (Brooke and Kaiser, 1970; Saltin et al., 1977). Capillaries were identified by use of the alpha-amylase PAS stain (Andersen, 1975). Fiber areas were determined planimetrically. The activity of the Krebs Cycle enzyme succinate dehydrogenase was determined fluorimetrically on a muscle homogenate according to the principles given by Lowry for NAD-NADP coupled reactions (Lowry and Passonneau, 1973).

## RESULTS

### Fiber Distribution

In all three muscles, the swimmers had a significantly higher proportion of ST fibers than was found in control muscles ($P < 0.001$) (Figure 1). Furthermore, in the upper body muscles of the swimmers, no FTb fibers were observed; this fiber type constituted 15–20% of total fiber population in control muscle. In the thigh muscles of swimmers, FTb fibers were present, but to a smaller extent than was seen in sedentary individuals ($P < 0.01$).

### Fiber Areas

Swimmers did not show any hypertrophy when compared with controls (Table 2). In fact both ST fibers and FTa fibers were smaller in

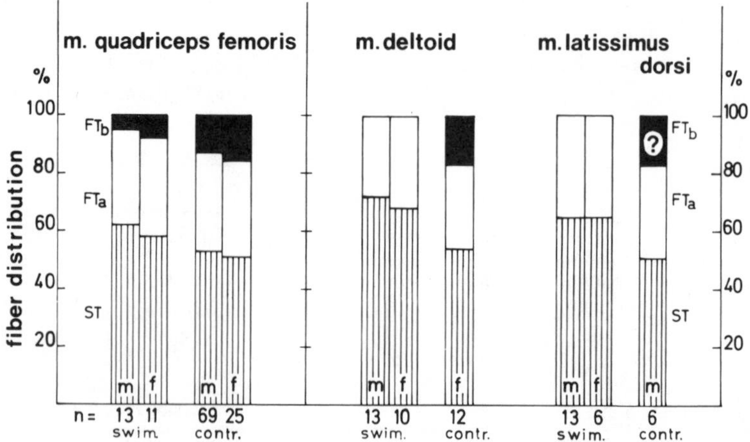


Figure 1. Fiber distribution in skeletal muscle is shown for sedentary subjects and elite swimmers. Of note is the high proportion of ST fibers and the absence of FTb fibers in the deltoid and latissimus dorsi muscles of the swimmers. m = males; f = females. For further details on sedentary subjects see Saltin et al., 1977. Control values on latissimus dorsi are from the study by Johnson et al., 1973. They did not subdivide the FT fibers, therefore a question mark is placed on the FT fibers.

Table 2. Fiber areas ($\mu m^2 \times 100$)

| | | M. quadriceps femoris | | | | M. deltoid | | | | M. latissimus dorsi | | | |
|---|---|---|---|---|---|---|---|---|---|---|---|---|---|
| | | (N)[a] | ST | FTa | FTb | (N) | ST | FTa | FTb | (N) | ST | FTa | FTb |
| Females | | | | | | | | | | | | | |
| Swimmers | Mean | (10) | 40 | 41 | 32 | (10) | 34 | 39 | 0 | (6) | 41 | 43 | 0 |
| | SD | | 8.5 | 4.4 | 8.2 | | 8.0 | 8.9 | | | 11.9 | 10.5 | |
| Controls | Mean | (15) | 39 | 36 | 22 | (8) | 41 | 48 | 38 | | 0 | 0 | 0 |
| | SD | | 7.4 | 8.2 | 6.1 | | 7.0 | 12.6 | 16.2 | | | | |
| Males | | | | | | | | | | | | | |
| Swimmers | Mean | (13) | 37 | 42 | 45 | (13) | 40 | 41 | 0 | (13) | 39 | 41 | 0 |
| | SD | | 7.6 | 7.1 | 9.6 | | 8.8 | 9.4 | | | 10.4 | 11.1 | |
| Controls | Mean | (5) | 39 | 50 | 36 | | 0 | 0 | 0 | | 0 | 0 | 0 |
| | SD | | 10.7 | 7.7 | 9.4 | | | | | | | | |

[a] Number of subjects.

swimmers than in controls ($P < 0.01$) (Figure 2). FTa fibers were larger than ST fibers in control subjects ($P < 0.05$); in swimmers, no difference was detectable between these two types of fibers.

## Capillary Supply

The number of capillaries was significantly higher in swimmers compared with sedentary subjects, whether expressed as the number of capillaries per fiber type, per fiber, or per mm$^2$ muscle tissue (Table 3 and Figure 3). Comparisons within the groups among the three muscles showed that in the female sedentary subjects, the thigh muscles had better capillarization (capillaries per mm$^2$) than was found in shoulder

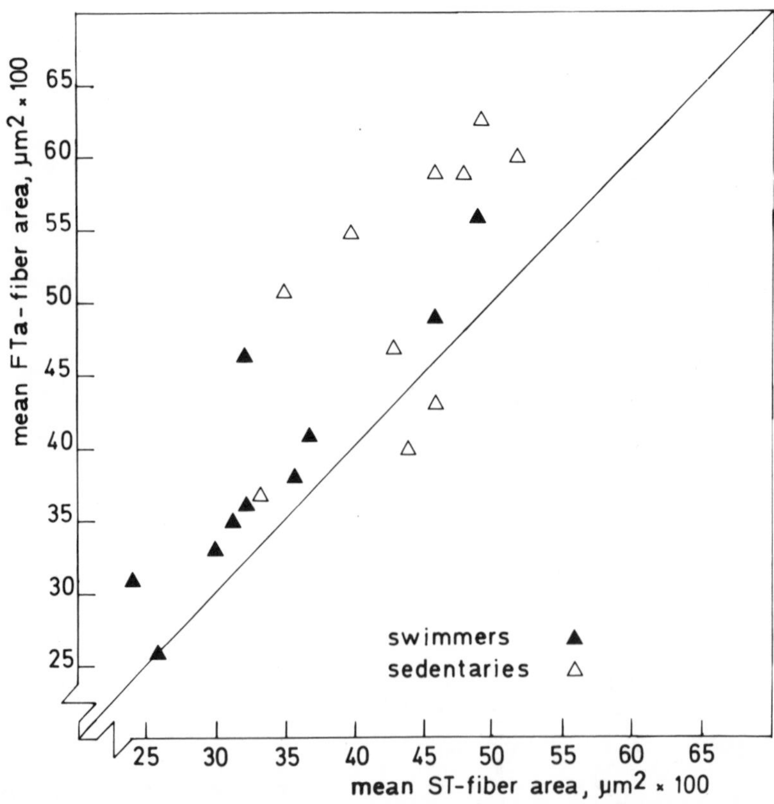


Figure 2. This is an identity diagram of the cross-sectional areas of ST fibers (x axis) and FTa fibers (y axis) in deltoid muscles of sedentary females (unfilled symbols) and swimmers (filled symbols). Both types of fibers are significantly smaller in the swimmers.

Table 3. Capillary supply

| | | M quadriceps femoris | | | | | | M. deltoid | | | | | | M. latissimus dorsi | | | | | |
|---|---|---|---|---|---|---|---|---|---|---|---|---|---|---|---|---|---|---|---|
| | | N[a] | /ST | /FTa | /FTb | /fib | /mm² | N[a] | /ST | /FTa | /FTb | /fib | /mm² | N[a] | /ST | /FTa | /FTb | /fib | /mm² |
| Females | | | | | | | | | | | | | | | | | | | |
| Swimmers | Mean | (11) | 4.8 | 4.6 | 3.8 | 1.8 | 400 | (10) | 5.1 | 5.2 | 0 | 2.0 | 465 | (6) | 5.8 | 5.6 | 0 | 2.3 | 556 |
| | SD | | 0.6 | 0.7 | 0.6 | 0.2 | 106 | | 0.7 | 0.8 | | 0.3 | 78 | | 1.0 | 1.1 | | 0.4 | 85 |
| Controls | Mean | (11) | 4.0 | 3.7 | 2.9 | 1.2 | 301 | (5) | 4.2 | 3.6 | 3.0 | 1.4 | 279 | | 0 | 0 | 0 | 0 | 0 |
| | SD | | 1.1 | 1.1 | 0.9 | 0.3 | 58 | | 0.6 | 0.7 | 0.7 | 0.3 | 56 | | | | | | |
| Males | | | | | | | | | | | | | | | | | | | |
| Swimmers | Mean | (13) | 5.2 | 5.1 | 5.4 | 1.9 | 465 | (13) | 5.8 | 5.8 | 0 | 2.3 | 526 | (13) | 5.5 | 5.5 | 0 | 2.1 | 526 |
| | SD | | 0.6 | 0.6 | 0.4 | 0.3 | 58 | | 0.9 | 1.0 | | 0.5 | 58 | | 0.4 | 0.3 | | 0.3 | 88 |
| Controls | Mean | | 3.9 | 4.2 | 3.0 | 1.4 | 329 | | 0 | 0 | 0 | 0 | 0 | | 0 | 0 | | 0 | 0 |
| | SD | | 0.5 | 0.6 | 0.6 | 0.2 | 33 | | | | | | | | | | | | |

[a] Number of subjects. Data give number of capillaries around each fiber type, number of capillaries per fiber and per mm².

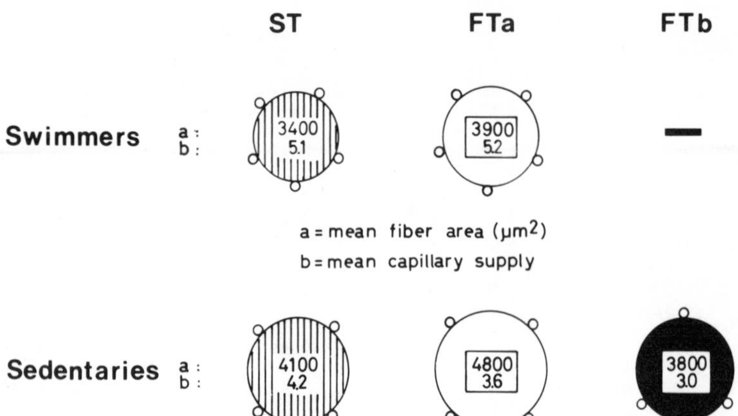


Figure 3. Fiber area and capillary supply in female deltoid muscles are illustrated. Of note are the small mean fiber areas and the large number of capillaries around the single fibers in swimmers as compared with sedentary subjects.

muscles ($P < 0.05$), while in female swimmers, capillarization was higher in the deltoids than in the quadriceps femoris muscles ($P < 0.05$), and in the latissimus dorsi muscles still higher than in the deltoid muscles ($P < 0.01$).

In the sedentary males, the situation was the same as in sedentary female subjects. In male swimmers, however, capillarization was identical in the deltoid and the latissimus dorsi muscles, and somewhat lower in the quadriceps femoris muscles ($P < 0.05$).

## Diffusion Distances

These two factors—fiber areas and capillary supply—were taken as indications of diffusion conditions expressed as fiber type area per capillary (Figure 4). A pronounced difference was again seen in the female deltoid, where 976 $\mu m^2$ (sedentary) and 667 $\mu m^2$ (swimmer) of the ST fibers was supplied by one capillary ($P < 0.001$). For the FTa fibers, the corresponding figures were 1333 $\mu m^2$ and 750 $\mu m^2$ for the two groups, respectively ($P < 0.001$).

## Krebs Cycle Activity

Swimmers had a higher succinate dehydrogenase activity than was found in controls (Table 4). The difference was most pronounced in the deltoid muscles with 4.6 and 5.6 $\mu$moles/g $\times$ min$^{-1}$ in male and female sedentary subjects, respectively, and 11.0 and 10.4 $\mu$moles/g $\times$ min$^{-1}$ in male and female swimmers ($P < 0.001$).

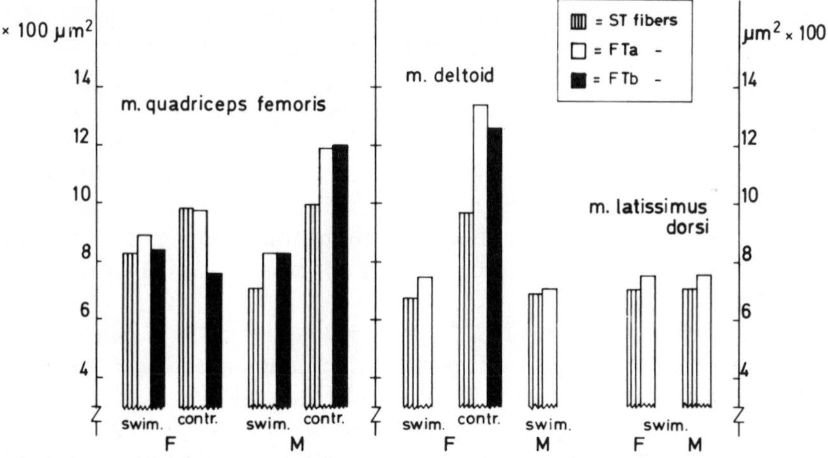


Figure 4. Fiber type area per capillary, indicative of diffusion distances, shows that diffusion conditions are much better in the well trained muscles of the swimmers than in the sedentary subjects'. F = female; M = male.

## DISCUSSION

### Fiber Distribution

The higher percentage of ST fibers in the trained muscles of the swimmers than in the controls' is in accordance with findings on successful athletes in various endurance events (Gollnick et al., 1972; Costill et al., 1976). As in longitudinal training studies, no changes have been observed in the ST/FT ratio (Eriksson, Gollnick, and Saltin, 1973; Gollnick et al., 1973; Thorstensson et al., 1976; Andersen and Henriksson, 1977; the observed high percentage of ST fibers has hitherto been explained as the result of natural selection for these specific

Table 4. Succinate dehydrogenase activity (µmoles/g × min$^{-1}$)

| | | M. quadriceps femoris | | M. deltoid | | M. latissimus dorsi | |
|---|---|---|---|---|---|---|---|
| | | Female | Male | Female | Male | Female | Male |
| Swimmers | Mean | 8.2 | 10.8 | 10.4 | 11.0 | 7.2 | 9.8 |
| | SD | 2.6 | 2.0 | 3.4 | 2.7 | 2.8 | 3.1 |
| | N[a] | (9) | (9) | (7) | (12) | (3) | (6) |
| Controls | Mean | 7.1 | 7.0 | 5.6 | 4.6 | | |
| | SD | 1.4 | 2.0 | 1.3 | 1.7 | | |
| | N | (22) | (24) | (8) | (2) | | |

[a] Number of subjects.

athletic disciplines. This explanation is based upon the plausibility of a high percentage of oxidative fibers being an advantage in the performance of physical work requiring endurance.

Because swimming involves upper body muscles to a greater extent than lower extremity muscles, and because the swimmers' ST/FT ratios in this study differed more from control values in the deltoid and latissimus dorsi muscles than in the quadriceps femoris muscle, it is suggested that training can affect the proportion of ST and FT fibers in the muscle. How this might be brought about is discussed later in this chapter.

The total absence of FTb fibers in the upper body muscles of the swimmers confirmed previous results on training-induced alterations in the subgroup pattern of FT fibers (Andersen and Henriksson, 1977). Because the fiber classification is based upon differences in the pH sensitivity of the myosin ATPase, and because this difference is related to the reactivity of sulphydryl groups of the myosin molecule (Brooke and Kaiser, 1970), structural changes of the myosin molecule, indicative of alterations in the contractile characteristics of the fibers, should constitute the basis for the conversion of FTb fibers to FTA fibers.

For this change to take place, one certain prerequisite is that the FTb fibers must be engaged in the activity. That this is the case with high intensity dynamic exercise has been shown through histochemical analysis of the glycogen depletion pattern (Secher and Nygaard, 1976).

## Fiber Areas and Capillary Supply

Results obtained on cross-sectional areas of the muscle fibers indicate that, in swimming, the more highly trained the muscles are, the smaller are the fibers. This finding is in contrast to previous studies that report on enlargements of the ST fibers with endurance training in long distance running and bicycling (Gollnick et al., 1973; Costill et al.; Andersen and Henriksson, 1977). Currently, no obvious explanation can be given for this discrepancy, although it may be suggested that changes in fiber area are determined through a balance between the specificity of the contraction (tension, speed of contraction, etc.) and the metabolic needs.

## Diffusion Distances

The observed facilitation of oxygen transport in swimmers, i.e., the short diffusion distances as a function of small fibers and a high number of capillaries around the single fibers, was much more pronounced in the deltoid and latissimus dorsi muscles than in the rectus femoris muscle. The smaller fibers in the more highly trained muscles conformed to the findings of Plyley and Groom (1975) on the question of distribution of capillaries in mammalian skeletal muscle: "Nature seems to prefer to increase $O_2$ supply by decreasing the diameter of a muscle fiber, rather than by increasing the primary sources of $O_2$ (viz. capillaries) around the perimeter of the fiber." Results from other animal studies, however, indicate that skeletal muscle reacts to increased levels of activity by forming new capillaries, and that increase in mitochondrial capacities is a later step in the adaptations (Brown et al., 1976). A time course study of adaptational events in skeletal muscle of man shows a parallel increase in capillary density and fiber areas, each increasing as much as 20% of pretraining values during an 8-week training period while the oxidative enzymes rose by 40% of pretraining values during the same period (Andersen and Henriksson, 1977).

The findings of this study support the conclusion that the metabolism of skeletal muscle in man is highly adaptable to increased demands for oxidation. In order to evaluate fully the adaptability and especially the time course of events, longer training periods should be used because some of the changes may not occur within an 8-week period. In addition, the type of endurance training should be specified; surely the demands on the organism to provide energy are totally different in endurance events such as running and swimming.

**Total Amount of Muscle Fibers**

The rather bulky muscle mass of the swimmers gives rise to the question as to whether, in the light of the small fibers, muscle fiber proliferation has taken place. Of course, it might be argued that in this case a natural selection has taken place on the basis of genetically determined small and numerous fibers. However, indications of fiber splitting are given through the large individual variations in the cross-sectional areas of muscle fibers in swimmers through the presence of extremely small fibers between the fibers of normal size. Furthermore, the observation of incisions in the cell membrane, almost dividing one cell into two, supports the concept of fiber splitting as an adaptational phenomenon in human skeletal muscle.

On the basis of glycogen depletion patterns, the ST fibers seem to be utilized more in swimming than are the FT fibers (Houston, 1978). It might be speculated that this fiber type would react the most to adaptational changes, and accordingly be the more involved in splitting processes. Consequently, the proportion of ST fibers would increase at the expense of FT fibers; this constitutes an alternative explanation for the high proportion of ST fibers found in the muscles of endurance athletes.

## REFERENCES

Andersen, P. 1975. Capillary density in skeletal muscle of man. Acta Physiol. Scand. 95:203–205.

Andersen, P., and Henriksson, J. 1977. Capillary supply of the quadriceps femoris muscle of man. Adaptive response to exercise. J. Physiol. (London) 270:677–690.

Bass, A., Vondra, K., Rath, R., Vitek, V., Teisinger, J., Mackova, E., Sprynarova, S., and Malkovaks, M. 1976. Enzyme activity patterns of energy supplying metabolism in the quadriceps femoris muscle (vastus lateralis). Pflügers Arch. 361:169–173.

Bergström, J. 1962. Muscle electrolytes in man. Scand. J. Clin. Lab. Invest. Suppl. 68.

Brodal, P., Ingjer, F., and Hermansen, L. 1976. Capillary supply of skeletal muscle fibres in untrained and endurance trained men. Acta Physiol. Scand. Suppl. 440:178.

Brooke, M. H., and Kaiser, K. 1970. Three myosin ATPase systems: The nature of their pH lability and sulphhydryl dependence. J. Histochem. Cytochem. 18:670–672.

Brooke, M. H., and Kaiser, K. K. 1970. Muscle fiber types: How many and what kind? Arch. Neurol. (Chicago) 23:369–379.

Brown, M. D., Cotter, M. A., Hudlicka, D., and Vrbova, G. 1976. The effects of different patterns of muscle activity on capillary density, mechanical properties, and structure of slow and fast rabbit muscles. Pflügers Arch. 361:241–250.

Costill, D. L., Daniels, J., Evans, W., Fink, W., Krahenbuhl, G., and Saltin, B. 1976. Skeletal muscle enzymes and fiber composition in male and female track athletes. J. Appl. Physiol. 90:149–154.

Eriksson, B., Gollnick, P., and Saltin, B. 1973. Muscle metabolism and enzyme activities after training in boys 11–13 years old. Acta Physiol. Scand. 87:485–497.

Gollnick, P. D., Armstrong, R. B., Saubert C. W., IV, Piehl, K., and Saltin, B. 1972. Enzyme activity and fiber composition in skeletal muscle of untrained and trained men. J. Appl. Physiol. 33:312–319.

Gollnick, P. D., Armstrong, R. B., Saltin, B., Saubert C. W., IV, Sembrowich, W. L., and Shepherd, R. E. 1973. Effect of training on enzyme activity and fiber composition of human skeletal muscle. J. Appl. Physiol. 34:107–111.

Henriksson, J., and Reitman, J. 1977. Time course of changes in human skeletal muscle succinate dehydrogenase, cytochrome oxidase activities, and maximal oxygen uptake with physical activity and inactivity. Acta Physiol. Scand. 99:91–97.

Hermansen, L., and Wachtlova, M. 1971. Capillary density of skeletal muscle in well trained and untrained men. J. Appl. Physiol. 30:860–863.

Houston, M. E. 1978. Metabolic responses to exercise, with special reference to training and competition in swimming. In: B. Eriksson and B. Furberg (eds.), Swimming Medicine IV, pp. 207–232. University Park Press, Baltimore.

Johnson, M. A., Polgar, D., Weightman, D., and Appleton, D. 1973. Data on distribution of fibre types in thirty-six human muscles: An autopsy study. J. Neurol. Sci. 18:111–129.

Lowry, O. H., and Passonneau, J. V., 1973. A Flexible System of Enzymatic Analysis. Academic Press, New York.

Plyley, M. J., and Groom, A. C. 1975. Geometrical distribution of capillaries in mammalian striated muscle. Am. J. Physiol. 228:1376–1383.
Saltin, B., Henriksson, J., Nygaard, E., Andersen, P., and Jansson, E. 1977. Fiber types and metabolic potentials of skeletal muscles in sedentary man and endurance runners. Ann. N. Y. Acad. Sci. 301:3–29.
Secher, N. H., and Nygaard, E. 1976. Glycogen depletion pattern in types I, II-A and II-B muscle fibers during maximal voluntary static and dynamic exercise. Acta Physiol. Scand. 96 (suppl. 440):287.
Thorstensson, A., Hultén, B., von Döbeln, W., and Karlsson, J. 1976. Effect of strength training on enzyme activities and fiber characteristics in human skeletal muscle. Acta Physiol. Scand. 96:392–398.

# Thermoregulation

# Physiology of Thermoregulation During Swimming

**B. Nielsen**

Because man is naturally a tropical land dweller, by invading the wet elements, the capability of many of his physiological regulatory mechanisms are challenged. This article deals mainly with the effects of water as an environment on the thermoregulatory system of the human body.

The temperature of the body core is maintained at approximately 37°C at rest. This is accomplished through the integrated action of the heat loss and heat conservation mechanisms, which are governed by the temperature centers in the brain. During exercise, body temperature increases to higher levels, depending on the severity of the work. The exercise plateau level is increased in proportion to the relative workload of the subject (% $\dot{V}_{O_2}$ max) (Saltin & Hermansen, 1966) but not to absolute oxygen consumption, workload, or heat production. During exercise in air, the core temperature is independent of environmental temperatures over a range of more than 20°C (between 5°C and 30–35°C air temperature ($T_a$)). This is made possible mainly through the great capacity of the sweating mechanism, which in trained individuals can produce sweat at rates up to 3-5 liters/hr. From 20 to 30 times the resting heat production can be eliminated through the evaporation of sweat. In water, this mechanism for temperature regulation is useless; it is therefore not surprising that the range of surrounding temperatures into which one can be immersed without an effect on core temperature is much smaller in water than in air (Figure 1).

This can be explained further by a closer look at the conditions for heat exchange in water compared with those in air. The body temperature is controlled by a balance between the heat produced in the body and the heat losses via conduction, convection, radiation and evaporation. If a balance cannot be reached through the thermoregulatory

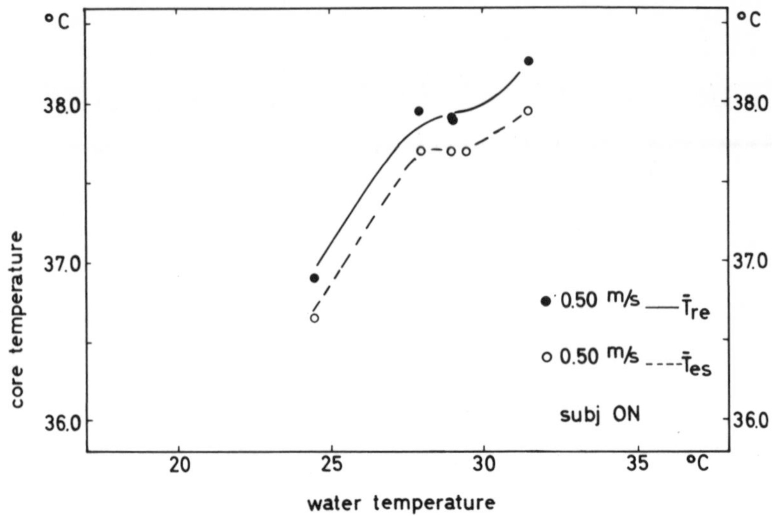


Figure 1. Rectal and esophageal temperature are shown after 60 min of swimming in water at different temperatures.

mechanisms, i.e., shivering, vasomotor reactions, and sweating, the body heat stores and the body temperature will change: it will increase if heat losses are smaller than heat production and decrease if heat losses are larger than the heat production.

Except for evaporative heat loss, the amount of heat exchanged by the different avenues for heat loss in air and water depends on the temperature difference between the body surface and the surroundings. Figure 2 shows the heat loss per degree for convective + radiative heat exchange in air, $h_o$, and for conduction + convection heat loss in water, $h_w$. The $h_o$ is about 15–20 W/m² × °C, while $h_w$ is about 600 W/m² × °C. The coefficients in water have been determined in model experiments (Bullard and Rapp, 1970; Winterspoon, Goldman, and Breckenridge, 1971) and measured in subjects resting and swimming in water at different speeds (Nadel et al., 1974). These values are 580 W/m² × °C for swimming (independent of speed), 230 resting in still water, increasing to 460 W/m² × °C during rest in flowing water. The reason for the large difference between heat transfer coefficients in air and water is the different physical properties of the two media. The heat conductance and the specific heat of water are about 25 and 1000 times greater, respectively, than those of air.

The skin temperature ($T_s$) in water will therefore be very close to the water temperature. $T_s$ in water has been measured in different studies (Burton and Bazett, 1936; Keatinge, 1959 and 1961; Boutelier,

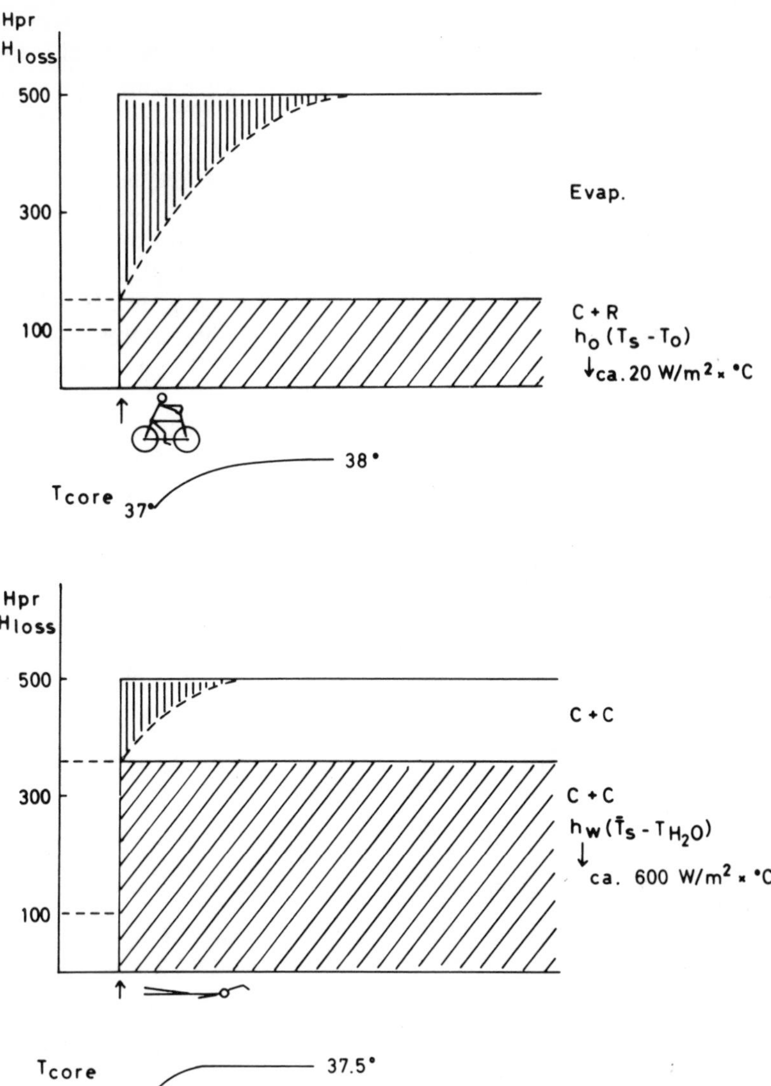


Figure 2. This figure illustrates heat transfer coefficients in air ($h_o$) and in water ($h_w$), and the heat loss in air (above) and in water (below) for a subject with a heat production of 500 W and a mean skin temperature of 30°C in each environment. "Forced heat loss" (loss caused solely by the difference between the skin and surrounding temperatures) is much greater in water. The latency in the activation of the sweating and the evaporative heat loss in air cause the greater heat storage and the greater core temperature increase during exercise in air compared with water.: ▨ = forced heat loss; ▥ = heat storage. (Based on data from Nielsen and Davies, 1976.)

1973; Nadel et al.). It varies with duration of exposure, water movements, swimming speed, and, to a certain extent, the site of measurement. Nadel et al. found the difference between average skin temperature ($\bar{T}_s$) and water temperature to be 0.25–0.75 °C during swimming and up to 2° during resting in still water.

In water, the physiological mechanism for varying the heat loss thus depends largely on the internal mechanisms for limiting the heat flow to the skin, that is, the variation in skin blood flow and the tissue insulation. The ease with which heat passes through the skin can be expressed as conductance $K = H/(T_{re} - \bar{T}_s)A_{Du}$, where H is heat loss through the skin, $T_{re}$ and $\bar{T}_s$ rectal and skin temperatures, and $A_{Du}$ the surface area. K is the heat transfer per degree difference between body core and body surface, measured in $W/m^2 \times °C$.

Conductance varies with two factors: skin blood flow and the amount of fat in the subcutaneous tissue. The skin blood flow is controlled from the temperature centers. Studies on the variation in heat

$$K = \frac{H_{SKIN}}{(T_{RE} - T_S) \times A_{DU}} \quad W/^{0}C \times M^2$$

$$K_{MAX} \sim 100\ W/^{0}C \times M^2$$

EXAMPLE I

$V_{O_2}$ =3 L/MIN ~1000 W OR 500 W/M$^2$

$T_{RE}$ =37.5°C
$T_S$ =32.5°C  } 5°C

HEAT TRANSFER PER DEGREE $\frac{500}{5}$ = 100 =$K_{MAX}$

EXAMPLE II

$T_{RE}$ =37.5°C
$T_S$ =35.0°C  } 2.5°C

HEAT PRODUCTION 500 W/M$^2$
MAX HEAT TRANSFER 2.5 × 100=250 W/M$^2$
STORAGE (IN 50 KG "CORE") 250 W/M$^2$

$T_{CORE}$ INCREASE 0.97°C PER KG PER WH

$\sim \frac{0.97 \times 500}{50}$ = 9.7°C IN ONE HOUR

Figure 3. Given here are examples of heat transfer by conductance and increase in rectal temperature ($T_{re}$) from swimming in warm water.

transfer across the skin demonstrate that it can increase 6–10 times over a minimal value, and that the blood stream can provide for the maximal transfer of about 100 W/m² × °C. A subject swimming with an oxygen uptake of 3 liters/min will produce heat at a rate of approximately 1000 W or 500 W/m². A maximal heat transfer by the skin blood flow of 100 W/m² per degree difference between core and body surface implies that swimming cannot go on for long at water temperatures above 32°C. If the water temperature is more than 34°C, the body temperature will rise and reach dangerous levels in about 30 min (Figure 3).

The minimum value for tissue conductance is related to the fat layer in the skin expressed as skinfold thickness, specific gravity, or calculated fat in percent of body weight. In Figure 4, the data from Carlson et al. (1958) are redrawn. The fatter subjects are better able to keep warm, because of the smaller heat transfer across the skin per degree difference between body core and skin or water temperature. In a study by Canon and Keatinge (1960), the fattest subject could tolerate a water temperature 10°C below his core temperature without shivering during rest, while the thinnest could tolerate no more than 3.8°C below his body temperature before he started to shiver.

After skin blood flow has been shut down, the next line of defense against cooling is to increase heat production by shivering and thereby

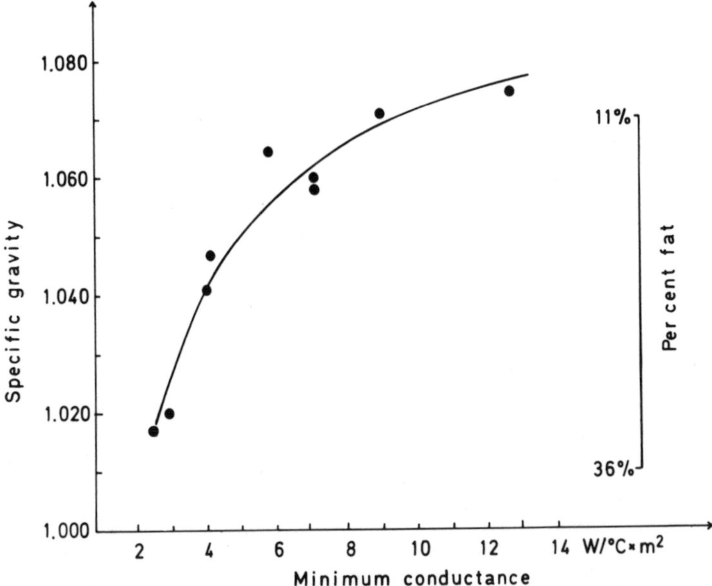


Figure 4. The relationship between minimum conductance and body fat is here expressed as a specific gravity and fat in percent of body weight (after Carlson et al., 1958).

maintain the heat balance. Shivering heat production is added to the heat production of any ongoing activity, e.g., swimming. In Subject R (Figure 5), the oxygen uptake can increase 0.5 liter by shivering both in rest and during swimming.

Figure 6 shows the events during an experiment. During swimming in the 16°C cold water, core temperatures fell; after about 15 min, the decrease was almost linear. Oxygen uptakes measured at 10-min intervals increased from the first to the second samples, and leveled off despite the continuous fall in core temperature. The subject then walked to a climatic chamber and started to exercise on a bicycle ergometer. When the core temperature began to rise, shivering stopped and oxygen uptake returned to normal, although the core temperature was still very low, below the normal exercise temperature. In a resting subject (Figure 7), the core temperature changed very little in cold water; the subject was shivering, however, and thereby increasing his oxygen uptake about 1 liter/min. In the warm (40°C) climatic chamber, the core temperature began to fall faster. These "reversed" core temperature changes are attributable to the shift in heat stores between "core" and shell, caused by the vasodilation in the skin in the warm environment. In the warm air, shivering ceased almost immediately when the skin became warm.

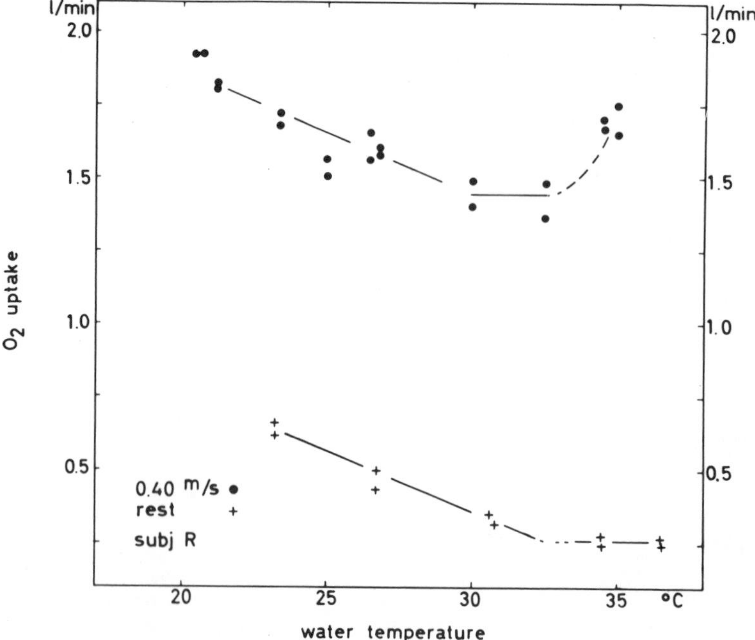


Figure 5. Oxygen uptake is given in liters/min during rest and swimming 0.4 m/sec at different water temperatures (from Nielsen, 1973).

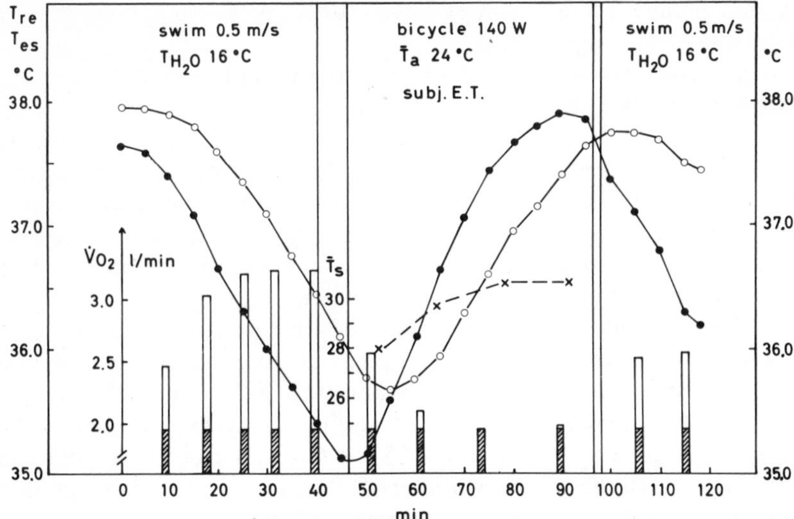


Figure 6. Core temperatures, mean skin temperature, and oxygen uptake are shown for swimming at 16° water temperature and bicycling at 24° air temperature ($T_{re}$ = o, $T_{es}$ = • , $\overline{T}_s$ = x). Shading on the oxygen uptake bars denotes the oxygen uptake at the given activity in thermoneutral environmental conditions (from Nielsen, 1976).

The water temperature at which a swimmer begins to shiver depends upon the activity level, i.e., heat production during swimming, and also on the individual's subcutaneous fat layers. It is worth mentioning that in six subjects swimming at constant speeds, each at 60–65% of their $\dot{V}_{O_2}$ max and at 21, 27, and 33°C, each had his lowest

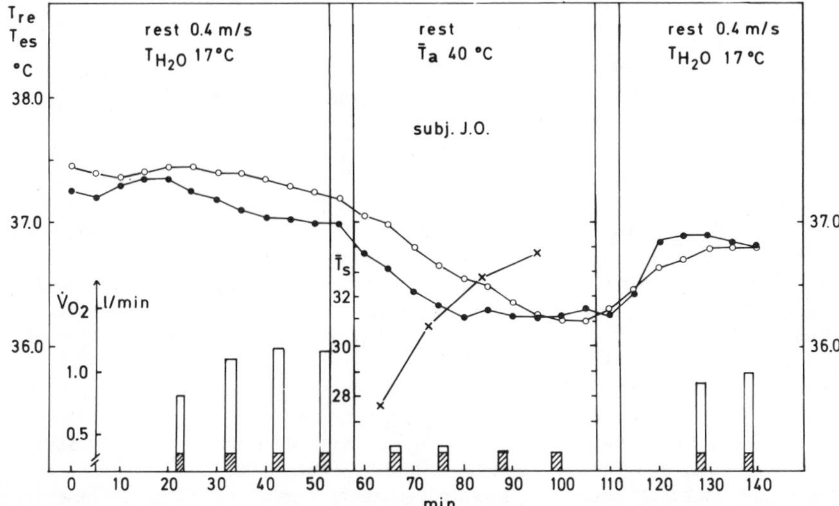


Figure 7. Data comparable to those depicted in Figure 6 are given here for a subject resting at 17° water temperature and 40° air temperature (from Nielsen, 1976).

oxygen uptake but his highest heart rate at 33°C water temperature (Houston et al., in preparation).

Shivering is elicited from the thermoregulation center when the core temperature tends to fall. However, even with very low core temperatures (34°C), shivering is abolished if the skin is warmed to above 30–32°C. The precise relationship between thermal stimulus and the response, shivering, is very difficult to establish because different body parts cool and rewarm at different rates, and thermosensitive nerve endings from all these areas may contribute sensory information to the temperature centers and modify their action.

Despite vigorous shivering, the body temperature of a swimmer will fall in cold water. The time required for the decrease in temperature will vary, depending on the temperature of the water, the activity level of the swimmer, and his/her insulating fat layers. Eventually, the core temperature will sink below 35°, where symptoms like euphoria and loss of reason are early warnings of the approaching disintegration of physiological and behavioral thermoregulation.

## REFERENCES

Boutelier, C. 1973. Echanges thermiques du corps humain dans l'eau. Thése.

Bullard, R. W., and Rapp, G. M. 1970. Problems of body heat loss in water immersion. Aerospace Med. 41:1269–1277.

Burton, A. C., and Bazett, H. C. 1936. A study of the average temperature of the tissues, of the exchange of heat and vasomotor responses in man by means of a bath calorimeter. Am. J. Physiol. 117:36–54.

Canon, P., and Keatinge, W. R. 1960. Metabolic rate and heat loss of fat and thin men in heat balance in cold and warm water. J. Physiol. 154:329–344.

Carlson, L. D., Hsieh, A. C. L., Fullington, F., and Elsner, R. W. 1958. Immersion in cold water and body tissue isolation. J. Aviation. Med. 29:145–152.

Houston, M., Nielson, B., Nygaard, E., and Saltin, B. Metabolic and hormonal responses to submaximal swimming at three different water temperatures. In preparation.

Keatinge, W. R. 1959. The effects of work. clothing, and adaptation on the maintenance of the body temperature in water and on reflex responses to immersion. Doctoral thesis. University of Cambridge.

Keatinge, W. R. 1961. The effect of work and clothing on the maintenance of the body temperature in water. Q. J. Exp. Physiol. 46:69–82.

Nadel, E. R., Holmér, I., Bergh, U., Åstrand, P.-O., and Stolwijk, J. A. J. 1974. Energy exchange of swimming man. J. Appl. Physiol. 36:465–471.

Nielsen, B. 1973. Metabolic reactions to cold during swimming at different speeds. Arch. Sci. Physiol. 27:A207–A211.

Nielsen, B. 1976. Metabolic reactions to changes in core and skin temperature in man. Acta Physiol. Scand. 97:129–138.

Nielsen, B., and Davies, C. T. M. 1976. Temperature regulation during exercise in water and air. Acta Physiol. Scand. 98:500–508.

Saltin, B., and Hermansen, L. 1966. Esophageal, rectal, and muscle temperature during exercise. J. Appl. Physiol. 21:1757–1762.

Winterspoon, J., Goldman, R. F., and Breckenridge, J. R. 1971. Heat transfer coefficients of humans in cold water. J.Physiol. (Paris) 63:459–462.

# Cold Immersion: Survival and Resuscitation

**W. R. Keatinge**

Most competitive swimming takes place in water that is warm enough to cause no thermal problems for the swimmer. However, long distance and recreational swims often take place in natural lakes or in the open sea, where water temperatures are usually low enough to cause death by hypothermia if the individual is of slim build and the swim is unduly prolonged. An ability to maintain body temperature at a safe level is therefore essential for anyone embarking on swims of this kind. Much of the information about the factors that determine whether a particular individual will maintain body temperature in water was obtained to assist survival after shipwreck, but it applies to swims of prolonged duration, as well.

The main background fact is that water carries heat away from the body much more effectively than air does, by both conduction and convection. The result is that once people are immersed in water without external protection, insulation outside the body virtually disappears. Body heat loss then depends on the amount of internal insulation, and this in turn depends mainly on the thickness of the layer of fat under the skin. Pugh and Edholm (1955) found, for example, that channel swimmers were relatively fat, and cold immersion experiments showed a close correlation between people's body cooling rates and their subcutaneous fat thicknesses. The reason for this was that blood flow through the skin and fat was rapidly shut off when the cold immersion started. The skin and the subcutaneous fat under it therefore became an almost inert layer of insulation, and the rate of body heat loss then depended largely on how thick this layer was. As a result, with immersions in water at 15°C, the thinnest people cooled as much as 2°C (4°F) in 30 min, while the fattest lost virtually no heat at all.

The effect of exercise also became clear from immersion studies of this kind, although it was somewhat more complicated. Exercise increased body temperature in water warmer than 24°C just as it does in air, but in colder water it accelerated body cooling. The reason was that, although exercise increased heat production by about the same amount at all water temperatures, it decreased tissue insulation by increasing blood flow: the colder the water, the more heat the blood carried to the surface of the body. Exercise therefore caused a net increase in the rate of body cooling when the water was cold enough. The main practical conclusion from a long series of experiments of this kind was that when anyone, fat or thin, was in water too cold for body temperature to stabilize, exercise always accelerated body cooling. Exercise never helped survival and often did harm.

The other major piece of information from such experiments was that when temperature was very cold, below about 12°C, there was a partial failure of vasoconstriction. Fat men, whose fat could theoretically provide plenty of subcutaneous insulation, in practice started to increase heat loss from the extremities after about 40 min in water at 5°C. Once this had happened, they cooled steadily in spite of increased heat production through shivering. This loss of vasoconstriction is called cold vasodilation and is caused by cold paralysis of the peripheral blood vessels. No way has yet been found to stop the blood vessels from becoming paralyzed at low temperatures, but they can be prevented from cooling to the critical level by quite small amounts of external insulation. Ordinary clothes do not provide much insulation in the water, but the little that they do provide generally kept skin temperature above the level at which the vessels become paralyzed. Clothing therefore greatly reduced body cooling, usually by well over 50%, despite the rather small amount of insulation that it provided in water.

These results, therefore, produced the practical advice that survivors do better to put on thick clothes in addition to life jackets before going into the water, and that, if they have to wait long for rescue, they should float in the life jackets rather than swim about. If this advice is given at the right time, more can probably be accomplished by it than in any other way to reduce deaths from accidents at sea. The Lakonia survey showed that without advice people generally did the wrong thing: they took off clothing and exercised in the water to try to keep warm. Hayward and his colleagues (1973) have more recently shown that heat loss can be further reduced by hunching up in the water, and by keeping the group of survivors close together.

Children are particularly at risk. It was found that during training swims in water at 20°C, the youngest children cooled fastest, and the boys cooled faster than did the girls, because the younger children were generally thinnest and boys were generally thinner than girls; these differences varied with age and sex and were not simply a result of the smaller body size of the youngest children. It was interesting that they began to shiver seriously only when body temperatures fell below 35–36°C. These low body temperatures do no harm in themselves, but children, particularly small boys, are clearly very much at risk during any accident in water in which they cannot leave the water as they cool down. Any child adrift in the water, even one wearing a life jacket or clinging to a float, should be considered a major emergency requiring immediate rescue.

After rescue, it should be emphasized first that the treatment in acute immersion hypothermia is different not only from the treatment for drowning, but also from the treatment of cases of prolonged exposure in the hills. The main reason that healthy people die when they are cooled in water to near 20°C within 1–2 hr is a decrease in the output of the heart with slowing of its rate and the inadequate filling of its ventricles. This eventually leads to death from tissue anoxia. If the temperature of the heart falls to about 10°C, its activity ceases altogether. The important point about these events in regard to treatment is that for a time they are reversible. Provided the patient is rewarmed before there is permanent tissue damage from lack of oxygen, everything can return to normal. The most remarkable case reported involved a woman who was cooled to 9°C, suffered complete cardiac arrest for 1 hr, and recovered to an apparently normal state when warmed.

The other major hazard to life during hypothermia is ventricular fibrillation. Its causes are complex, but a reduced energy supply to the heart muscle in the cold seems to be the main factor. Treatment principles are simple: rewarm the patient out of the danger zone as soon as possible without doing anything that can precipitate fibrillation. This ideally means getting the patient into a hot bath, as hot as is tolerable to the hand, as soon as it is certain that he/she is suffering from cold rather than drowning. People with body temperatures near or below 30°C can usually be recognized without a thermometer because they are confused and have slow pulse and respiration rates. One thing to avoid is any unnecessary manipulation of the throat such as the insertion of a laryngeal airway or an esophageal probe. These cause reflex vagal slowing of the heart and are likely to precipitate ventricular fibrillation. The airway must be clear, of course, but if its clearing is necessary, it must be done with the greatest care. It is also important not to give cardiac massage or artificial ventilation merely because the spontaneous heart and respiration rates are slow; sudden overventilation and trauma to the heart are also likely to precipitate fibrillation, as can manipulation of the limbs, probably by overloading the heart with a rapid return of acid blood from the periphery. The only circumstances in which cardiac massage and artificial ventilation may be beneficial in hypothermia are when it is certain that the heart has stopped or is already in ventricular fibrillation. Even then, rewarming without cardiac massage will sometimes restore normal function.

Therefore, the best treatment is usually to put the hypothermia victim into a hot bath, clear the airway if necessary, and otherwise disturb him/her as little as possible. If it is impossible to get a hot bath quickly, the next best solution is a warm room and dry blankets. One of the devices available for warming inspired air can also help a little if the patient cannot be taken to a warm room. In any case, it is safest not to continue a hot bath longer than approximately 20 min, provided the patient is obviously improving by that time; otherwise, there is some risk of a serious fall in blood pressure. For the same reason the patient should be kept prone after leaving the hot bath.

Once equipment is available, it is important to have a reliable measure of body temperature. Mouth temperature is not reliable in the cold. Temperature can be measured by a rectal probe, but the rectal reading lags seriously when the body temperature is changing fast. For prolonged monitoring in conscious people, a probe in the external auditory meatus is preferred, with a simple servocontrolled battery heating unit over the ear to eliminate external cooling. The probe is packed lightly 10 mm into the meatus with cotton wool, and an earpiece over the head keeps the temperature outside the ear at the same level as is recorded in the meatus. The device takes some minutes to stabilize, but then tracks cardiac temperature almost as well as esophageal probes do. At a later stage it is useful to monitor the ECG and blood chemistry, but usually the patient is either recovering rapidly or irretrievably dead by the time these methods can be made available. It is the immediate treatment that will normally have determined whether or not the patient survives.

Many of the deaths in inland waters occur too rapidly for hypothermia to be responsible. A few of them can be explained by sudden ventricular fibrillation of the heart during the first few minutes of immersion, caused by intense reflexes from the cooled skin. However, the great majority of rapid deaths in cold water are attributable to drowning, even in good swimmers. Breathing is severely disturbed during the first few minutes of cold immersion, to such a degree that many people find it impossible to control their breathing voluntarily during that time. Any pattern of swimming that involves the head going under water is impossible while this lasts, and total immersion by a wave can cause immediate drowning.

Even in calm water, good swimmers were unable to swim far in water at 4.7°C (Figure 1). Swimming clothed, one of them suddenly floundered, sank, and had to be rescued after only 1.5 min and all four that were studied had to give up and be pulled out within 12 min. The

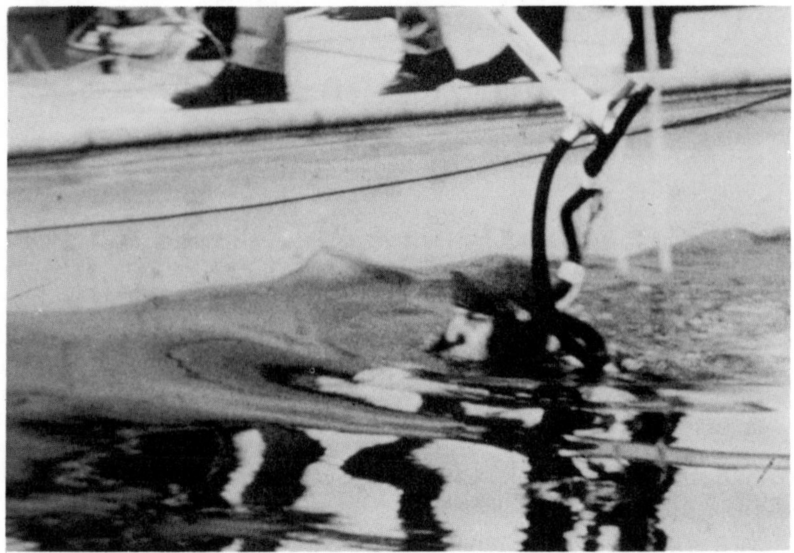

Figure 1. Respiration, body temperature, and electrocardiogram are monitored in a cold swim experiment.

main reason for their collapse was exhaustion caused by the high viscosity of cold water that makes swimming more tiring than in water at higher temperatures. The people who became exhausted and collapsed first were the thinnest and fittest, because, being thin, they had a high specific gravity and had to swim hard to keep above water. In the viscous, cold water, this exhausted them quickly, while the fat people with their greater bouyancy could swim at a slower rate that could be sustained longer. The practical conclusions, of course, are that it is dangerous to try to swim even short distances in very cold water without support. Accidental deaths of this type can be almost entirely prevented if small boat enthusiasts always wear life jackets, particularly in winter.

## REFERENCES

Hayward, J. S., Collis, M., and Eckerson, J. D. 1973. Thermographic evaluation of relative heat loss areas of man during cold immersion. Aerospace Med. 44:708–711.

Keatinge, W. R. 1969. Survival in Cold Water. Blackwell Scientific Publications.

Pugh, L. G. C., and Edholm, O. G. 1955. The physiology of channel swimmers. Lancet 2:761–768.

Sloan, R. E. G., and Keatinge, W. R. 1973. Cooling rates of young people swimming in cold water. J. Appl. Physiol. 35:371–375.

Treatment of Immersion Hypothermia. 1976. London University Audiovisual Centre, London. Videotape.

# Sudden Cold Water Immersion

**R. C. Goode, T. T. Romet, J. Duffin, R. R. Bechbache, D. A. Cunningham, and W. O'Hara**

Drowning is one of the major causes of accidental death, and cold water can hasten this process (Cold Water Symposium, 1976). Exhaustion and fatal drownings are known to occur in the first few minutes of exposure. While much information is available on long term exposure (Burton and Edholm, 1955; Keatinge, 1969; Hayward, Eckerson, and Collis, 1975) little information is available on the acute respiratory and circulatory effects of sudden cold water immersion, and no information is available on the acute effects of complete immersion on unclothed man.

The study of the first few minutes of immersion provides data not available from prolonged immersion studies, especially because all such previous studies have involved gradual immersion and not an abrupt change such as that involved in a fall into cold water.

## PROCEDURE AND RESULTS

In the first of two series of experiments this chapter describes (Goode et al., 1975), 26 experiments were performed on eight men aged 20–34 years. The subjects were dressed in bikini style bathing suits (both series) and climbed down a ladder to a point just above the water level. After 2–3 min, they dropped into the water on a signal from the experimenter. Once the subject was immersed, the water level would reach the neck while the subject was standing. Water temperatures for test and control experiments in the incomplete and complete immersion studies were 8–10°C and 30°C, respectively. The subjects were told the water temperature before immersion. None of the subjects had been immersed into such cold water before.

---

This work was supported by a grant from the Defense Research Board of Canada.

Figures 1a and 1b show a segment of the record from one experiment. The arrow indicates when the subject entered the water. In Figure 2, breath-by-breath inspired ventilation (volume of inspiration/ time for inspiration + time for expiration) for a 60-sec period as plotted against breath number is graphically shown. There was a substantial ($P < 0.001$) change in ventilation on immersion in cold water. The mean ventilations for all eight subjects on the first three breaths following cold water immersion were 94.5, 71.3, and 94.6 liters/min, compared with 60.0, 36.3, and 38.5 liters/min for warm water immersion. Alveolar $CO_2$ decreased from a pre-immersion value of 36.4 to 23.9 mm Hg on the gasp breath (initial breath on immersion), and was less than 30 mm Hg for the next nine breaths. While all subjects showed large increases in ventilation and decreases in $P_{ACO_2}$, Subject 101 showed the smallest change in ventilation (60.2, 72.6, and 43.4 liters/min on the first, second, and third breaths during immersion in cold water). The subject stated that he had been taught to reduce his ventilation on immersion in cold water in a wet suit when breathing by means of scuba apparatus and had attempted the same maneuver in this experiment. The apparent success of this subject would suggest that the initial drive to breathe can be overriden and with the relatively decreased ventilation there will be comparatively less change in the $P_{ACO_2}$.

In the second series (complete immersion), 10 experiments were performed on five volunteer subjects 22– 35 years of age. Four of the five were unaware of the purpose of the experiment. The subjects sat in a boswain's chair while breathing through respiratory apparatus. Blood pressure was measured automatically by a cuff technique at 15-sec intervals (Duffin, 1977).

Fifty ml of venous blood was drawn from the forearm for the catecholamine assay (Griffiths, Leung, and McDonald, 1970) immediately prior to the placing of the chair directly above the water by means of a small crane and winch arrangement. When the ventilation and heart rate were steady, the subject was dropped abruptly by releasing the lock on the winch. The subject was completely immersed within 6–8 sec such that the top of the head was approximately 6 inches below the water surface (Figure 3). After 1.5 min of immersion, the subject was brought to the surface and an additional 50 ml of venous blood was drawn.

Figures 4a and 4b show a segment of the record for the complete immersion experiment. Blood pressure and heart rate are shown on the top records, heart rate being indicated by a vertical movement of the pen. Systolic and diastolic blood pressure were determined from the first and last heart rates, respectively, after each inflation of the cuff

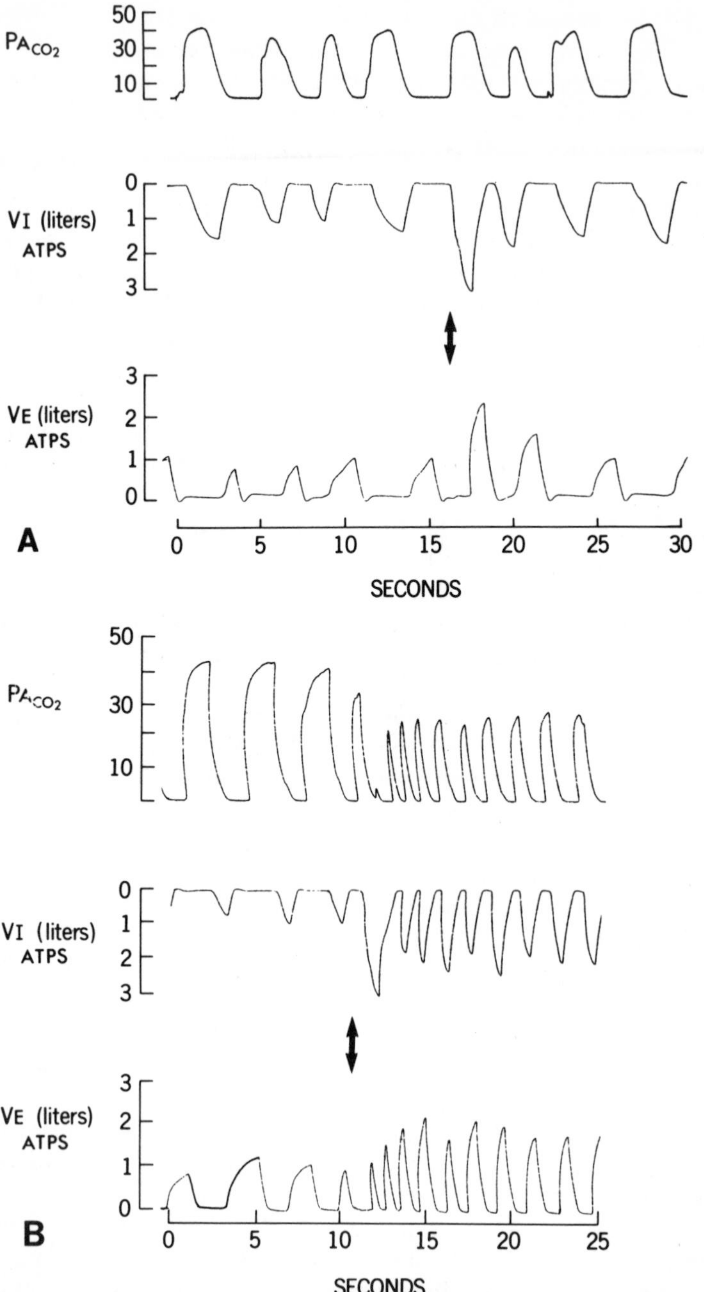


Figure 1. Shown are experimental records of alveolar $P_{CO_2}$ and breath-by-breath inspired and expired ventilation in warm water (28°C) Figure a, and cold water (10°C) Figure b for immersion to neck level. The arrow indicates when the subject dropped into the water.

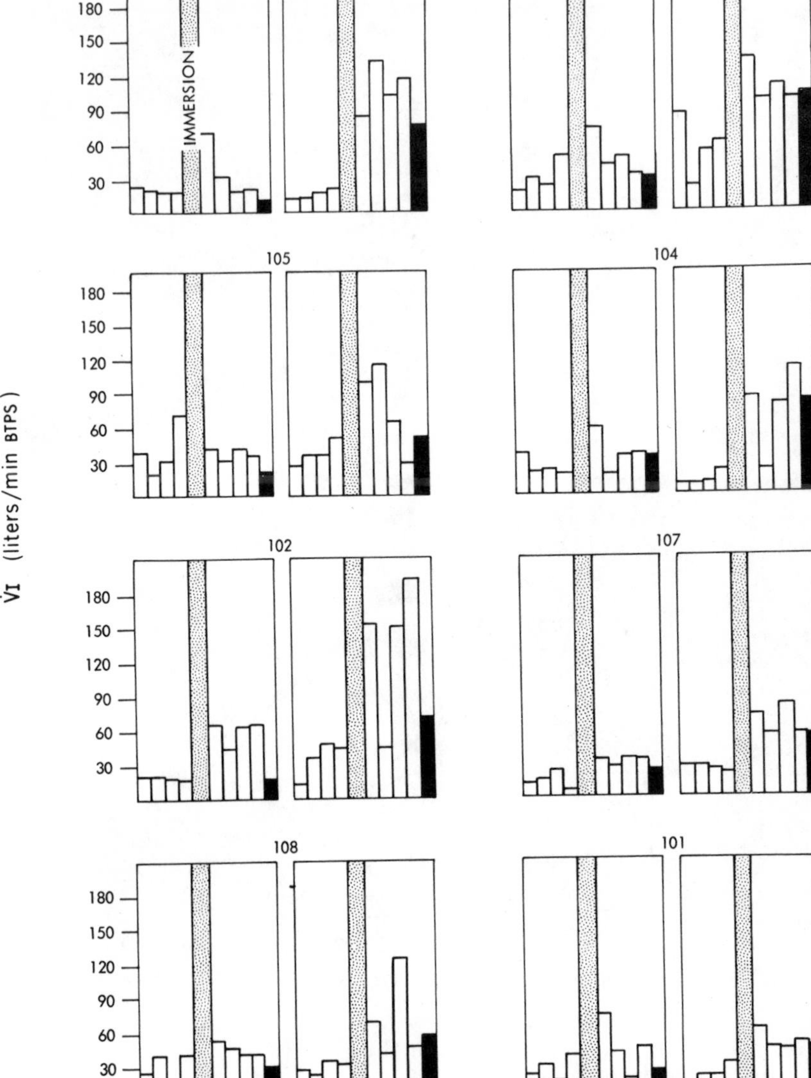


Figure 2. Breath-by-breath ventilation is given for before and after immersion to the neck level (Temperatures: control, 28°C; test 10°C). Hatched line indicates when the drop occurred. Solid black bars represent the mean ventilation in breaths 5–9.

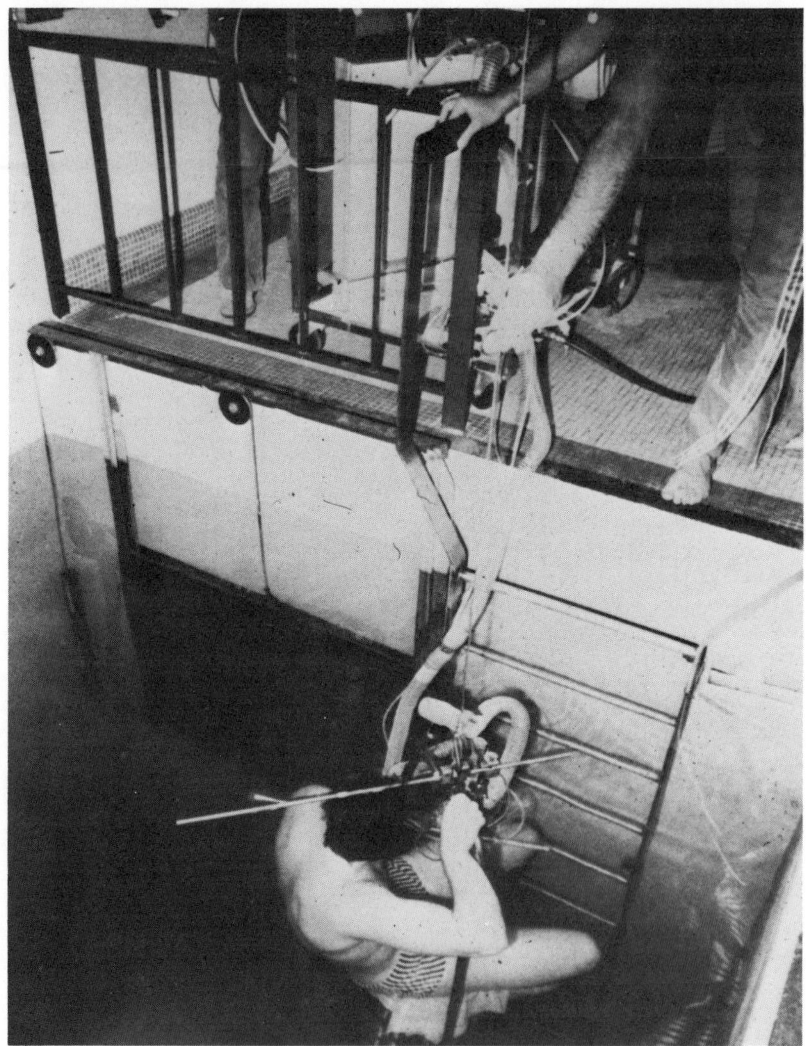

Figure 3. This photograph shows a subject immersed 6 inches below the water surface.

(Geddes, 1970). $P_{ACO_2}$ is shown on the middle tracings and inspired ventilation on the bottom lines.

Resting heart rates were slightly elevated for three subjects prior to immersion and showed an increase upon immersion, with the greatest increase observed after cold water immersion. The two subjects who had the highest recorded maximal oxygen uptakes (53 and 51 ml/Kg/min) had significantly lower resting heart rates and showed no

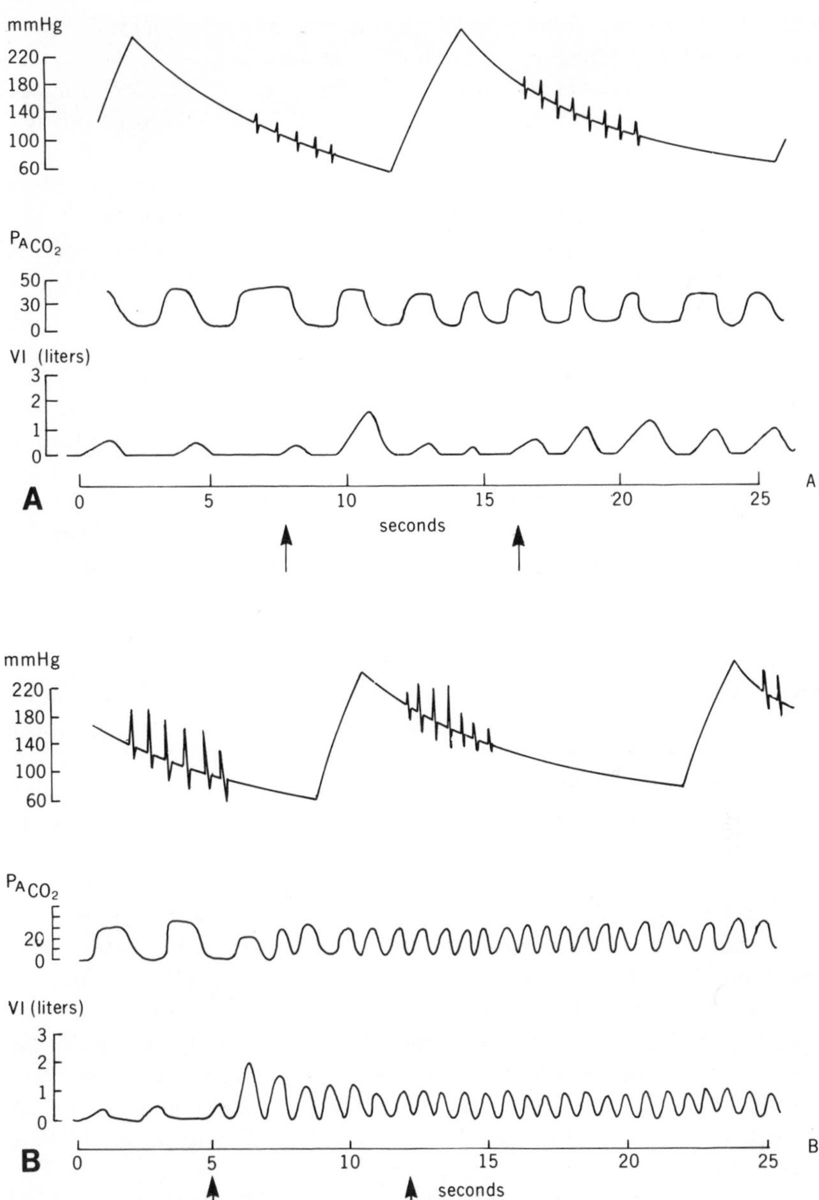


Figure 4. Given are experimental records of blood pressure, alveolar $P_{CO_2}$, and inspired breath-by-breath ventilation for controls (Figure 4A at 33°C) and test subjects (Figure 4B, at 8°C). Postimmersion blood pressure recordings require the subtraction of 40 mm Hg to accommodate the hydrostatic pressure increase induced by the external water column. The arrows indicate the time for immersion to occur.

change in heart rate in the control experiment and only a slight increase (approximately 10 beats/min) upon cold immersion.

Blood pressures at rest were normal for all subjects except Subject 105, who was mildly hypertensive. Blood pressure showed no change in warm immersion except for the previously mentioned two fit subjects who showed a slight drop (110/65 to 100/40 and 120/65 to 110/40 mm Hg). Systolic pressures showed significant increases upon cold immersion without change in diastolic pressure. The mildly hypertensive subject (105) showed the highest systolic value (180 mm Hg) but also had the highest initial heart rate and lowest $\dot{V}O_2$ max (26 ml/Kg/min).

As observed in the first series, cold immersion produced significantly higher ventilations. The average ventilation during the immersion phase (approximately 7 sec) in the cold water was significantly higher than control values (87.2 liters/min versus 30.2 liters/min). Ventilation in the control series returned to near resting levels within 30 sec. In the cold immersion, ventilation was elevated throughout (78 liters/min average of the five last breaths before removal) (Figure 5).

## DISCUSSION

The large, abrupt increase in ventilation on sudden immersion in cold water as compared with the corresponding control immersion in warm water ($P < 0.001$) was statistically significant. Cold water immersion was associated with an immediate and prolonged decrease in alveolar $CO_2$ and, over a longer exposure period, considerable weakness, as compared with immersion in warm water.

Previous workers in similar experiments observed increases in ventilation with cold water immersion and cold showers (Schneider, 1957; Keatinge, McIlroy, and Goldfien, 1964). Those increases were substantially less than the ones observed in this study (28 liters/min as compared with 86.8 liters/min). This is most likely a result of previous investigators' averaging for a period of 1 min as compared with this study's calculation of ventilation on a breath-to-breath basis. The average ventilation for the first three breaths for 4 sec of exposure ($N = 8$) in the previous series (Goode et al.) was 86.8 $P_{ACO_2}$ 27 mm Hg for TORR, versus 94.0 in the present complete immersion series ($N = 5$). The large difference in ventilation between these results and those of earlier investigations are a result of the period over which the ventilation observed was measured and must be considered in estimating the potential drive to breathe caused by cold water immersion.

The initial ventilatory drive is neurogenic; the increase in ventilation occurred on contact with the water in all subjects. The response is

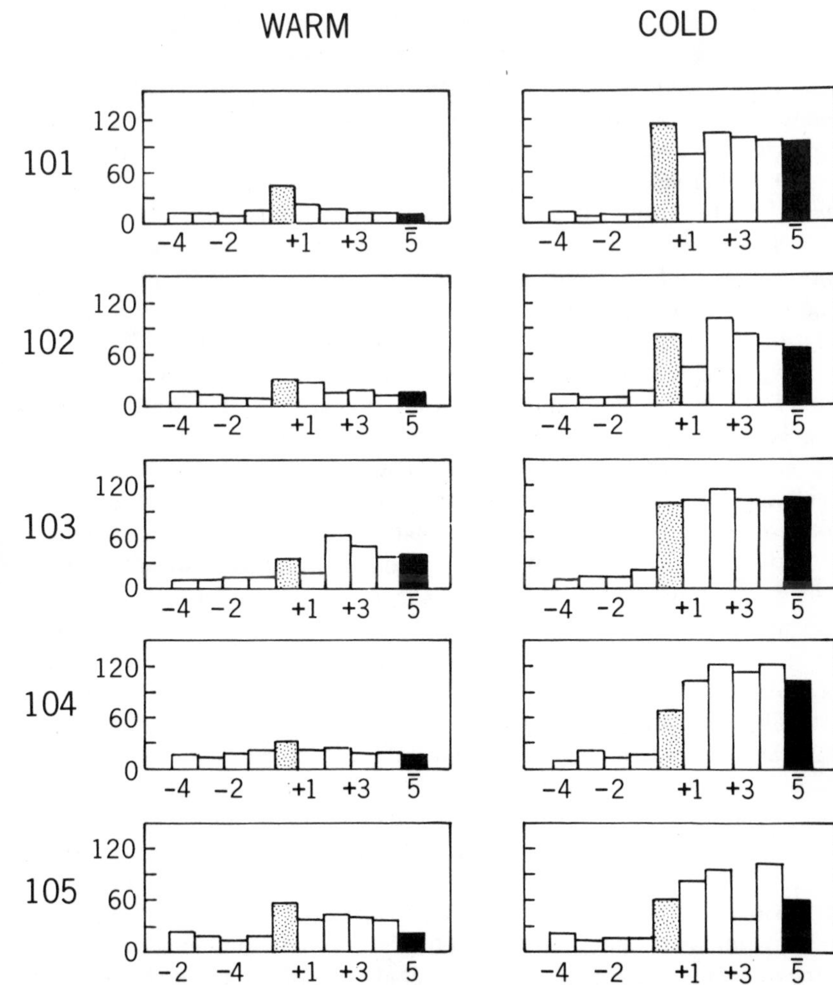


Figure 5. Breath-by-breath ventilation in liters/min for warm (33°C) and cold (8°C) immersion is given for five subjects. The hatched bar represents the mean ventilation during the 7-sec immersion period. Solid black bar represents the mean ventilation in breaths 5–9.

likely a consequence of reflex action from receptors in the skin affecting the respiratory center.

Sudden complete immersion in cold water results in large increases in systolic pressure. These increases, however, are not as large as those experienced in heavy exercise (~180 and higher mm Hg), and are also less than a previously unpublished value of 200 mm Hg. During cold water showers, Keatinge, McIlroy, and Goldfien observed systolic blood pressure rising to a mean of 175 mm Hg from a pretest level of 134 mm Hg, using an indwelling arterial catheter. Systolic blood pressure rose by the first reading some 8 sec after immersion, and after 1 min had begun to plateau. In the present study, the mean systolic value rose to 160 mm Hg, some 12–15 mm Hg lower than that during cold water showers as reported by Keatinge et al. While diastolic blood pressure increased in the subjects reported by those authors (78 to 93 mm Hg), this study did not reveal a significant change.

Systolic blood pressure did not significantly change in warm water immersion, but diastolic pressure did. Diastolic blood pressure is known to be primarily dependent on total peripheral resistance. A 30% decrease in resistance was reported (Arborelius et al., 1972) under experimental conditions similar to those used here (i.e., warm water).

The increase in circulating noradrenaline with cold water immersion is suggestive of a large increase in sympathetic activity. This activity may account for some of the observed increases in heart rate, systolic blood pressure, and ventilation. Any increases in diastolic blood pressure that occurred as a result of large increases in sympathetic activity may not be apparent because of the effects of adrenaline, which under physiological doses can cause a drop in diastolic pressure (Seeman and Sellers, 1975). The single subject (103) in whom there was an increase in diastolic pressure did not have an increase in the amount of adrenaline.

The adrenaline values before and after cold water immersion were well above resting values in two subjects. While it was reported (Keatinge, McIlroy, and Goldfien, 1964) that no important release of catecholamines occurs with partial cold water exposure, resting values were 10 times higher than reported in this study. Present results suggest that there is a large significant release of noradrenaline, and that adrenaline may be elevated prior to immersion as a consequence of anticipation and is likely to show a further increase following cold water exposure. With the stimulus of severe cold, it is not surprising the elevated adrenaline values were maintained throughout the experiment.

Venous blood samples for the estimation of plasma catecholamines reflect primarily the local concentration at the site from which they are sampled. While it is not possible to estimate the circulating catecholamine levels accurately from venous samples, it is possible to indicate changes in direction. There is no apparent reason to believe other peripheral regions are acting differently in these cold water experiments.

## PROLONGED EXPOSURE

Two subjects were dropped into neck high water at 8°C. Compared with results of brief exposure experiments at 11.1°C, there was no substantial difference in the magnitude of gasp breath or breaths 2–5 following immersion. In the first minute, ventilation reached an average value of 48.8 liters/min; during the second minute, it fell to 29.0 liters/min and then climbed to ~35 liters/min for the next 3–5 min.

A further stimulus to respiration is the increase in shivering, which was quite evident in the 4th and 5th min of prolonged exposure for one subject. Both subjects had difficulty in climbing out of the tank, experienced much physical weakness and local areas of pain in the legs (end of 3 min and 5 min). A change in grip strength of 1.8% per min after 5 min was reported by Cooper (1976). This change does not seem sufficient to account for the obvious weakness experienced by present subjects. Cooper suggests the reduction in muscular strength could be related to the nerve-muscle temperature. The conducting velocity in the ulnar nerve is decreased with cold water immersion, and the delay between direct electrical stimulation of a muscle and the occurrence of the muscular twitch is prolonged.

The marked increase in desire to breathe upon immersion (whether immersed completely or to the neck) is likely to interfere greatly with the presently taught survival technique called drownproofing (Lanoue, 1963), in which the head is immersed and the body maintained in a relaxed position until a breath is required. The prolonged exposure experiment in which the subjects were stationary suggests it would be most difficult to continue drownproofing where a considerable urge to breathe is combined with local areas of pain in the limbs. Collis (1976) reported that rectal temperature fell more quickly (1°C in 0.5 hr) in a group performing drownproofing compared with a group treading water with heads above the surface. The fact that the head was not immersed and the increased metabolic rate as a consequence of the treading activity presumably interacted to prevent the same amount of decline in the water treading group (final rectal temperature after 30 min: 36.3°C, treading water; 35.4°C drownproofing). In addition, the activity associated with treading water is likely to promote blood flow in the limbs, increasing skin and muscle temperature and possibly reducing the incidence of pain. As a result of these findings, the Royal Life Saving Society does not recommend drownproofing be used as the primary survival technique and has recommended treading water be taught instead. In addition, the increased metabolic activity is likely to promote an increase in blood flow to the limbs with a resulting increase in temperature that might be sufficient to offset, fully or partially, some of the physical weakness observed. More work is required to establish these points.

With such a drive to breathe (40 liters/min at the end of 1 min, increasing to ~35 liters/min at 5 min in a motionless subject with head above water), it would be difficult to assume a relaxed swimming posture with the face in the water (e.g., as in the front crawl). Observations of two swimmers in cold water during the first minute support this. This inappropriate posture, that is, face and usually most of the head out of the water, prevents proper body position (body and head parallel to the surface of the water). An erect head position does not permit adequate displacement of water and its increase in the buoyant force that would partially or wholly offset the effects of gravity on the head. Energy is thus wasted in keeping the head erect. These factors, accompanied by an increase in the viscosity of water with a decline in temperature (0.83 centipoises at 28°C; 1.00 cp at 20°C; 1.3 cp at 11°C) and possible general muscular weakness, would interfere with the ability to swim any distance in cold water. Collis, without considering the above factors, but solely concerned with core temperature, observed a decline in body temperature of 1°C for each 0.25 mi of swimming with kapok flotation at a water temperature of 10°C. At a core temperature of approximately 33.5°C, coordinated swimming movements become progressively difficult. Using clothed swimming subjects, it was reported (Keatinge, 1976) that rescue had to take place in one subject after 1.5 min in cold water, an interval much shorter than the projected 1 hr with flotation. Thus, deep body temperature, for some individuals, is only one factor in survival time. The drive to breathe on exposure to cold is most likely a major contributing factor toward the inability of skin divers to stay under cold water as long as they can under warm conditions.

In addition to the possibility of exhaustion in cold water, three other mechanisms associated with the large increase in ventilation on immersion in cold water may bring about death. Sudden death has been attributed to vagal arrest of heart action following the inhalation of cold water in the nasopharynx and glottis (Simpson, 1958). A second mechanism involves the inhalation of water leading to death by drowning (Timperman, 1962; Neidhart and Greendyke, 1967). And third, large falls in arterial carbon dioxide pressure, such as observed here, are also associated with ventricular fibrillation in man and in dogs (Brown and Miller, 1952; Miller et al., 1952; and Gerst, Fleming, and Malm, 1966; Rose, 1969). Arrhythmias are common on initial exposure to cold water and it is possible that the large change in $P_{ACO_2}$ may play a role in these changes. The failure to see such a large change in ventilation and in $P_{ACO_2}$ in one subject, who successfully prevented large changes in tidal volume and frequency by controlling his breathing, suggests that it is possible to a great extent to override the urge to breathe on contact with cold water. This would prevent large changes in $P_{ACO_2}$ and could diminish the likelihood of arrhythmias occurring.

## ACKNOWLEDGMENTS

The authors thank the Defense and Civil Institute for Environmental Medicine in Toronto, Canada, for use of their facilities.

## REFERENCES

Arborelius, M., Jr., Balldin, U. I., Lilja, F., and Lundgren, C. E. 1972. Hemodynamic changes in men during immersion with the head above water. Aerospace Med. 43:592–593.

Brown, E. B., and Miller, F. 1952. Ventricular fibrillation following a rapid fall in alveolar carbon dioxide concentration. Am. J. Physiol. 169:56–60.

Burton, A. C., and Edholm, D. G. 1955. Man in a Cold Environment. Edward Arnold Ltd., London. pp. 200–222.

Cold Water Symposium 1976. Survival behaviour in cold water immersion. Cold Water Symposium, Toronto. pp. 25–27.

Collis, M. 1976. Survival behaviour in cold water immersion. Cold Water Symposium, pp. 25–27. Toronto.

Cooper, K. E. 1976. Respiratory and thermal responses to cold water immersion. Cold Water Symposium, Toronto. pp. 23–24.

Duffin, J. 1977. Fluidics and pneumatics principles and applications in anesthesia. Can. Anesth. Soc. J. 24:126–141.

Geddes, L. A. 1970. Direct and Indirect Measurement of Blood Pressure. Year Book Medical Publications, Ltd., Chicago.

Gerst, P. H., Fleming, M. D., and Malm, J. R. 1966. Increased susceptibility of the heart to ventricular fibrillation during metabolic acidosis. Circ. Res. 19:65–70.

Goode, R. C., Duffin, J., Miller, R., Romet, T. T., Chant, W., and Ackles, K. 1975. Sudden cold water immersion. Resp. Physiol. 23:301–310.

Griffiths, J. C., Leung, F. Y. T., and McDonald, T. J. 1970. Fluorimetric determination of plasma catecholamines: Normal human epinephrine and norepinephrine levels. Clin. Chim. Acta 30:395–405.

Hayward, J. S., Eckerson, J. D., and Collis, M. 1975. Thermal balance and survival time predication of man in cold water. Can. J. Physiol. Pharmacol. 53:21–32.

Keatinge, W. R., McIlroy, M. B., and Goldfien, A. 1964. Cardiovascular responses to ice-cold showers. J. Appl. Physiol. 19:1145–1149.

Keatinge, W. R. 1969. Survival in Cold Water. Blackwell Scientific Publications, Ltd., Oxford.

Keatinge, W. R. 1976. The concept of hypothermia. Cold Water Symposium, Toronto. pp. 15–18.

Lanoue, F. 1963. Drownproofing. Prentice Hall, Inc., Englewood Cliffs, N.J.

Miller, F. A., Brown, E. B., Buckely, J. J., Van Bergen, F. H., and Varco, R. L. 1952. Respiratory acidosis: Its relationship to cardiac function and other physiologic mechanisms. Surgery 32:172–183.

Neidhart, D. A., and Greendyke, R. M. 1967. The significance of diatom demonstration in the diagnosis of death by drowning. Am. J. Clin. Pathol. 48:377–382.

Rose, K. D. 1969. Telemetry in the study of the heart in athletes. Part II. In: C. F. Reynolds, G. T. Aitken, M. B. Coventry, and C. V. Heck (eds.), American Academy of Orthopaedic Surgeons Symposium on Sports Medicine, pp. 51-61. C. V. Mosby, St. Louis.

Schneider, U. 1957. Kalter Hautreig and Atmung. Hippokrates 28:433–435.

Seeman, P., and Sellers, E. M. (eds.). 1975. Principles of Medical Pharmacology. University of Toronto Press, Toronto.

Simpson, C. K. 1958. Forensic Medicine, 34th Ed. Edward Arnold Ltd., London.

Timperman, J. 1962. The detection of diatoms in the marrow of sternum as evidence of death by drowning. J. Forensic Med. 9:134–136.

# Aerobic Power During Exercise at Varying Body Temperatures

**U. Bergh and B. Ekblom**

It has previously been demonstrated that low body temperature (hypothermia), may lower physical performance considerably, partly because of a reduction in maximal aerobic power and an increased energy cost of submaximal work (Nadel et al., 1974; Holmér and Bergh, 1974; Davies et al., 1975). Because information regarding quantitative aspects and individual responses to different levels of hypothermia is not available, these experiments were conducted to study the effects of different skin, core, and muscle temperatures on physiological responses to submaximal and maximal exercise with large muscle groups. Some preliminary data are presented in this chapter.

## METHODS

In five well trained male subjects, different levels of core and muscle temperatures were obtained by swimming in cold water. After cooling, the subjects moved to a bicycle ergometer constructed for combined arm and leg work, where they performed submaximal or maximal exercise. Skin temperature was varied through different room temperatures. Body temperatures were measured by thermocouples. Core temperature ($T_{es}$) was monitored in the esophagus at the level of the heart. Mean skin temperature ($=\overline{T}_{sk}$) was calculated from measurements made at six different skin loci. The temperature in the vastus lateralis muscle ($T_m$) was measured with a needle probe immediately after the exercise. Maximal oxygen uptake ($\dot{V}_{O_2}$ max) was determined with the Douglas bag method. $O_2$ and $CO_2$ concentrations were analyzed in a mass spectrometer.

The $T_{es}$ varied between 33 and 37.5°C, $T_{sk}$ between 26 and 33°C, and $T_m$ between 33.5 and 38.4°C.

## RESULTS

During submaximal exercise, $\dot{V}_{O_2}$ was elevated when $T_{es}$ was lower than 36°C. This increase in $\dot{V}_{O_2}$ at lower $T_{es}$ was elevated by a lower $\bar{T}_{sk}$ and diminished by an elevated $\bar{T}_{sk}$ (Figure 1). Despite these variations in $\dot{V}_{O2}$, heart rate (HR) was the same at the standard submaximal rate of work when $T_{es}$ was between 33 and 35.8°C. At $T_{es}$ above 36°C, HR was higher at higher $\bar{T}_{sk}$, although $V_{O2}$ was unchanged (Figure 1). Furthermore, the increase in $\dot{V}_{O2}$ at lower $T_{es}$ was less at higher than at lower rates of submaximal work (comparison at the same $\bar{T}_{sk}$). Because the $\bar{T}_{sk}$ did not affect any of the physiological parameters during maximal exercise, only data in relation to $T_{es}$ and $T_m$ are discussed below.

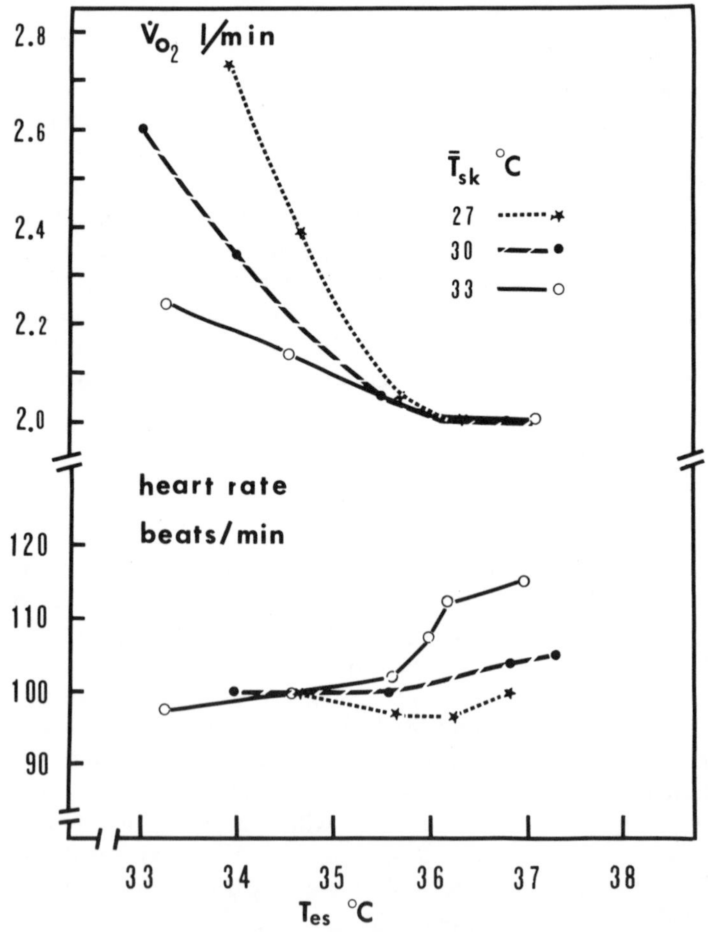


Figure 1. This graph presents heart rate and oxygen uptake during submaximal exercise (150 W) at different core ($T_{es}$) and skin ($\bar{T}_{sk}$) temperatures (N = 1).

The work time at the standard maximal rate of work ("physical performance") was reduced with lowered $T_{es}$ (Figure 2). The $\dot{V}_{O_2}$ was linearly related to the $T_{es}$. Thus, from $T_{es}$ 37.5° and lower, the decrease in aerobic power was about 7%/°C decrease in $T_{es}$ (N = 5).

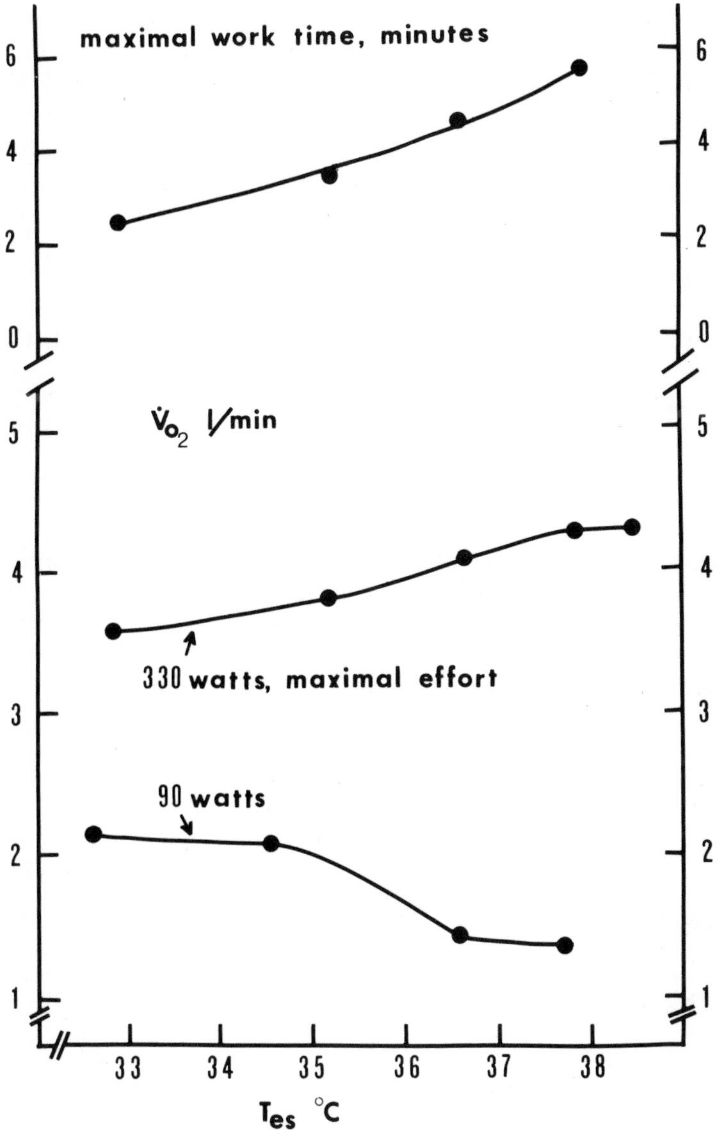


Figure 2. Maximal work time, and oxygen uptake during submaximal (bottom part of the figure) and maximal (middle part of the figure) exercise are shown as functions of esophageal temperature ($T_{es}$) (N = 1).

## DISCUSSION

It may be suspected that the decrease in aerobic power with lower $T_{es}$ was caused by a change in the acceleration of the $\dot{V}_{O_2}$. However, after 2.5 min of exercise, there were no differences in $\dot{V}_{O_2}$ at different $T_{es}$, thus indicating that the reduction in aerobic power during hypothermia was not merely an effect of a slower acceleration of the oxygen uptake. It is interesting to note that none of the subjects was able to attain maximal aerobic power at $T_{es}$ and $T_m$ lower than 37.5 and 38.0°C, respectively. Thus, it is evident that there are large individual variations in the capability to avoid body cooling (i.e., through differences in body fat content), while the effects of hypothermia on maximal aerobic power and physical performance are similar in different subjects.

HR at the end of the maximal exercise was also linearly related to $T_{es}$ and $T_m$ within the range of temperatures measured. This was not an effect of the difference in work time; HR was the same after 1 min of exercise. However, after 2 min of exercise, there were significant differences. The physiological explanation of this HR reduction with lowered $T_{es}$ is not known, but it might be explained by direct or indirect temperature effects on the heart (speed of contraction), on the autonomic nervous system, etc.

During maximal exercise, then, aerobic power, physical performance, and heart rate decreased with decreasing core and muscle temperatures but were unaffected by different skin temperatures. During submaximal exercise, oxygen uptake at a given rate of work increased with decreasing core and skin temperatures. Heart rate at a given submaximal work intensity was unaffected by changes in oxygen uptake, core, and skin temperatures, at core temperatures ranging from 33–35.8°C.

## REFERENCES

Davies, M., Ekblom, B., Bergh, U., and Kanstrup, I.-L. 1975. The effects of hypothermia on submaximal and maximal work performance. Acta Physiol. Scand. 95:201–202.

Holmér, I., and Bergh, U. 1974. Metabolic and thermal response to swimming in water at varying temperatures. J. Appl. Physiol. 37:702–705.

Nadel, E. R., Holmér, I., Bergh, U., Åstrand, P.-O., and Stolwijk, J. A. J. 1974. Energy exchange in swimming man. J. Appl. Physiol. 36:465–471.

# Metabolic Responses to Swimming at Three Different Water Temperatures

**M. E. Houston, N. J. Christensen, H. Galbo, J. J. Holst, B. Nielsen, E. Nygaard, and B. Saltin**

The responses of human subjects to swimming in water at varying temperatures have been previously studied (Nielsen, 1973; Holmér and Bergh, 1974; Nadel et al., 1974; Nielsen, 1976). These studies focused on muscle, skin, esophageal, and core temperature responses to cold and warm water, in addition to such physiological parameters as oxygen uptake ($\dot{V}_{O_2}$) and heart rate (HR).

The effects of submaximal exercise on the plasma and blood concentrations of metabolites and hormones have also been studied during bicycle exercise and treadmill running (Hartley et al., 1972; Ahlborg et al., 1974; Lassarre et al., 1974; Rennie and Johnson, 1974; Galbo, Holst, and Christensen, 1975; Bloom et al., 1976; Galbo et al., 1976). However, detailed hormonal and metabolic responses to swimming exercise have not been reported. Because the thermal conductivity of water is approximately 25 times that of air, the possibility of imposing a severe temperature stress in addition to an exercise stress suggests that a unique adaptive response would be required.

The purpose of the present investigation was to investigate the hormonal and metabolic responses to submaximal swimming with or without an added temperature stress. (A more detailed description of this study has been submitted for future publication elsewhere.)

## METHODS

Six male subjects swam continuously for 1 hr using the breast stroke in a swimming flume at a speed calculated to require 65% of their swimming $\dot{V}_{O_2}$ max. Each subject swam on three occasions, separated by at least 1 week, in water at a temperature of 21°C, 27°C, and 33°C.

Blood was drawn from a superficial arm vein through an inserted cannula and attached manometer line at various times before, during, and after swimming (Figure 1). Hormonal and metabolic analyses were performed as previously described (Galbo, Holst, and Christensen). Core and esophageal temperatures were recorded continuously (Nielsen, 1976) and the temperatures of the deltoid and quadriceps muscles were measured before and immediately after swimming.

Expired air was collected in Douglas bags, before and at intervals during swimming, and was analyzed as previously described (Nielsen, 1976). Heart rate was measured at rest and during swimming using a specially constructed telemetric system (Nielsen, 1976). In all cases, experiments were performed in the morning, and subjects fasted for at least 12 hr.

## RESULTS

Core and esophageal temperatures, in general, tended to rise approximately 0.80°C during the hour of swimming at 27°C, decreased by the same magnitude at 21°C, and rose by 1.6°C at 33°C. With the exception of the postswim deltoid temperature at 21°C, all muscle temperatures were elevated immediately after swimming, the increase in temperatures being directly related to the water temperature.

Heart rates during swimming gradually increased with time for the 33°C and 27°C water temperatures. For the 21°C swim, the heart rate fell initially, then remained steady for the balance of the swim. During the last minute of swimming, mean heart rates were 143, 137 and 127 beats/min for the 33°C, 27°C, and 21°C, respectively.

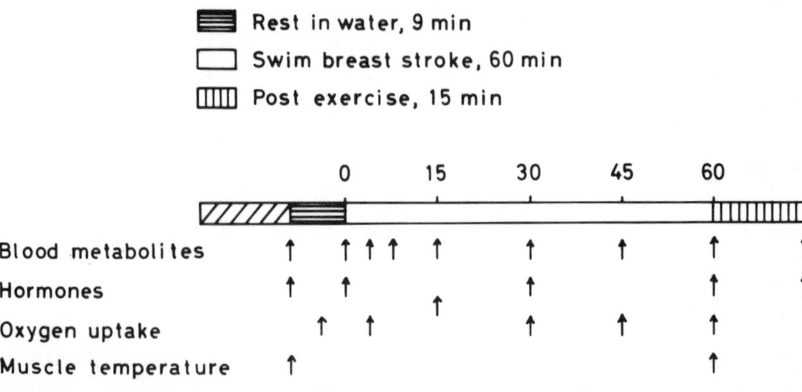


Figure 1. A schematic outline of the experimental protocol for the 60 min of submaximal swimming, as well as the essential pre- and postexercise periods. The arrows indicate when the different measurements were made.

In contrast to heart rate, $V_{O_2}$ (Figure 2) was lowest at the warmest water temperature, both during the swim and while resting in the water prior to commencing the swim. Respiratory exchange ratios (R values) declined with time, the values during swimming being inversely related to water temperature.

Mean blood lactate levels were generally low, the highest values being recorded after 10 min of swimming. For all subjects, the highest values were recorded during swimming at 21°C. No significant differences were noted for glycerol and free fatty acid values under the three water temperature conditions, and both metabolites increased with time.

Glucose and insulin (Figure 3) tended to follow the same pattern of change with time: an initial decline was followed by generally steady levels, then a rise during the postexercise period. No significant tem-

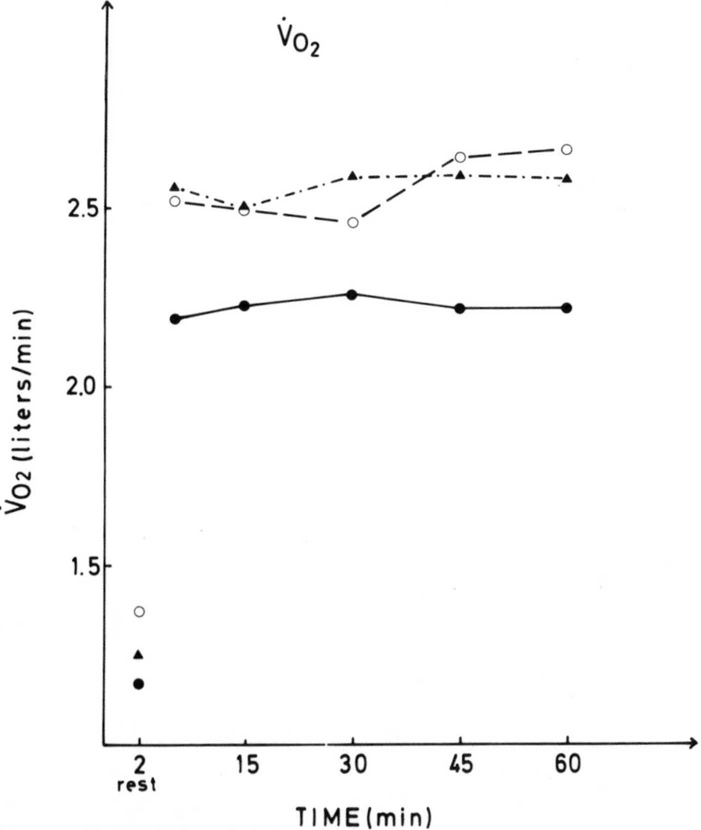


Figure 2. Oxygen uptake ($\dot{V}_{O_2}$) during rest in water and at different times during 60 min of submaximal swimming in 21°C (○- - -○), 27°C (▲·—·▲), and 33°C (●—●) water.

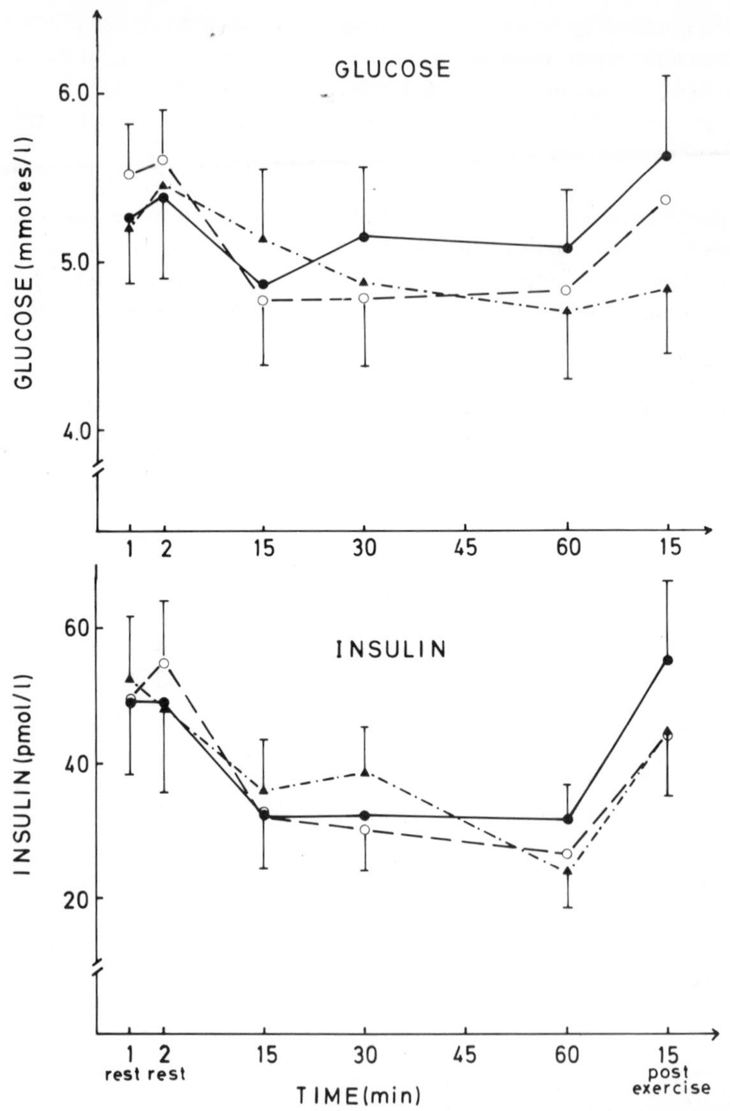


Figure 3. Plasma glucose and insulin concentrations (mean ±SE) were obtained during rest and during 60 min of submaximal swimming in 21°C (○- - -○), 27°C (▲· — ·▲), and 33°C (●— ●) water.

perature effects for either insulin or glucose were observed. Glucagon concentrations did not change significantly with time or temperature, except for a sharp rise in glucagon during the postexercise period after the swim at 33°C. Noradrenaline and adrenaline increased during the first 30 min of exercise; the increases over the values obtained during resting in the water were 182, 152, and 58% for the 33°C, 21°C, and 27°C temperatures, respectively.

## DISCUSSION

The subjects had little difficulty swimming for 1 hr at the moderate workload selected (approximately 65% of $\dot{V}_{O_2}$ max), although some discomfort was experienced at the lowest and highest water temperatures. The effect of water temperature on the heart rate and $\dot{V}_{O_2}$ responses noted in this study were similar to those previously reported during submaximal swimming (Holmér and Bergh; Nadel et al.) and arm-leg cycle ergometry in water (McArdle et al., 1976). Both resting and exercise $\dot{V}_{O_2}$ values were higher in the coldest water environments. Conversely, HR during swimming was directly related to water temperatures, as well as core and esophageal temperatures.

The blood metabolites, glucose, lactate, glycerol, and free fatty acids (FFA) responded in a manner typical for continuous submaximal bicycle (Ahlborg et al., 1974; Bloom et al., 1976; Essén, Hagenfeldt, and Kaijser, 1977) and running (Rennie and Johnson, 1974; Galbo, Holst, and Christensen, 1976) exercises. No significant temperature effects were noted, with the exception of a greater initial increase in lactate concentration at the two colder temperatures. The low R values (approximately 0.84 at the end of exercise at all three water temperatures), plus the rising FFA and glycerol levels suggest that lipid was the major fuel for swimming exercise of this intensity.

The decline in plasma insulin during swimming was consistent with what has been previously observed for submaximal running (Rennie and Johnson; Galbo, Holst, and Christensen) and bicycle (Ahlborg et al.) exercises. There was no significant effect of water temperature on either the insulin or glucagon responses to exercise. The swimming exercise resulted in an increase in plasma levels of both noradrenaline and adrenaline, a response typical for submaximal exercise (von Euler, 1974; Galbo et al., 1976). A more marked increase in both catecholamines was detected after 30 min of swimming in the warmest and coldest water environments. This latter effect seemed to be particularly related to the temperature stress on the subjects. Moreover, the elevated catecholamine levels at 21°C and 33°C were not related to any significant alterations in the venous concentrations of FFA, glycerol, and glucagon, although such an effect could be expected (Iversen, 1973; von Euler).

The major observation from these experiments is that thermal stress at 18°C and 33°C resulted in a greatly increased sympathoadrenal response compared with what was observed in the more thermoneutral water environment. For moderate intensity swimming, the thermal stress apparently dominates the exercise stress. Moreover, despite the increased catecholamine levels, swimming heart rates were lowest at the coldest temperature, and were accompanied by the highest $\dot{V}_{O_2}$ values near the end of exercise. For maximal swimming, Holmér and Bergh have reported lower $\dot{V}_{O_2}$ values and shorter performance times at 18°C than at warmer water temperatures, an effect most pronounced for leaner subjects. For swim training, where many hours are spent in the water each day, the imposition of a mild thermal stress in addition to an exercise stress could augment the training stimulus, although there is little data to support this, at least for swimming. As the metabolic responses to swimming are so poorly understood at present (Houston, pp. 207–232) such a suggestion is primarily conjecture. For recreational swimming, where energy expenditure is lower than in these present experiments, a water temperature warmer than 27°C seems most advisable for maintaining thermal balance and hence reducing the catecholamine levels.

## REFERENCES

Ahlborg, G., Felig, P., Hagenfeldt, L., Hendler, R., and Wahren, J. 1974. Substrate turnover during prolonged exercise in man. Splanchnic and leg metabolism of glucose, free fatty acids, and amino acids. J. Clin. Invest. 53:1080–1090.

Bloom, S. R., Johnson, R. H., Park, D. M., Rennie, M. J., and Sulaiman, W. R. 1976. Differences in the metabolic and hormonal response to exercise between racing cyclists and untrained individuals. J. Physiol. 258:1–18.

Essén, B., Hagenfeldt, L., and Kaijser, L. 1977. Utilization of bloodborne and intramuscular substrates during continuous and intermittent exercise in man. J. Physiol. 265:489–506.

Galbo, H., Holst, J. J., and Christensen, N. J. 1975. Glucagon and plasma catecholamine responses to graded and prolonged exercise in man. J. Appl. Physiol. 38:70–76.

Galbo, H., Holst, J. J., Christensen, N. J., and Hilsted, J. 1976. Glucagon and plasma catecholamines during beta-receptor blockade in exercising man. J. Appl. Physiol. 40:855–863.

Hartley, L. H., Mason, J. W., Hogan, R. P., Jones, L. G., Kotchen, T. A., Mougey, E. H., Wherry, F. E., Pennington, L. L., and Ricketts, R. P. 1972. Multiple hormonal response to prolonged exercise in relation to physical training. J. Appl. Physiol. 33:607–610.

Holmér, I., and Bergh, U. 1974. Metabolic and thermal response to swimming in water at varying temperatures. J. Appl. Physiol. 37:702–705.

Iversen, J. 1973. Adrenergic receptors and the secretion of glucagon and insulin from the isolated, perfused canine pancreas. J. Clin. Invest. 52:2102–2116.

Lassarre, C., Girard, F., Durand, J., and Raynaud, J. 1974. Kinetics of human growth hormone during submaximal exercise. J. Appl. Physiol. 37:826–830.

McArdle, W. D., Magel, J. R., Lesmes, G. R., and Pechar, G. S. 1976. Metabolic and cardiovascular adjustment to work in air and water at 18, 25, and 33°C. J. Appl. Physiol. 40:85–90.

Nadel, E. R., Holmér, I., Bergh, U., Åstrand, P.-O., and Stolwijk, J. O. 1974. Energy exchanges of swimming man. J. Appl. Physiol. 36:465–471.

Nielsen, B. 1973. Metabolic reactions to cold during swimming at different speeds. Arch. Sci. Physiol. 27:A207–A211.

Nielsen, B. 1976. Metabolic reactions to changes in core and skin temperature in man. Acta Physiol. Scand. 97:129–138.

Rennie, M. J., and Johnson, R. H. 1974. Alteration of metabolic and hormonal responses to exercise by physical training. Eur. J. Appl. Physiol. 33:215–226.

von Euler, U. S. 1974.Sympatho-adrenal activity in physical exercise. Med. Sci. Sports 6:165–173.

# Physiological Response of A World Class Distance Swimmer During Cold Water Immersion

**W. B. McCafferty, R. D. Rochelle, B. L. Drinkwater, and S. M. Horvath**

Long distance ocean swimming imposes considerable physiological stress from both the exercise and the environment, with swims of long duration and/or low ambient temperature often reported. The subject of this study has recently swum the Strait of Magellan, a swim in 5°C ocean water for over an hour. Year-long ocean training and an acclimatization period of 1 week in the 5–7°C water are two of the possible factors responsible for this successful swim.

Maintenance of optimal body temperature is of critical importance to channel swimmers. The primary responses to cold environments are blood flow shifts and heat production by shivering (Horvath, 1960). The active exercise of swimming provides heat during this activity.

The primary environmental problem faced by the channel swimmer is heat loss. Water has a greater heat transfer coefficient than air, with heat loss to cold water 2–4 times heat loss to air (Smith and Hanna, 1975). One of the factors considered important in preventing heat loss in this type of activity is the presence of subcutaneous fat. This has been found to be the case both at rest (Canon and Keatinge, 1960) and during exercise (Holmér and Bergh, 1974).

Long distance swimming is an endurance activity. It has been suggested that women may in fact have a physiological edge in endurance swimming events. For example, the record for a 50-mi swim is held by a woman. Greta Anderson performed this swim, ahead of the closest male by five hours. Until the summer of 1976, the female subject of this study held both the men's and women's records for the English Channel crossing. Her record was broken by a woman. A partial reason for the success of women in long distance swimming may lie in the relatively higher percentage of body fat, providing both hydrostatic and insulatory benefits.

The training of one of the world's foremost distance swimmers at the University of California provided researchers a unique opportunity to assess the physiological response of this athlete to an acute cold stress of 19°C water immersion.

## METHODS

Lynne Cox, a world class female distance swimmer, served as the subject for this case study. (The nature and purpose of the study and the risks involved were explained verbally and given on a written form to the subject prior to her voluntary consent to participate. The protocol and procedures for this study have been approved by the Committee on Activities Involving Human Subjects of the University of California, Santa Barbara.) Swims completed by Ms. Cox are presented in Table 1. Preliminary examinations, including a resting 12-lead ECG and pulmonary function evaluation, were performed on the subject before experimentation. Physical characteristics of the subject are listed in Table 2. Body fat was determined by the method of Brozek et al. (1963).

The subject, 12 hr postabsorptive, participated in a 60-min immersion in 19°C fresh water. The subject was monitored during a 15-min rest period, the 60-min immersion, and a 15-min recovery period. Heart rate, minute ventilation, oxygen uptake, and skin and rectal temperatures were measured each minute according to the procedure of Rochelle and Horvath (in preparation). Blood samples were taken during the final 2 min of rest and immediately following removal from the water. Before and after blood samples were both analyzed for hematocrit, by the microhematocrit method, and hemoglobin, by the

Table 1. Subject's channel swimming record

| | | Distance (mi) | Time (hr:min.sec) | Temperature °C |
|---|---|---|---|---|
| 1971 | Catalina Channel, USA | 27 | 12:36 | 13.3 |
| 1972 | English Channel | 28 | 9:57 | 14.4 |
| 1973 | English Channel | 28 | 9:36 | 14.4 |
| 1974 | Catalina Channel, U.S.A. | 27 | 8:48 | 16 |
| 1975 | Cook Straits, New Zealand | 12 | 12:02.5 | 14–16 |
| 1976 | Denmark to Sweden | 12 | 5:09 | 16 |
| 1976 | Norway to Sweden | 15 | 6:16 | 16 |
| 1976 | Strait of Magellan, Chile | 4.5 | 1:01.2 | 5 |
| 1977 | Aleutian Islands | 8 | 2:06 | 6.6 |
| 1977 | Cape of Good Hope | 8 | 3:21 | 14–16 |

Table 2. Subject's characteristics

| | |
|---|---|
| Age, years | 19 |
| Sex | F |
| Wt before, kg | 90.3 |
| Wt after Post, kg | 90.0 |
| Ht, cm | 165.6 |
| BSA, $m^2$ | 1.98 |
| Body fat, % | 36 |
| $\dot{V}_{O_2}$ max, liters | 3.65 |
| $\dot{V}_{O_2}$ max, ml/kg | 39.6 |
| $\dot{V}_{O_2}$ max, ml/kg LBW | 60.9 |

cyanmethemoglobin technique. Shifts in plasma, blood and red cell volumes were calculated according to the method of Dill and Costill (1974). Blood samples were analyzed for cortisol by radioimmunoassay technique (Campuzano et al., 1973) and corrected for hemoconcentration. The subject was instructed beforehand to signal the onset of shivering and the observer noted this time as well as the onset of visible shivering. The intensity of shivering was recorded by the observer on a scale of 0–5 (0 = no shivering, 1 = reported by subject but not visible, 2 = slight but visible, 3 = mild, 4 = moderate, 5 = heavy).

Experimental protocol would have effected removal of subject if her rectal temperature had fallen 2°C. Urine collected before and after immersion was analyzed for volume, pH, and specific gravity. Weight was measured following the 15-min recovery period.

## RESULTS

During the course of the 60-min immersion in the 19°C water, the rectal temperature decreased from 37.8°C to 37.2°C. Average decline in rectal temperature of male subjects in a concurrent study was 2.2°C (Rochelle and Horvath, in preparation).

The subject exhibited a typical immersion response; however, a diminished response was then observed for the duration of the exposure period. An approximately two-fold rise in oxygen uptake and ventilation (BTPS) occurred during the first minutes of immersion, but by minute 3 they had returned to control levels, where they remained throughout the exposure period. The subject had no significant change from rest in the respiratory exchange ratio (R), while that of the male subjects rose to 1.00. Heart rate rose from 67 beats/min at rest to 102 beats/min at minute 1 before falling to and remaining near control levels. While male subjects exhibited a similar early response in heart rate,

Table 3. Subject's physiological responses during rest (R) and immersion (I) in 19°C water

| Event | Duration | V BTPS | ml $0_2$/kg | HR | Mean skin temperature | Mean body temperature | Body heat kcal/m² | Radiation kcal/m²-HR | Tissue conductivity | Rectal temperature |
|---|---|---|---|---|---|---|---|---|---|---|
| R | 9–13 | 7.98 | 3.92 | 67 | 30.73 | 35.33 | 1337.18 | 35.73 | 7.27 | 37.8 |
| I | 1 | 15.85 | 8.40 | 102 | 23.80 | 32.83 | 1242.90 | 18.12 | 7.92 | 37.7 |
| I | 2 | 15.31 | 7.41 | 65 | 22.16 | 32.20 | 1218.78 | 11.58 | 6.30 | 37.6 |
| I | 3 | 11.26 | 4.84 | 69 | 21.97 | 32.13 | 1216.20 | 10.81 | 4.14 | 37.6 |
| I | 4 | 10.39 | 5.05 | 65 | 21.77 | 32.06 | 1213.61 | 10.04 | 4.19 | 37.6 |
| I | 5 | 7.76 | 3.81 | 65 | 21.57 | 31.99 | 1210.96 | 9.25 | 3.13 | 37.6 |
| I | 6–10 | 8.31 | 3.74 | 59 | 21.16 | 31.85 | 1205.47 | 7.62 | 3.01 | 37.6 |
| I | 11–15 | 7.54 | 3.54 | 58 | 20.37 | 31.57 | 1195.00 | 4.53 | 2.71 | 37.6 |
| I | 16–20 | 8.20 | 3.72 | 58 | 19.93 | 31.35 | 1186.78 | 2.84 | 2.80 | 37.5 |
| I | 21–25 | 7.11 | 3.41 | 54 | 19.77 | 31.30 | 1184.66 | 2.22 | 2.51 | 37.5 |
| I | 26–30 | 9.40 | 4.43 | 54 | 19.66 | 31.26 | 1183.20 | 1.79 | 3.25 | 37.5 |
| I | 31–35 | 7.22 | 3.48 | 55 | 19.57 | 31.16 | 1179.55 | 1.45 | 2.58 | 37.4 |
| I | 36–40 | 7.33 | 3.46 | 53 | 19.52 | 31.14 | 1178.82 | 1.23 | 2.55 | 37.4 |
| I | 41–45 | 7.22 | 3.44 | 52 | 19.52 | 31.08 | 1176.36 | 1.23 | 2.54 | 37.3 |
| I | 46–50 | 7.98 | 3.60 | 55 | 19.36 | 30.96 | 1171.78 | 0.62 | 2.68 | 37.2 |
| I | 51–55 | 7.54 | 3.79 | 51 | 19.36 | 30.96 | 1171.78 | 0.62 | 2.76 | 37.2 |
| I | 56–60 | 7.22 | 3.64 | 53 | 19.31 | 30.94 | 1171.11 | 0.42 | 2.66 | 37.2 |
| R | 0–5 | 11.37 | 5.42 | 50 | 20.12 | 31.16 | 1179.45 | −7.75 | 4.20 | 37.1 |
| R | 6–10 | 8.53 | 4.24 | 53 | 20.95 | 31.32 | 1185.46 | −4.53 | 3.48 | 36.9 |
| R | 11–15 | 8.75 | 3.98 | 55 | 21.36 | 31.46 | 1190.96 | −2.90 | 3.37 | 36.9 |

their levels continued to rise to 20 beats/min above resting during the exposure.

Mean skin temperature dropped to near ambient temperature during the course of the exposure, while the mean body temperature remained above 30°C. Body heat content dropped 166 kcal/m$^2$ during the exposure.

The subject exhibited a rise in hematocrit (43.0 before, 44.0 after), hemoglobin (9.7 before, 10.1 after), and plasma protein (6.7 before, 7.2 after) as a consequence of the cold exposure. The plasma cortisol concentration of the subject fell from 15.51 to 14.61 ($\mu$g/mM Hb) but still seemed to differ from the normal morning circadian rhythm of a fall in plasma cortisol concentration. A decrease in plasma volume of 7.2% accompanied these changes. Diuresis occurred with a postexposure urine volume of 165 ml and a urine flow rate of 1.3 ml/min.

The subject reported the test conditions as having been mild and at no time felt cold, while the majority of male subjects reported the conditions as severe. In addition, the subject never reported any shivering. Visible shivering, although slight, was noted at minute 50 of the immersion. The average onset of visible shivering in the male subjects was 10 min.

## DISCUSSION

This subject was characterized by a remarkable diminished stress response to cold water, which may be a factor in her success in long distance swimming. It is likely that this diminished stress response was attributable to a combination of the subject's hereditary characteristics, her training state, and an adaptation to cold.

Following immediate increases upon immersion, physiological parameters such as heart rate, ventilation, and oxygen uptake returned to near rest levels for the duration of the exposure. This transient change in physiological parameters was in agreement with results of previous investigations (Keatinge and Evans, 1961; Cooper et al., 1975; Goode et al., 1975). The hemoconcentration observed agrees with previous reports (Wilkerson et al., 1974; Rochelle and Horvath). Diuresis concurrent with this hemoconcentration also agrees with earlier reports (Arnett and Watts, 1960; Suzuki, 1967; Wilkerson et al.) approximating the loss in plasma volume in this subject.

This subject seemed to minimize heat loss effectively through apparent vasoconstriction. During the first minute of immersion, her mean skin temperature dropped to 23.8°C, while that of male subjects in a concurrent study dropped only to 27.5°C. From the first minute of immersion, this female subject, because of the smaller skin-to-water temperature gradient, had the advantage of losing less heat to the environment. Both this subject and the male subjects dropped to similar low levels as exposure progressed. During the following 60 min of immersion, the drop in mean skin temperature indicated this subject had effectively decreased circulation to the skin, thus minimizing heat loss to the surrounding water. Tissue conductance thus dropped to a low level in this subject, while the male subjects experienced increased conductance during immersion, possibly as a result of shivering. However, while the male subjects may have produced heat through shivering, this process may also have increased their conductive heat loss.

It is likely that the high percent of body fat (36%) of this subject was responsible for the diminished stress response to cold water. As suggested by previous investigations of channel swimmers (Pugh and Edholm, 1955) and others (Keatinge, 1966; Holmér and Bergh; Nadel et al., 1974), the most important factor in reducing body cooling is the thickness of subcutaneous fat. Several investigators have noted that the rate of fall of rectal temperature is proportional to the subcutaneous fat thickness (Carlson et al., 1958; Canon and Keatinge, 1960; Keatinge, 1966; Rochelle and Horvath, in preparation). In addition to the insulatory benefits of this subject's subcutaneous fat level, there may have been some hydrostatic advantage. Because the drag component appears to be important in decreasing resistance (di Prampero et al., 1974), the high percent of body fat may have been important in reducing the effective drag of this subject while swimming. A notable exception to this thesis was Florence Chadwick, who at 5′6″ and 140 pounds swam sixteen channels in her career, including the first crossing of the English Channel by a woman. Further study on women subjects would be especially helpful in determining the relative importance of the layer of subcutaneous fat in this subject.

Because cold acclimatization decreases the stress response, especially shivering (Rennie et al., 1962; Hong, 1963; Lapp and Gee, 1967; Skreslet and Aarefjord, 1968; Hong et al., 1969; Hanna and Hong, 1972), this subject's virtual absence of a shiver response may have been the result of daily training in ocean water at Santa Barbara, California (1975 mean temperature: 14.4°C, range 9–20°C). Her max $\dot{V}_{O_2}$ level (60.9 ml/kg LBW) indicated a highly trained state comparable with that of other endurance athletes. One training swim of 4 hr duration in 15°C ocean water showed an increase in this subject's rectal temperature of 0.2°C. Her minimal heat loss through vasoconstriction and insulation and heat gain from swimming exercise provided a temperature balance favorable for long distance swimming in cold water.

Several months prior to the subject's recent swims in Scandinavia and South America, a tethered swim in 5°C and 9°C water was attempted by the subject at the Institute of Environmental Stress. In both, the subject's rectal temperature rose slightly, while swimming at approximately 65% of $\dot{V}_{O}$ max. The subject swam at 9°C for 60 min; she terminated the 5°C tethered swim, however, after 15 min. It is interesting to note that the duration of the first training immersion in the 5°C water at the Strait of Magellan was also 15 min. The subject progressed from a 15-min training immersion the first day to 2 hr duration after 1 week. Acclimatization thus appears to be beneficial in channel swimming.

There may have been a greater heat loss in this subject while ocean swimming than during the experimental immersion because of two factors. First, because the head is a major site of heat loss in the cold (Froese and Burton, 1957), this may be a factor while swimming. The insulation provided by long hair confined in a polyurethane cap is unknown. Secondly, the amount of heat loss will be accelerated while swimming because of the relative velocity of the water (Nadel et al.). In this respect, an elevated $\dot{V}_{O_2}$ in a given submaximal exercise in temperatures colder than 26–28°C has been reported by several investigators (Holmér and Bergh; Costill, Cahill, and Eddy, 1967; Craig and Dvorak, 1968; Nadel et al.).

It appears that a multiplicity of factors was responsible for this subject's success in long distance swimming. These included her physiological characteristics, her training state, and her adaptation to cold water. It is likely that her training in cold ocean water was a specific stress that insured adaptations beneficial for channel swimming.

## REFERENCES

Arnett, E. L., and Watts, D. T. 1960. Catecholamine excretion in men exposed to cold. J. Appl. Physiol. 15(3):499–500.

Brozek, J., Grande, F., Anderson, J., and Keys, A. 1963. Densitometric analysis of body composition: Revision of some quantitative assumptions. Ann. N.Y. Acad. Sci. 110:113–140.

Campuzano, H. C., Wilkerson, J. E., Raven, P. B., Schabram, T., and Horvath, S. M. 1973. A radioimmunoassay for cortisol in human plasma. Biochem. Med. 7:350–362.

Canon, P., and Keatinge, W. R. 1960. Metabolic rate and heat loss of fat and thin men in heat balance in cold and warm water. J. Physiol. 154:329–344.

Carlson, L. D., Hsieh, A. C., Fullington, F., and Elsner, R. W. 1958. Immersion in cold water and body tissue insulation. J. Aviat. Med. 29:145–152.

Cooper, K. E., Martin, S., and Riben, P. 1975. Respiratory and other responses in subjects immersed in cold water. J. Appl. Physiol. 40(6):903–910.

Costill, D. L., Cahill, P. J., and Eddy, D. 1967. Metabolic responses to submaximal exercise in three water temperatures. J. Appl. Physiol. 22:628–632.

Craig, A. B., Jr., and Dvorak, M. 1968. Thermal regulation of man exercising during water-immersion. J. Appl. Physiol. 25:28–35.

Dill, D. B., and Costill, D. L. 1974. Calculation of percentage changes in volumes of blood, plasma, and red cells in dehydration. J. Appl. Physiol. 37(2):247–248.

di Prampero, P., Prendergast, D., Wilson, D., and Rennie, D. 1974. Energetics of swimming in man. J. Appl. Physiol. 37:1–5.

Froese, G., and Burton, A. C. 1957. Heat losses from the human head. J. Appl. Physiol. 10:235–241.

Goode, R. C., Duffin, J., Miller, R., Romet, T. T., Chant, W., and Ackles, K. 1975. Sudden cold water immersion. Resp. Physiol. 23:301–310.

Hanna, J. M., and Hong, S. K. 1972. Critical water temperature and effective insulation in scuba divers in Hawaii. J. Appl. Physiol. 33(6):770–773.

Holmér, I., and Bergh, U. 1974. Metabolic and thermal response to swimming in water at varying temperatures. J. Appl. Physiol. 37(5):702–705.

Hong, S. K. 1963. Comparison of diving and nondiving women of Korea. Fed. Proc. 22(3):831–833.

Hong, S. K., Lee, C. K., Kim, J. K., Song, S. H., and Rennie, D. W. 1969. Peripheral blood flow and heat flux of Korean women divers. Fed. Proc. 28:1143–1148.

Horvath, S. M. 1960. Man in Cold Environments. Paper presented at American Society of Mechanical Engineers meeting, November 27, New York.

Keatinge, W. R. 1966. Effect of subcutaneous fat and of previous exposure to cold on the body temperature, peripheral blood flow, and metabolic rate of men in cold water. J. Physiol. 153:166–178.

Keatinge, W. R., and Evans, M. 1961. The respiratory and cardiovascular response to immersion in cold and warm water. Q. J. Exp. Physiol. 46:83–94.

Lapp, M. C., and Gee, G. K. 1967. Human acclimatization to cold water immersion. Arch. Environ. Health 15:568–579.

Nadel, E. R., Holmér, I., Bergh, U., Åstrand, P.-O., and Stolwijk, J. A. J. 1974. Energy exchanges of swimming man. J. Appl. Physiol. 36:465–471.

Pugh, L. G. C., and Edholm, O. G. 1955. The physiology of channel swimmers. Lancet 2:761–768.

Rennie, D. W., Covino, B. G., Howell, B. J., Song, S. H., Kong, B. S., and Hong, S. K., 1962. Physical insulation of Korean diving women. J. Appl. Physiol. 17:961–966.

Rochelle, R. D., and Horvath, S. M. Thermoregulatory and metabolic responses during cold water immersion. In preparation.

Skreslet, S., and Aarefjord, F. 1968. Acclimatization to cold in man induced by frequent scuba diving in cold water. J. Appl. Physiol. 24(2):177–181.

Smith, R. M., and Hanna, J. M. 1975. Skinfolds and resting heat loss in cold air and water: Temperature equivalence. J. Appl. Physiol. 39(1):93–102.

Suzuki, M. 1967. Initial response of human thyroid, adrenal cortex, and adrenal medulla to acute cold exposure. Can. J. Physiol. Pharmacol. 45:423.

Wilkerson, J. E., Raven, P. B., Bolduan, N. W., and Horvath, S. M. 1974. Adaptation in man's adrenal function in response to acute cold stress. J. Appl. Physiol. 36(2):183–189.

# Body Temperature Response to a Long Distance Swimming Race

U. Bergh, B. Ekblom, I. Holmér, and L. Gullstrand

In recent years, the interest in physical fitness has increased considerably. As a result, more and more people take part in so-called fitness races. Some of these competitions are long distance swimming races, which often take place at water temperatures below 20°C. It has been demonstrated that such temperatures might produce body cooling, at least in lean subjects (Keatinge, 1969; Holmér and Bergh, 1974; Nadel et al., 1974). Therefore, hypothermia is likely to occur in some of the participants in these races.

An excellent opportunity to study the frequency and the degree of body cooling during such activities was provided when a 3.2 km swimming race took place in the city of Stockholm.

## MATERIALS AND METHODS

The subjects were 41 males and 8 females of various ages (range: 13–63 years) and training status (200–70,000 m of swimming per week). Only 15 of the subjects were competitive swimmers.

Rectal temperature ($T_r$) was measured with mercury thermometers 10–20 min before the start (N = 34) and within 5 min after the end of the race (N = 49). Mean skin fold thickness ($\overline{SF}$) was calculated from measurements at the abdomen, above the triceps brachii and above the patella.

The water temperature was 19°C and the weather was sunny with very little wind.

## RESULTS AND DISCUSSION

The above mentioned differences in training status and age produced large variations in the time needed to finish the race (range: 37–150 min; mean: 72 min).

Mean $T_r$ values before and after the race were 37.7°C and 36.4°C, respectively. The comparatively high body temperature before the start was due to warmup activities, e.g., jogging and calisthenics. Despite this increased heat content of the body, only 19 subjects had a $T_r$ above 37°C at the finish; thus, the majority of the subjects become more or less hypothermic (Figure 1), and 10 of them attained a body temperature below 35°C. Furthermore, five of the participants were unable to complete the race and had to be helped out of the water. Their symptoms included shivering and cramps and, in some cases, dizziness. Evidently, moderately cold water can produce hypothermia in most subjects within 1–2 hr.

In contrast, some of the subjects raised their $T_{rs}$; one of them had a $T_r$ of 39.1°C at the end of the race, thus illustrating the great differences in the body temperature responses.

These differences were related both to $\overline{SF}$ and to the exposure time (i.e., time spent in water). The lean subjects had a faster cooling rate then the fat subjects, in whom even elevated body temperatures were observed. At equal $\overline{SF}$, fast swimmers cooled less than did slow swimmers. $\overline{SF}$ seemed to be more important than the exposure time; all

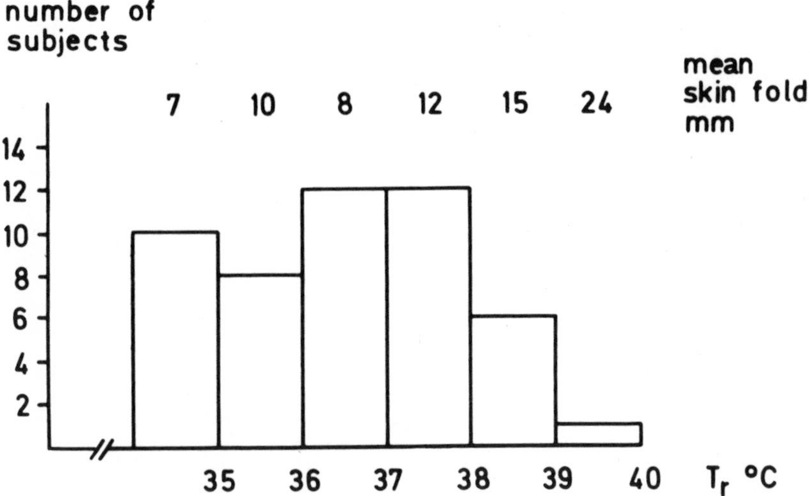


Figure 1. The number of subjects that attained each of the different levels of rectal temperature ($T_r$) at the end of the race. The numbers given in the upper part of the figure denote average mean skinfold values for the subjects in each of the $T_r$ intervals.

subjects with $\bar{SF}$ less than 10 mm showed a fall in $T_r$, and all subjects whose SF was more than 20 mm maintained or raised their $T_r$ without regard to the large variations in exposure time.

These data indicate that hypothermia may occur quite frequently in this type of activity. It has been shown that hypothermia decreases physical performance by reducing the maximal aerobic power and by the increased energy cost of submaximal exercise (Holmér and Bergh; Nadel et al.; Davies et al., 1975). These effects were related to the degree of hypothermia. That condition might induce a vicious cycle: as the individual cools, his physical performance worsens, he is forced to reduce his swimming speed, and exposure time increases, which leads to further body cooling. If the hypothermia becomes severe, heart failure and death may occur. Other effects of body cooling are diminished judgment and loss of motor skill.

In summary, the change in body temperature when covering a given distance at a given water temperature is related to both $\bar{SF}$ and swimming ability, the former being the more important factor. Even in moderately cold water, most people are unable to avoid the body cooling that in some cases might become severe and thereby endanger health.

## REFERENCES

Davies, M., Ekblom, B., Bergh, U., and Kanstrup, I.-L. 1975. The effects of hypothermia on submaximal and maximal work performance. Acta Physiol. Scand. 95:201–202.

Holmér, I., and Bergh, U. 1974. Metabolic and thermal responses to swimming in water at varying temperatures. J. Appl. Physiol. 37:702–705.

Keatinge, W. R. 1969. Survival in Cold Water. Blackwell, Oxford.

Nadel, E. R., Holmér, I., Bergh, U., Åstrand, P.-O., and Stolwijk, J. A. J. 1974. Energy exchange in swimming man. J. Appl. Physiol. 36:465–471.

# Biomechanics

# Analysis and Comparison of Swimming Starts and Strokes

**R. C. Nelson and N. L. Pike**

World records for competitive swimming events continue to be broken on a regular basis. This is the result of a number of interacting factors, including an increased number of participants, better nutrition and training methods, and improvements in starting techniques and stroke mechanics. Interest in the latter two areas has stimulated investigations of the biomechanical aspects of starting and stroking. The results of this research are being applied by coaches and swimmers as a means of enhancing swimming performances.

The purpose of this chapter is to review the more pertinent research that has been done on swimming in the last few years. The major emphasis will be on: swimming starts, fluid mechanics, comparison of strokes, tethered swimming, and mathematical modeling of swimming strokes. Other topics of interest in swimming have previously been reviewed by Miller (1975).

## SWIMMING STARTS

Starting techniques for the freestyle, breast stroke, and butterfly are reasonably similar. Execution of the start is of considerable importance, especially in the shorter events. Until recently, it was assumed that some form of arm swing was necessary to produce the best starting technique. As a consequence, earlier studies were concerned with various types of arm actions. For example, Maglischo and Maglischo (1968) compared three arm actions described as straight backswing, circular backswing, and arms back. The first two were performed from the same static position, with arms and hands forward of the starting blocks. The first method involved a short backswing, while the second used a circular arm swing. The third technique was executed with the arms back in the set position, followed by a direct thrust forward. The results indicated that the circular backswing technique was superior to the other two.

In recent years, the grip or grab start has become increasingly popular. In this technique, the swimmer grasps the front edge of the starting block with both hands placed just outside the feet. The swimmer was then thought to pull his body downward, causing his arms to assist his legs in thrusting the body forward. This body position not only allowed the center of gravity to be moved further forward at the time the gun was fired, but it also offered added stability, reducing the tendency to false start.

Hanauer (1967) first compared the grab start with the conventional arm swing starts previously discussed. The one subject he used left the starting block sooner and entered the water sooner, but did not travel as far horizontally when employing the grab start.

Roffer (1971), utilizing one female and eight male swimmers, compared the grab and conventional racing starts as to time off the block, time of flight, and time to cover 12 feet. He found statistically significant differences in favor of the grab start for time off the block and total time to cover the 12-foot distance. However, the two starts were similar in time of flight, contradicting the results reported by Hanauer.

Other studies comparing the conventional and grab starts were performed by Hanauer (1972), Jorgensen (1972), and Bowers (1973). All three of these authors found the grab start to be superior to the conventional start. Hanauer and Bowers both ascertained that this superiority was attributable to the lesser time spent on the starting block. The research by Bowers found the block time differences to be the result of faster reaction and movement times by the grab starters. She also established that the two starts were similar in their angles of take-off, horizontal distances travelled, and times of flight.

Although the grab start has been shown superior to the conventional start, the exact mechanics employed in its execution are not known. Cavanagh, Palmgren, and Kerr (1975) used a strain-gauged starting block in an attempt to determine the magnitude and direction of forces exerted by the hands in the grab start. The one subject utilized by these researchers showed a steady force production during the set position. He was then observed anticipating the starting gun by rapidly increasing his force output at a time preceding his normal reaction time delay.

Figure 1 shows the position of the swimmer and the horizontal and vertical forces acting on him due to the action of his hands. The forces exerted by the hands on the bar are opposite to those shown, resulting in retardation of the horizontal acceleration of the swimmer. The advantage achieved by the grab start seems to be in the ability of the swimmer to pretense his leg muscles, providing a greater resultant impulse.

Thomsen (1975) ascertained the temporal components and forces exerted on the starting block by the feet in both the conventional and grab starts. His one subject was 0.11 sec faster utilizing the grab start. This difference was due to the shorter block times registered during the performance of the grab start. The resulting time differential recorded at the end of a 12.5 m swim was still 0.10 sec in favor of the grab start.

Thomsen also found that the location of the center of gravity of the swimmer when in contact with the starting block fluctuated more in the conventional start than in the grab start. These observable fluctuations were caused by the forces being exerted on the swimmer. Both horizontal and vertical forces in the conventional start showed greater variability in their production than did the forces in the grab start. For example, the vertical force generated in the grab start remained close to the body weight of the swimmer, while the horizontal force exhibited a more uniform build-up.

The angles of center of gravity take-off for the grab and conventional starts were −8.0° and −11.2°, respectively. These angles were

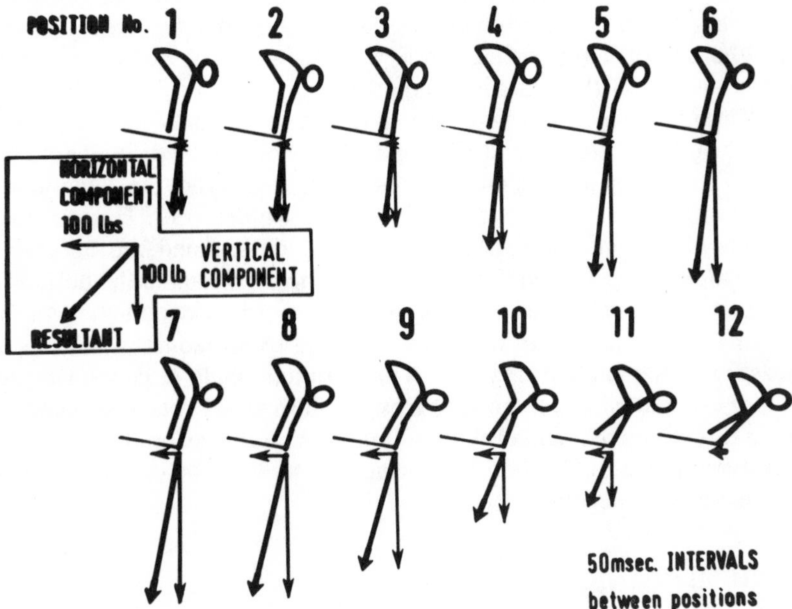


Figure 1. Reaction forces at the hands during the performance of the grab start (from Cavanagh, Palmgren, and Kerr, 1975).

significantly different while all other measured angles—angles of body at take-off and at water entry and angle of center of gravity at water entry—were not found to be different. The combination of angle of center of gravity at take-off and time of force application proved to be the reason that the conventional start recorded higher horizontal and vertical velocities at take-off despite the grab start's demonstration of a significantly larger horizontal displacement of the center of gravity during the flight phase (1.369 m versus 1.293 m).

To obtain an even greater horizontal impulse during the force production phase of the racing start, a bunch and a track start are now being proposed. The bunch start combines the placement of the hands in the grab start with a forward-backward separation of the feet. The track start is similar to the bunch start except that the back leg is supported.

Ayalon, Van Gheluwe, and Konitz (1975) used untrained subjects to compare the conventional, grab, bunch, and track starts. They found the track start to be significantly better than the other three types of starts, its superiority attributable to the reduced time spent on the starting block. Conventional and grab starts were not significantly different from each other, while the bunch start was the slowest of the four methods studied. Therefore, the support of the back leg favors the track style, allowing the swimmer to obtain the lower starting position that is beneficial in the production of a strong horizontal force at take-off. The use of a supporting block for the back foot, however, precludes the use of this start in competition.

The ideal angle of take-off for a racing start has been studied by several authors. Heusner (1959) analytically determined this angle to be 13°. The theoretical equation he used minimized the total swimming time with respect to the angle of take-off ($dt/d\theta = 0$). Groves and Roberts (1972) and Bowers experimentally determined the optimum angle using collegiate swimmers. These authors calculated the horizontal and vertical velocities of the center of gravity of each swimmer at take-off. The ratio of the velocities, vertical to horizontal, provides a measure of the angle of take-off. The optimum angle in each of these studies was calculated to be 13° below the horizontal. The discrepancy in the directions of angle of take-off among these three studies is probably attributable to Heusner's ignoring negative results obtained in his minimization procedures.

## FLUID MECHANICS

How does a swimmer propel himself through water? In the past, it was generally agreed that propulsion was created by the drag force the swimmer produced. Lately, swimming experts have hypothesized that lift is the mechanism of propulsion (Brown and Counsilman, 1971; Counsilman, 1971; Firby, 1973; Schleihauf, 1974).

Hydrodynamic lift and drag forces are direct consequences of Bernoulli's principle: the faster a fluid flows around an object, the greater is the pressure differential. This is accomplished in swimming by "pitching" the hand as it moves through the water. This is why many outstanding swimmers perform a sculling motion with their hands. Barthels and Adrian (1975) and Scheuchenzuber (1975) found positive relationships between the amount of lift and the performance of their swimmers (butterfly and front crawl, respectively).

Counsilman (1971) also suggests that efficient propulsion in swimming is achieved by having the swimmer displace a large amount of water a short distance, rather than displacing a small amount a great distance. Research projects on this topic by Schleihauf (1974) and Tendy (1974) produced differing results. The male world record holder used by Schleihauf was observed to retract his hand from the water in front of its entry point. The collegiate female swimmers in the study by Tendy exhibited "slippage" of the hand that was displaced backwards during the stroke. Thus, more research must be initiated to determine accurately the displacement of the hand and, ultimately, the amount of water being displaced.

## COMPARISON OF STROKES

Only one published study was found that showed the relationships among swimming velocity, stroke length, and stroke frequency. East (1970) filmed all the 110-yard events, both preliminaries and finals, at the 1969 New Zealand National Swimming Championships. He analyzed them with regard to the number of strokes and time taken to complete the event.

East found that faster times in the front crawl for men were characterized by increases in stroke frequency in conjunction with slight decreases in stroke length. Male backstroke and butterfly swimmers exhibited negligible changes in their stroke frequency with concomittant increases in stroke length. Female butterflyers tended to increase both their stroke frequency and stroke length with decreased swimming times. When male and female swimmers were compared across all strokes, they were found to have the same stroke frequencies with differences in performance times being a function of their stroke lengths. Female times were always greater (Table 1).

Craig (personal communication) found results at the United States Olympic swimming trials similar to those reported by East. His data

Table 1. Mean values of stroke rate and length for male and female competitive swimmers[a]

| | Males | | Females | |
|---|---|---|---|---|
| Event | Stroke rate (cycles/sec) | Stroke length (m/stroke) | Stroke rate (cycles/sec) | Stroke length (m/stroke) |
| Freestyle | 0.85 | 1.90 | 0.86 | 1.66 |
| Breast stroke | 0.96 | 1.26 | 0.96 | 1.16 |
| Backstroke | 0.77 | 1.85 | 0.70 | 1.81 |
| Butterfly | 0.90 | 1.61 | 0.91 | 1.38 |

[a] Modified from D. J. East (1970)

also included comparisons among different distances swum using the same stroke. These results indicated that as the distance increased, the stroke rate decreased, regardless of the stroke being performed. The male swimmers exhibited increased stroke lengths for the front crawl, breast stroke, and back crawl strokes when 100- and 200-m events were compared. The women exhibited similar increases in stroke lengths for the breast and back strokes. Both males and females reduced their stroke lengths when the 100- and 200-m butterfly events were analyzed. The women failed to show any discernable pattern when stroke lengths for the front crawl were compared. These changes in stroke lengths are graphically represented in Figure 2.

Further comparisons were made for the freestyle events from 100–1500 m. The results seen in Figure 3 indicate that the men's stroke lengths increased for event distances up to 400 m and then declined while the women exhibited no changes with increasing distances. Male stroke rates decreased sharply over distances from 400–800 m and then leveled off, while the female swimmers showed a much more gradual decline. These patterns suggest that the females must tolerate higher turnover rates because of their inability to increase their stroke lengths. This suggests a different optimization strategy is being employed.

The females were able to maintain a higher percentage of their initial 100-m stroke frequencies than the men for all strokes except the breast stroke. This outcome, in conjunction with the lower swimming velocities exhibited by the women (Figure 4), further emphasizes the discrepancies in stroke length between the two sexes. Anthropometric differences between men and women have been proposed as the reason for the observable differences in stroke lengths and swimming velocities.

Table 2. Stroke rates, lengths, and velocities for US Olympic competitive swimmers[a]

| | Males | | | Females | | |
|---|---|---|---|---|---|---|
| Event | Stroke rate (strokes/min) | Stroke length (m/stroke) | Velocity (m/sec) | Stroke rate (strokes/min) | Stroke length (m/stroke) | Velocity (m/sec) |
| Freestyle | | | | | | |
| 100 | 57.0 | 2.03 | 1.92 | 58.2 | 1.76 | 1.69 |
| 200 | 46.4 | 2.27 | 1.74 | 54.6 | 1.75 | 1.58 |
| 400 | 44.4 | 2.28 | 1.67 | 51.6 | 1.78 | 1.52 |
| Breast stroke | | | | | | |
| 100 | 60.9 | 1.46 | 1.48 | 61.0 | 1.28 | 1.29 |
| 200 | 52.3 | 1.58 | 1.36 | 51.2 | 1.42 | 1.21 |
| Backstroke | | | | | | |
| 100 | 45.7 | 2.24 | 1.70 | 46.3 | 1.94 | 1.49 |
| 200 | 39.3 | 2.40 | 1.57 | 41.8 | 2.02 | 1.40 |
| Butterfly | | | | | | |
| 100 | 53.6 | 1.99 | 1.78 | 54.5 | 1.70 | 1.53 |
| 200 | 51.1 | 1.91 | 1.62 | 53.2 | 1.61 | 1.43 |

[a] From data provided by A. Craig (personal communication).

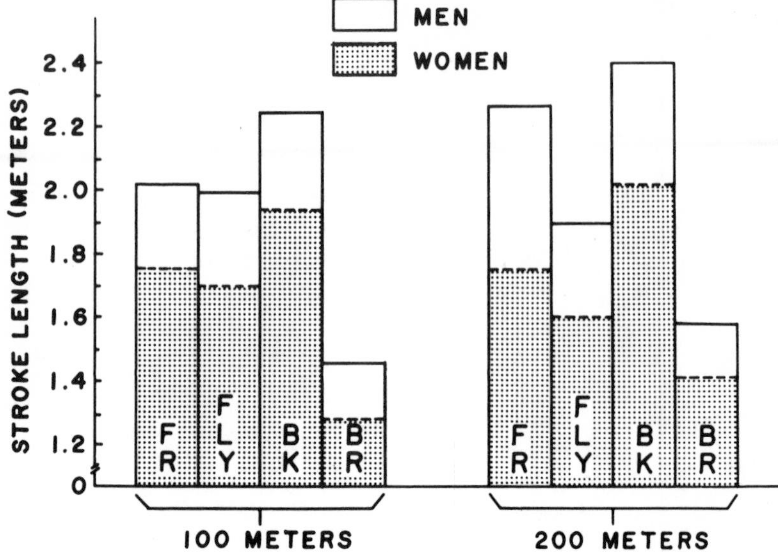


Figure 2. Stroke lengths and rates for men and women in competitive freestyle events. (Based on data provided by A. Craig, personal communication.)

It must be emphasized that these results were obtained between subjects and may not apply within subject variations associated with increased swimming speeds. More research is needed in assessing the mechanisms utilized by swimmers to increase their swimming speeds over a wide range.

## TETHERED SWIMMING

Most of the information that is available on forces produced during the propulsive phases of swimming has been obtained from experimentation utilizing tethered swimmers. Unlike free swimming where the swimmer progresses through the water, a tethered swimmer is held in place by means of a pulley or cable system to which a force measuring device is attached.

Goldfuss (1970) used such a system to analyze the phases of the front crawl arm stroke during a 2-min, all out swimming performance. He found that the maximum force produced by either arm occurred during the entry phase of the opposite arm, and the left arm produced the greatest maximum force. The time to complete a stroke cycle was found to increase progressively during each of the four data collection periods. This increase in time was attributed to the underwater phase of the arm stroke because the duration of the recovery phase was not

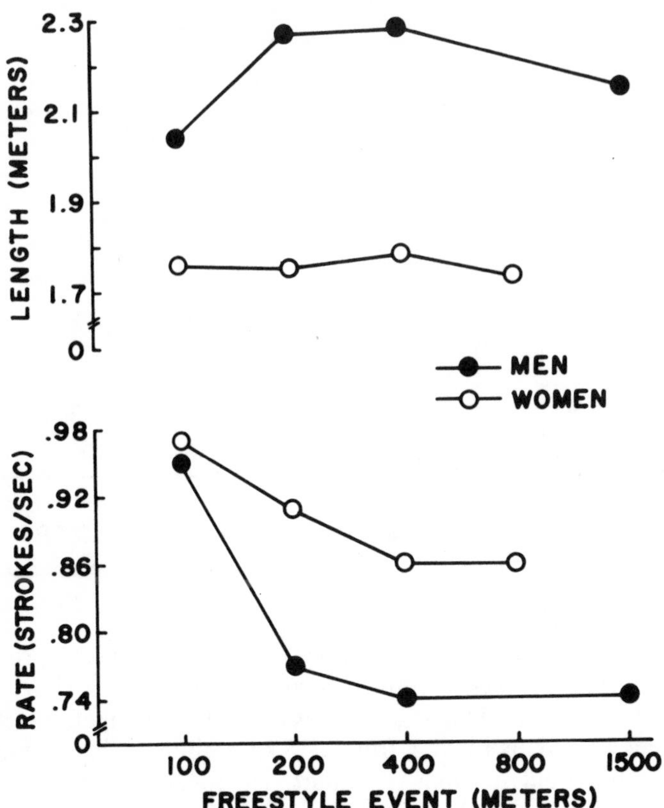


Figure 3. Lengths of competitive swimming strokes for men and women. (Based on data provided by A. Craig, personal communication.)

altered throughout the testing session. Other factors that characterized the fatigue state in the swimmer were increases in time for the left arm to execute the entry phase and the progressive reduction in the magnitude of the force produced by both arms.

Goldfuss did caution that the differences in force production by the two arms could be a bias of his testing procedure in that swimming at zero velocity may accentuate differences in propulsive force that may not be present in free swimming. He also suggested that the greater force recorded by the left arm could have been caused by his subjects breathing on the left side. He argued that this breathing pattern may have placed the right arm in an unfavorable position for applying force. Because data were obtained only for a stroke cycle encompassing breathing, the asymmetry exhibited between the two arms may disappear or even be reversed in a nonbreathing cycle.

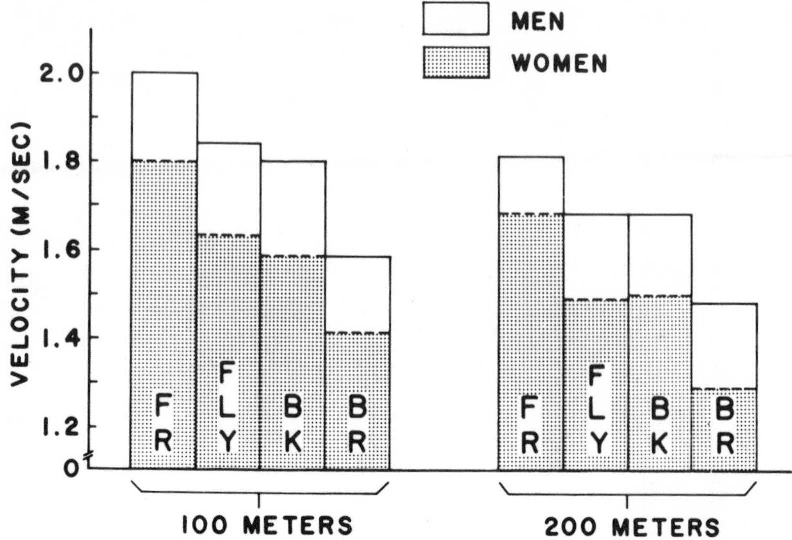


Figure 4. World record velocities for competitive swimming strokes performed by men and women.

Magel (1970) used a tethering system to measure the propelling forces exerted by highly trained swimmers during maximal 3-min swims. His study involved the analysis of the four competitive strokes at varying workloads ranging from 4.55 kg until the subject reached a load that he could no longer support. He found that breast stroke swimmers recorded the highest force output values, while front crawl, back crawl, and butterfly swimmers did not differ in the amounts of force they produced. The least variation in the propulsive and recovery phases of the swimming stroke occurred in the back crawl, while the front crawl and butterfly showed the greatest variation. Magel, in addition, ascertained that the major producers of propulsion forces in the breast stroke were the legs, while the arms provided the force in the front and back crawls. The arms and legs were found to contribute equally to propulsion in the butterfly.

Although the breast stroke exhibited the highest force output and the back crawl the least variation in the propulsion and recovery phases of the four competitive strokes, the front crawl and butterfly strokes were both faster. This apparent disagreement in results is attributable to the increased water resistance met during execution of the breast stroke and back crawl. In fact, the water resistance is so great during the recovery phase of the breast stroke that the velocity of the breast stroke swimmer may approach zero (Kent and Atha, 1975). This increased water resistance is a result of the underwater recovery phases of both the arms and legs, which causes a disturbance in the amount of water being displaced backwards (Miyashita, 1974). The backstroker is at a further disadvantage in terms of resistance because his back glide position is less efficient than the prone positions of the front crawl and butterfly. Magel proposed that back crawlers are also handicapped because of their slower starting and turning times.

The purpose of tethered swimming experiments is to gather data, otherwise difficult if not impossible to obtain, that is directly applicable to free swimming. Scheuchenzuber determined the relationships between measurements of palmar-dorsal pressure differentials during tethered and nontethered performance of the arm action in the front crawl stroke. The results he obtained during tethered performances were not found to be related to the free swimming condition and cast reasonable doubt on the applicability of tethered swimming studies to the free swimming situation. Other studies utilizing all four competitive strokes will have to be performed to evaluate accurately the relationship between tethered and nontethered swimming. Also, more research should be performed employing the water treadmill, a device where water is forced past a swimmer at a regulated rate. Again, the objective would be to compare the water treadmill outcomes with those of free swimming.

## MODELING

Mathematical modeling has been proposed as a method whereby the optimal mechanics of swimming can be obtained. Utilizing Newtonian mechanics and standard periodic functions as input, models ranging from the very simple to the very complex are possible.

Seireg and Baz (1971) developed a first approximation to the front crawl. Their model assumed no flexion of the torso, arms, or legs. Propulsive forces were assumed to be caused by the rotation of the straight arms and the kicking of the straight legs. The legs were assumed to be moving opposite to each other, while the motion of the arms depended upon the period during which they were in the air and water. The action of the arms in the front crawl was also dependent on the constant angular displacement (phase shift) between the two arms.

This model, as well as all the swimming models to be discussed, accounted for the drag, buoyancy, inertial, and hydrodynamic forces exerted on the body. This particular model produced results that indicated that the contribution of the leg action in propulsion was small compared with that of the arms; this agreed with results obtained by several authors (Counsilman, 1968; Watson, 1969; Bruce, 1974; Bucher, 1975), who believed the legs are used only for stabilization in swimming. Cyclic variations were found to occur for the motion of the arms and the center of gravity, indicating symmetry of motion. Because human motion is not normally characterized by symmetry and because the elbow joint is not considered fixed in full extension, both of these factors can be considered as major limitations of this particular model.

A better approximation of the true arm stroke in the front crawl was reported by Jensen and Blanksby (1975), who developed a three-segment, rigid body model for comparing straight and flexed arm strokes. Their results indicated that the greatest horizontal propulsive force was produced at the wrist of the swimmer, with a limited contribution by the upper arm. The flexed elbow stroke was found to be superior because it required the development of smaller muscular forces and moments.

A more complex swimming model that can be applied to the four competitive strokes was proposed by Gallenstein and Huston (1973). This model incorporated 15 rigid body segments that were assumed to be frustra of elliptical cylinders or cones. The authors used this model to simulate the flutter and breast stroke kicks as well as the complete breast stroke. All the input parameters to the model were sinusoidal in nature. The generated results demonstrated the supremacy of the bent-knee flutter kick over the straight-legged kick. The authors also ascertained that the resultant output of the arms and kick together in the breast stroke was slightly less than the sum of the separate outputs of arms and legs. This analytical result agrees with experimental velocity data collected by Bucher on front crawl swimmers.

A major deficiency of this model was the negative velocities calculated for the center of gravity of the body during the recovery phase of the stroke. This would indicate that the swimmer was travelling in a direction opposite to that desired. This negative outcome is probably a consequence of the prescribed symmetric inputs to the model. These parameters should be determined experimentally and the generated functions should then be used as the input to the model. Belokovsky (1971) examined the pulling action of the arms during the front crawl and classified the strokes into three categories—exponential, trapezoidal, and sinusoidal—based upon the pressure being exerted against the palms of the hands.

## SUMMARY

Selected studies dealing with certain biomechanical aspects of swimming starts and strokes have been presented. Although the answers to some fundamental and practical questions have been forthcoming, it is clear that research in this area is in the early stages of development. It can be anticipated that biomechanics research related to swimming will increase markedly in the years ahead. Hopefully, the results of this work will be of major importance to continue improvement in competitive swimming performances.

## REFERENCES


Ayalon, A., Van Gheluwe, B., and Konitz, M. 1975. A comparison of four styles of racing starts in swimming. In: J. P. Clarys and L. Lewillie (eds.), Swimming II. International Series on Sport Sciences, Vol. 2, pp.233–240. University Park Press, Baltimore.

Barthels, K. M., and Adrian, M. J. 1975. Three-dimensional spatial hand patterns of skilled butterfly swimmers. In: J. P. Clarys and L. Lewillie (eds.), Swimming II. International Series on Sport Sciences, Vol. 2, pp. 154–160. University Park Press, Baltimore.

Belokovsky, V. 1971. An analysis of pulling motions in the crawl arm stroke. In: L. Lewillie and J. P. Clarys (eds.), First International Symposium on Biomechanics in Swimming, pp. 217–221. Universite Libre de Bruxelles, Brussels.

Bowers, J. E. 1973. A biomechanical comparison of the grab and conventional sprint starts in competitive swimming. Unpublished master's thesis, Pennsylvania State University.

Bowers, J. E., and Cavanagh, P. R. 1975. A biomechanical comparison of the grab and conventional sprint starts in competitive swimming. In: J. P. Clarys and L. Lewillie (eds.), Swimming II. International Series on Sport Sciences, Vol. 2, pp. 225–232. University Park Press, Baltimore.

Brown, R. M., and Counsilman, J. E. 1971. The role of lift in propelling the swimmer. In: J. M. Cooper (ed.), Biomechanics. Proceedings of the C.I.C. Symposium on Biomechanics, pp. 179–188. The Athletic Institute, Chicago.

Bruce, J. 1974. Paired movements between pull and kick in 6-beat backstroke and freestyle crawl. Swimming World 15:48–49.

Bucher, W. 1975. The influence of the leg kick and the arm stroke on the total speed during the crawl stroke. In: J. P. Clarys and L. Lewillie (eds.), Swimming II. International Series on Sport Sciences, Vol. 2, pp. 180–187. University Park Press, Baltimore.

Cavanagh, P. R., Palmgren, J. V., and Kerr, B. R. 1975. A device to measure forces at the hands during the grab start. In: J. P. Clarys and L. Lewillie (eds.), Swimming II. International Series on Sport Sciences, Vol. 2, pp. 43–50. University Park Press, Baltimore.

Counsilman, J. E. 1968. The Science of Swimming. Prentice Hall, Englewood Cliffs, N.J.

Counsilman, J. E. 1971. The application of Bernoulli's principle to human propulsion in water. In: L. Lewillie and J. P. Clarys (eds.), First International Symposium on Biomechanics in Swimming, pp. 59–71. Universite Libre de Bruxelles, Brussels.

East, D. J. 1970. Swimming: An analysis of stroke frequency, stroke length, and performance. N. Z. J. Health, Phys. Educ., and Recr. 3:16–27.

Firby, H. 1973. The breast stroke kick. Swimming World 14:40–41.

Gallenstein, J., and Huston, R. L. 1973. Analysis of swimming motions. Hum. Factors 15:91–98.

Goldfuss, A. J. 1970. A temporal and force analysis of the crawl arm stroke during tethered swimming. Unpublished masters thesis, Pennsylvania State University.

Groves, R., and Roberts, J. A. 1972. A further investigation of the optimum angle of projection for the racing start in swimming. Res. Q. 43:167–174.

Hanauer, E. S. 1967. The grab start. Swimming World 8:5 and 42.

Hanauer, E. S. 1972. Grab start faster than conventional start. Swimming World 13:8–9 and 54–55.

Heusner, W. W. 1959. Theoretical specifications for the racing dive: Optimum angle of take-off. Res. Q. 30:25–37.

Jensen, R. K., and Blanksby, B. 1975. A model for upper extremity forces during the underwater phase of the front crawl. In: J. P. Clarys and L. Lewillie (eds.), Swimming II. International Series on Sport Sciences, Vol. 2, pp. 145–153. University Park Press, Baltimore.

Jorgensen, L. W. 1972. A cinematographic and descriptive comparison of three selected freestyle racing starts in competitive swimming. Dissert. Abstr. Int. 3761-A.

Kent, M. R., and Atha, J. 1975. Intracycle kinematics and body configuration changes in the breast stroke. In: J. P. Clarys and L. Lewillie (eds.), Swimming II. International Series on Sport Sciences, Vol. 2, pp.125–129. University Park Press, Baltimore.

Magel, J. R. 1970. Propelling force measured during tethered swimming in the four competitive swimming styles. Res. Q. 41:68–74.

Maglischo, C. W., and Maglischo, E. 1968. Comparison of three racing starts used in competitive swimming. Res. Q. 39:604–609.

Miller, D. I. 1975. Biomechanics of swimming. Exercise and Sport Sciences Reviews, Vol. 3, pp. 219–248. Academic Press, New York.

Miyashita, M. 1974. Method of calculating mechanical power in swimming the breast stroke. Res. Q. 45:128–137.

Persyn, U., DeMaeyer, J., and Vervoeche, H. 1975. Investigation of hydrodynamic determinants of competitive swimming strokes. In: J. P. Clarys and L. Lewillie (eds.), Swimming II. International Series on Sport Sciences, Vol. 2, pp. 214–222. University Park Press, Baltimore.

Roffer, B. J. 1971. A comparison of the grab and conventional racing starts in swimming. Unpublished masters thesis, Pennsylvania State University.

Scheuchenzuber, H. J., Jr. 1975. Kinetic and kinematic characteristics in the performance of tethered and nontethered swimming of the front crawl arm stroke. Dissert. Abstr. Int. 6498-A.

Schleihauf, R. E. 1974. A biomechanical analysis of freestyle. Swimming Technique 89–96.

Seireg, A., and Baz, A. 1971. A mathematical model for swimming mechanics. In: L. Lewillie and J. P. Clarys (eds.), First International Symposium on Biomechanics in Swimming, pp. 81–103. Universite Libre de Bruxelles, Brussels.

Tendy, S. M. 1974. A biomechanical analysis of the freestyle arm stroke. Unpublished masters thesis, Pennsylvania State University.

Thomsen, E. A. 1975. Comparison of the conventional and grab starts in crawl swimming. Tidsskrift for Legemsøvelser 39:130–138.

Watson, D. 1969. Variations in freestyle swimming. Swimming World 10:13.

# Time Relations: Running, Swimming, and Skating Performances

**I. Holmér**

It is well known that world swimming records are broken more frequently than world running records. Furthermore, a distance swimmer, as opposed to a sprint swimmer, can maintain a higher percentage of maximal velocity than can a distance runner, as opposed to a sprint runner. Attempts have been made to explain these differences between swimming and running (Jokl et al., 1976). To be relevant, such a comparison requires consideration of the physical factors determining work rate in the different types of exercise. Furthermore, a comparison must be based on similar physiological conditions. This means that the source of energy yield for the muscular contractions must be essentially the same.

## ENERGY YIELDING PROCESSES

During short-term, sprint type exercise (for about 10 sec), the energy for muscular contractions is provided by high energy phosphate compounds (ATP and CP). It is possible that oxygen bound to myoglobin can play a role for the energy yielding processes during the first seconds of muscular work (Åstrand et al., 1960). When maximal work time is prolonged, a resynthesis of ATP is necessary and is provided by anaerobic and aerobic energy yielding processes. The relative importance of these two processes in relation to maximal work time is rather well developed. In a 1-min maximal exercise period, the anaerobic processes may account for approximately 70–80% of the total energy yield, while in maximal work periods greater than about 2 min, the aerobic processes are responsible for more than 50% of the energy yield (Åstrand and Rodahl, 1970). As a result of this shift of energy yielding processes, the power output of the human muscle is significantly reduced with increasing time (Hill, 1927; Wilkie, 1960; Margaria, 1968).

## TIME/VELOCITY RELATIONSHIP

Taking into account these fundamental metabolic properties of human muscular functioning, it is evident that work times should be as close as possible when comparing maximal performance in the different types of exercise. For this purpose, swimming 50 yards in 20.6 sec compares favorably with running 200 m in 19.8 sec. Corresponding velocities in m/s are defined as maximal velocities (100%) for that particular type of exercise. Swimmers do not compete over shorter distances. In work times less than 10 sec, the start is a substantial part of the race, and calculated mean velocity may not be very representative of that work time. Actually, the 200-m run in 19.80 sec is faster (10.10 m/s) than the 100-m race in 9.95 sec (10.05 m/s). The percentage of maximal velocity attained in events of longer distances are plotted in Figure 1, where men's world records of 1976 have been used. Also included are the 1976 swimming records of US swimmers (distances in yards).

A similar curve for speed skating has been plotted using 1976 world records. Here, however, extrapolation back to a work time of about 20 sec is necessary because 500 m (37.00 sec) is the shortest distance of competition. Assuming a reduction in maximal velocity from 20–40 sec of work similar to that in swimming and running (about 8%), the maximal velocity (100%) is 14.59 m/s, i.e., 286 m in 20 sec. An underestimation of this value by 5% (15.36 m/s) will result in values approximately 4% lower at longer distances. It appears that the decrease in velocity with increased work time in speed skating is similar or even less pronounced than in swimming (Figure 1).

Runners lose speed at rates about 50% greater than do swimmers. Within about 4 min, runners lose 30%, swimmers 22%, and skaters 18% of their maximal velocities attained during a 20 sec race. This difference between running on the one hand and swimming and speed skating on the other is probably explained by physiological factors. A closer examination of the mechanical load factors and of the energy cost and efficiency of human locomotion seems appropriate.

## ENERGY COST OF WORK

Swimming, running, and skating are quite different types of locomotion and with different mechanical load factors; differences in efficiency of movement might be expected. However, comparing data for the energy

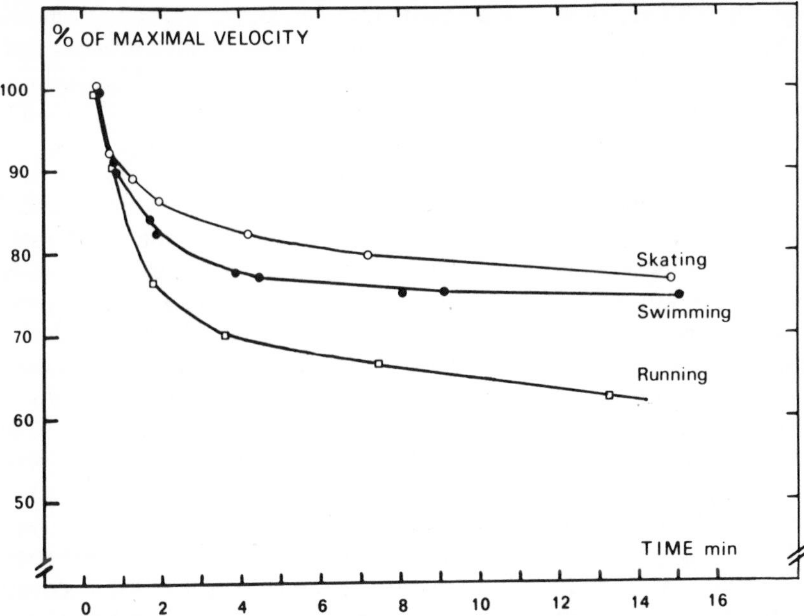


Figure 1. Decline of running, swimming, and skating velocities, with work times based on 1976 world records.

costs (E) of swimming, running, and skating yields an integrated measure of total mechanical work ($W_{tot}$) and efficiency (e) by definition:

$$E = \frac{W_{tot}}{e} \tag{1}$$

When a body moves through a fluid medium (e.g., water or air), a force reacts against it, resisting its motion. This force is known as drag (D). The amount of drag depends on the medium and on the size, shape, and speed (v) of the body.

Drag is proportional ($\propto$) to the square of the velocity:

$$D \propto v^2 \tag{2}$$

Drag of the human body passively towed in water at different velocities satisfies Equation 2 (Karpovich 1933; Clarys, 1976).

The concept of active drag (di Prampero et al., 1974) probably does not affect this general relationship between drag and velocity. In swimming, work against drag constitutes almost the entire mechanical work load. Vertical work and energy spent in acceleration of the body limbs can probably be neglected in this context. It can be assumed that energy expenditure rate ($\dot{E}_{sw}$) is approximately proportional to the square of the velocity ($v^2$), although the data developed by di Prampero et al. (in preparation) yield a slightly smaller exponent.

In running, drag (wind resistance) is of much less importance (Pugh, 1971). Mechanical work in running can be divided into external and internal work. External work is that fraction of total mechanical work necessary to sustain the displacements of the center of gravity; internal work is that fraction that is required to overcome muscle viscosity and joint friction, to sustain isometric contractions, and to produce those movements of the limbs that do not lead to a displacement of the center of gravity (Cavagna, Saibene, and Margaria, 1964). According to these authors, the total mechanical work, external and internal, per km seems to be independent of speed. As a consequence, energy expenditure rate ($\dot{E}_r$) is reported to be linearly related to velocity (Margaria et al., 1963). However, work against wind resistance does contribute to the total mechanical work at higher running velocities. The energy cost of overcoming air resistance is calculated at 7.5% of the total energy cost at middle distance speed and 13% at sprint speed (Pugh).

Di Prampero et al. (1976) recently published an extensive analysis of speed skating. A speed skater has to overcome work against wind resistance (drag) and work against other forces (vertical displacement of the center of gravity, acceleration and deceleration of the limbs, and friction between the skate blades and the ice). Because of the higher velocities in skating, wind resistance is a significantly greater loading factor than in running. According to di Prampero et al. (1976), the energy cost of skating ($\dot{E}_{sk}$) in liters of oxygen per min for a 70-kg man is described by the equation:

$$\dot{E}_{sk} = 3.2v + 0.028v^3 \tag{3}$$

where v is the speed in m/s. At 10 m/s, work against drag and work against nondrag forces are almost equal.

Table 1 schematically summarizes the relationships between energy expenditure rate and velocity for the three types of exercise as presented in the literature. Athletes in endurance events are distinguished by high maximal aerobic power without regard to the type of exercise involved (Saltin and Åstrand, 1967; Holmér, Lundin, and Eriksson, 1974). There seems to be no reason to assume that anaerobic

Table 1. Schematic illustration of the relationship between energy expenditure rate (E) and velocity (v) in swimming, running, and speed skating[a]

| Exercise | Relationship | Reference |
|---|---|---|
| Swimming | $\dot{E}_{sw} \propto v^2$ | di Prampero et al. (in preparation) |
| Running | $\dot{E}_r \propto v$ | Margaria et al. (1963) |
| Skating | $\dot{E}_{sk} \propto v + v^3$ | di Prampero et al. (1976) |

[a] Correction for wind resistance at higher velocities according to Pugh (1971).

power or muscular power should differ significantly among swimmers, runners, and speed skaters.

## TIME RELATION OF ENERGY EXPENDITURE RATE

Using $\dot{E}$ for the 20 sec event as 100% and calculating $\dot{E}$ for longer distances according to the relationship given in Table 1, a new set of curves can be drawn. As illustrated in Figure 2, the decrease in performance with increasing work time based upon the energy expenditure rate is almost identical in swimming, running, and skating. In other words, whatever the nature of the mechanical load factors, the rate of energy expenditure decreases with time in essentially the same way, an expected result considering the fundamental metabolic properties of human muscles. Consequently, the slower decrease in maximal velocity of swimmers compared with runners (Figure 1) can be explained by differences in mechanical work performed and efficiency of movement (Equation 1). The physiological adaptations to swimming are apparently of less importance.

The surprisingly steep increase in speed of running when work time is progressively reduced might be readily explained by the linear relationship between total mechanical work rate and velocity (Cavagna, Saibene, and Margaria). This linear relationship reveals an efficient

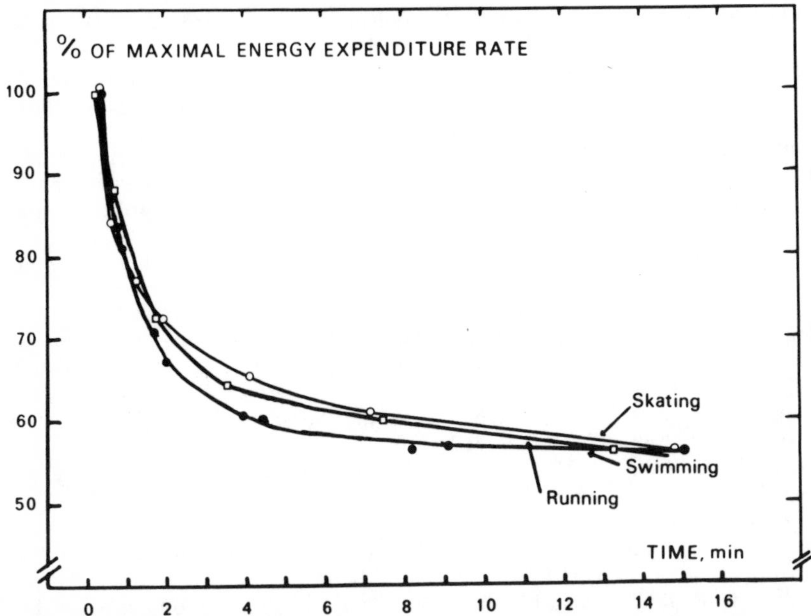


Figure 2. The decline of energy expenditure rates in running, swimming, and skating are shown with work times.

means of locomotion. Efficiency values of 50–60% have been calculated (Cavagna, Saibene, and Margaria; Pugh). One possible explanation for this phenomenon is that the elastic potential energy stored in the stretched contracted muscle is utilized during the subsequent positive work phase (Cavagna et al., 1971; Asmussen and Bonde-Petersen, 1974).

## REFERENCES

Asmussen, E., and Bonde-Petersen, F. 1974. Storage of elastic energy in skeletal muscles in man. Acta Physiol. Scand. 91:385–392.

Åstrand, I., Åstrand, P.-O., Christensen, E. H., and Hedman, R. 1960. Myohemoglobin as an oxygen-store in man. Acta Physiol. Scand. 48:454–458.

Åstrand, P.-O., and Rodahl, K. 1970. Textbook of Work Physiology. McGraw-Hill Book Company, New York.

Cavagna, G. A., Komarek, L., Citterio, G., and Margaria, R. 1971. Power output of previously stretched muscle. In: Biomechanics II. Medicine and Sport, Vol. 6, pp. 159–167. Karger, Basel.

Cavagna, G. A., Saibene, F. P., and Margaria, R. 1964. Mechanical work in running. J. Appl. Physiol. 19:249–256.

Clarys, J. P. 1976. Investigations on the hydrodynamic and morphological aspects of the human body. Vrije Universiteit Brussel, Brussels.

di Prampero, P. E., Cortili, G., Mognoni, P., and Saibene, F. 1976. Energy cost of speed skating and efficiency of work against air resistance. J. Appl. Physiol. 40:584–591.

di Prampero, P. E., Pendergast, D. R., Wilson, D. W., and Rennie, D. W. 1974. Energetics of swimming in man. J. Appl. Physiol. 37:1–5.

di Prampero, P. E., Pendergast, D. R., Wilson, D. W., and Rennie, D. W. Energy expenditure, body drag, and lactic acid production during high speed swimming in man. In preparation.

Hill, A. V. 1927. Muscular Movement in Man. Cornell University Press, Ithaca.

Holmér, I., Lundin, A., and Eriksson, B. O. 1974. Maximum oxygen uptake during swimming and running by elite swimmers. J. Appl. Physiol. 36:711–714.

Jokl, E., Jokl, P., Green, R., and Reinhardt, B. 1976. Running and swimming world records. Am. Corr. Ther. J. 30(5).

Karpovich, P. V. 1933. Water resistance in swimming. Res. Q. 4:21–28.

Margaria, R. 1968. Capacity and power of the energy processes in muscle activity: Their practical relevance in athletics. Int. Z. Angew. Physiol. 25:352–360.

Margaria, R., Cerretelli, P., Aghemo, P., and Sassi, G. 1963. Energy cost of running. J. Appl. Physiol. 18:367–370.

Pugh, L. G. C. E. 1971. The influence of wind resistance in running and walking and the mechanical efficiency of work against horizontal and vertical forces. J. Physiol. 213:255–276.

Saltin, B., and Åstrand, P.-O. 1967. Maximal oxygen uptake in athletes. J. Appl. Physiol. 23:353–358.

Wilkie, D. R. 1960. Man as a source of mechanical power. Ergonomics 3:1–8.

# The Influence of Selected Biomechanical Factors on the Energy Cost of Swimming

**D. R. Pendergast, P. E. di Prampero, A. B. Craig, Jr., and D. W. Rennie**

The biomechanical and physiological study of human performance is dependent upon valid and quantitative measurement methods. Cinematographic, mechanical, and physiological analyses are hampered by the environmental conditions imposed in swimming. The presence of water through which the swimmer must move and the inaccessibility of the swimmer while actually swimming limit the type of measurements that can be performed in standard swimming pools. Swimming analysis is possible in facilities specifically designed for swimming research such as an annular pool, the swimming flume, and ship towing tanks. These specialized facilities are not at the disposal of swimming teachers and coaches and consequently other methods of analysis must be used. By utilizing research performed in sophisticated facilities, it is possible for practitioners to analyze swimming performances quantitatively.

The first step in analyzing swimming performances is to examine the basic equations that govern the overall energetics of performance as they apply to swimming:

$$\dot{W} = D \times v \qquad (1)$$

$$W = \dot{E} \times e \qquad (2)$$

where $\dot{W}$ is the external power expressed in kg/m/min$^{-1}$, v is the average velocity in m/min$^{-1}$, D is body drag in kg, $\dot{E}$ is the total energy cost per unit time expressed as equivalent oxygen units, in liters/min$^{-1}$, and e is the net mechanical efficiency. An examination of these equations reveals the important factors in determining the energetics of swimming: body drag, velocity, energy cost, and efficiency.

By equating and rearranging Equations 1 and 2 as follows:

$$v = \dot{V}_{O_2} \times (e \times D^{-1}) \tag{3}$$

it can be demonstrated that the velocity of progression is determined by two factors. The first is the total energy input, which is the product of aerobic and anaerobic power, and the second is the ratio of efficiency and body drag, which is a reflection of the technical ability to swim. In running, D is negligible until very high speeds are reached, whereas, during swimming, D is a predominant variable throughout the entire range of velocities. The necessity to consider D while swimming and not while running, in combination with the fact that D is highly variable in swimming, complicates interpretation of comparisons of the changes in world record times for running and swimming. Furthermore, it is important to note that it is the ratio of efficiency to drag that is important in determining swimming velocity at any given oxygen consumption and not e or D independently. However, inasmuch as both e and D can vary independently, it is important to consider each variable in analyzing swimming performance. It is possible for two swimmers to achieve the same maximum swimming speed although one might have a high D, if his e compensates.

The purpose of this chapter is to discuss the ratio of e/D or the technical aspects of swimming. The importance of the e/D ratio can be emphasized by examining the potential performance improvement that would result from improvements of $\dot{V}_{O_2}$ and/or e/D. An individual can increase his $\dot{V}_{O_2}$ max only by about 10% while running. $\dot{V}_{O_2}$ max during swimming has been reported to be about 20% lower than for running (Holmér, 1974), a difference that can be eliminated by swim training that sets the maximum improvement in $\dot{V}_{O_2}$ max at 30%. Although this is a large improvement, an examination of data for the e/D ratio reveals a potential improvement of 100%. This analysis should not suggest that metabolic training is not beneficial, and it should suggest the importance of improving technical ability. In this analysis, the maximum potential changes in both $\dot{E}$ and the e/D ratio was used. The actual improvement in performance of a given swimmer depends on his initial and maximum potential for performance.

Although competitive swimming performance is commonly evaluated by maximum swimming velocity, this analysis is complicated by the determination of v by both $\dot{E}$ and e/D. The use of velocity as a measure does not allow discrimination of the effect of $\dot{E}$, e, or D, i.e., metabolic or technical ability. For purposes of biomechanical analysis, it is more appropriate to correct for $\dot{E}$ by rearranging Equation 3 as follows:

$$\frac{\dot{V}_{O_2}}{v} = \frac{\dot{V}_{O_2}}{d} = \frac{D}{e} \qquad (4)$$

where $\dot{V}_{O_2}$ and v have been factored for time. This set of equations provides a quantitative method of independently analyzing the biomechanical factors that influence the technical ability for swimming, D/e. In Equation 4, the energy cost per unit distance is expressed as the amount of oxygen consumed for a 1000-m swim in liters/km. As can be seen, the value of $V_{O_2}/d$ is equal to the ratio of D to e, assuming 1 liter of $O_2$ = 5 kcal and 1 kcal = 427 kg/m. Based on the equality of $V_{O_2}/d$ and D/e and the ease of measuring the $V_{O_2}$ required to swim a given d in any swimming pool (McArdle, Glasser, and Magel, 1971), analysis of the $V_{O_2}/d$ for any swimmer provides a quantitative measure of his technical ability. In Table 1, $V_{O_2}/d$ data are presented for men and women competitors and noncompetitors using the front crawl stroke. As can be seen from these data, there is a significant difference ($P \leq 0.05$) between the technical abilities of competitive men and women when compared with noncompetitive men and women. In addition, there is a significant difference ($P \leq 0.05$) between the $V_{O_2}/d$ of women and that of men of either skill level. It is also important to note the wide range of $V_{O_2}/d$ values for both men and women at each level of skill. The wide individual variability of $V_{O_2}/d$, even in the competitive group, emphasizes the potential improvement in performance that may result from improved technical ability.

In a separate study (Vaudry, 1976), 40 swimmers were evaluated by swimming instructors utilizing standard ARC criterion. Their $V_{O_2}/d$ values were measured while they swam the breast stroke and back crawl at 0.7 m/s. There was little relationship (r = 0.62) between the subjective evaluation and the $V_{O_2}/d$. The apparent inability of these instructors to

Table 1. Energy cost in liters of oxygen required to swim a given distance in km for competitive and noncompetitive male and female swimmers utilizing the front crawl

| | Women | | Men | |
|---|---|---|---|---|
| | Competitive | Noncompetitive | Competitive | Noncompetitive |
| Range | 16–50 | 28–82 | 30–62 | 41–99 |
| Mean | 36 | 40 | 49 | 56 |
| S.D. | 11 | 10 | 10 | 13 |
| N | 21 | 26 | 37 | 62 |

judge technical ability subjectively suggests the need for quantitative measurement. The $V_{O_2}$/d ratio is a valuable tool for evaluation and detection of improvements for swimmers. Based on the data from Table 1 and competitive swimming times for poor to world class swimmers, standards for evaluating $V_{O_2}$/d are proposed in Table 2. Any reduction of the $V_{O_2}$/d for a given swimmer would suggest a technical improvement.

Although the $\dot{V}_{O_2}$/d ratio provides a measure of technical ability, D, e, $\dot{E}$, and $\dot{V}_{O_2}$ at any velocity must be known for full understanding of the swimming performance. Assuming that v can be controlled, e can be calculated from measurements of $\dot{E}$ and D. The methods of measuring $\dot{E}$ were discussed previously by di Prampero which leaves only the measurement of D to analyze swimming performance on the basis of Equations 3 and 4.

A review of the literature on swimming reveals that body drag measurements were first reported by Karpovich (1933) and subsequently by many other authors (Alley, 1952; Councilman, 1955; Clarys et al., 1974; Jiskoot and Clarys, 1975). The method employed by these authors was to measure the force necessary to tow a swimmer through the water at a constant speed. In this situation, the swimmer must remain motionless because any propulsive force supplied by the swimmer would reduce the measured towing force.

The application of this type of body drag, called *passive drag,* to actual swimming is inappropriate because of the constantly changing body position and water flow characteristics around the moving body during swimming. Although passive drag apparently underestimates D during swimming, it has application for the evaluation of water resistance characteristics that are not affected by changes of body position and water flow characteristics.

In the 1950s, an alternative method of measuring drag was proposed (Alley). This method was a modified passive towing system that allowed the swimmer to swim at a set speed away from a tethering device while the force exerted by the swimmer was measured by a strain gauge. Although this method was convenient and allowed the

Table 2. Suggested values of $V_{O_2}$/d (economy) for evaluation of swimming proficiency

| | Women | Men |
|---|---|---|
| Competitive | 15–30 | 30–40 |
| Skilled | 30–35 | 40–50 |
| Average | 35–40 | 50–60 |
| Unskilled | 40–50 | 60–80 |
| Poor | 50–60 | 80–100 |

swimmer to swim, considering the average force exerted by the swimmer it may have under- or overestimated D.

A method has been developed to determine the overall effective D of a swimmer while actually swimming (di Prampero et al., 1974). The method is based on changes in aerobic metabolism caused by systematically varying the propulsive force required of the swimmer while moving at a constant velocity. This method can be used at speeds that exceed the subject's maximum aerobic swimming speed.

Based on this method, data have been obtained on the front crawl for men and women over a velocity range of 0.4–2.0 m/s. The D data for actual swimming are on the average two times greater than D determined by passive towing. D ranged from 2–24 kg between 0.4 and 2.0 m/s, with individual data widely distributed at any velocity because of variations in technical ability (di Prampero et al.; Rennie et al., 1974; Holmér, 1974 and 1975; Pendergast et al., in press). As a general trend, those swimmers who were less skilled (higher $V_{O_2}/d$) had a higher D value than did those who were more skilled (lower $V_{O_2}/d$). There were, however, exceptions to this generalization. Women had significantly less body drag on the average than men at all investigated speeds (Åstrand and Rodahl, 1970; di Prampero et al.; Rennie et al.; Pendergast et al.), a difference that was reduced but not eliminated by correcting the data for body size differences (di Prampero et al.; Pendergast et al.). In addition, correcting the $V_{O_2}/d$ for body size did not eliminate the significant difference in this value when women were compared to men (Rennie et al.; Pendergast et al.).

Active D increased as a function of v for all subjects and can be expressed by the following general equation:

$$D = k \times v^n \tag{5}$$

where the constant (k) and the exponent (n) are dependent upon individual technical ability and are consequently different for all individuals. The constant (k) is dependent upon geometric factors and the exponent (n) on hydrodynamic factors that may change during actual swimming but are constant during passive towing (Karpovich, 1933 and 1939; Counsilman; Clarys et al.). The values for k ranged from 5–12 kg and the exponents varied from 1.35–2.11; the actual value of each was dependent upon technical ability.

Given a value for D, the other factor that determines the energy cost of swimming at any velocity is e, $\dot{W}/\dot{V}_{O_2}$ (above rest). Previous studies (Karpovich, 1939; Alley; Counsilman; Clarys et al.) calculated efficiencies from 2–8% for swimming, depending upon the particular individual swimming and on the value of v. These values appear low when compared with muscle efficiencies of 25% and result from underestimation of D through the use of passive towing measurements. In three studies (di Prampero et al.; Rennie et al.; Pendergast et al.), efficiencies based on active D ranged from 2–18% for the front crawl. The actual observed value for e was dependent upon the subject and the swimming speed, with the highest values observed at 1.8 m/s in a competitive swimmer. On the average, e was higher in skilled than in unskilled swimmers and for women when compared with men at almost all speeds for both competitive and noncompetitive swimmers (de Prampero et al.; Rennie et al.; Pendergast et al.). In cases selected for both sex and skill level, lower e's were observed in women and in skilled subjects; however, because of an even lower D value, their $V_{O_2}/d$ values followed the pattern of lower values for women and skilled swimmers.

It has been shown that D and e vary independently for individual subjects and increase in all subjects as a function of v, the nature of which is dependent upon the subject's skill level. Because it is the ratio of D to e that determines the $V_{O_2}/d$ (Equation 4), any variation in $V_{O_2}/d$ can be explained by variations in either D or e or both. It has been reported (di Prampero et al.; Rennie et al.; Pendergast et al.) that $V_{O_2}/d$ is independent of swimming speed up to 1.2 m/s for skilled swimmers with an average value of 51 liters/km for men and 37 liters/km for women. This consistency can be explained by an increase in e that is proportionate to the increase in D that results when swimming velocity is increased. However, above a given speed, 1.1–1.4 m/s in the case of a skilled swimmer, D increases curvilinearly based on Equation 5, whereas e increased linearly, the result of which was an increased D/e ratio and a concomitant increase in $V_{O_2}/d$. $V_{O_2}/d$ was constant up to a speed that represented 75 and 30% of the individual swimmer's $v_{max}$ for skilled and unskilled subjects, respectively. In general, women could not swim to as high a percentage of their maximum speed without increased cost per unit distance when compared with men; as a result, their maximum v was less than would be predicted for their $E_{max}$.

At relatively high speeds, and at more than 75 and 30% of $V_{max}$ for skilled swimmers respectively, the increase in D was disproportionate when compared with the increase observed in e at all speeds. The result of an increase in D that is not offset by a proportionate increase in e is a progressive increase in $V_{O_2}/d$ with increasing speed up to maximum. In two athletes (Pendergast et al.) swimming at speeds greater than 1.8 m/s, there was a decrease in e that resulted in a dramatic increase in both D/e and $V_{O_2}/d$. The average value of $V_{O_2}/d$ at the individual swimmer's $v_{max}$ was twice the value observed for the same swimmer over the optimum velocity range (40–80 and 80–160 for skilled and unskilled swimmers, respectively).

As stated earlier, women expend about 30% less energy to swim a given distance than their male counterparts at any given velocity. Examination of the components of $V_{O_2}/d$—D and e—reveals that women have significantly less D at all investigated speeds (di Prampero et al.; Rennie et al.; Pendergast et al.) and equal or greater e values, depending upon the specific velocity. The differences in both $V_{O_2}/d$ and D were reduced but were still significant when corrected for body surface area differences. This suggests that women are technically better swimmers than men, even when corrections are made for body size. This conclusion is an apparent contradiction to the observation that all competitive swimming times are better for men than for women. This apparent contradiction is resolved by the observation that the metabolic power of men is sufficient to compensate for their higher $V_{O_2}/d$; consequently, they swim faster than women. However, under conditions where the metabolic power differences between men and women are minimized and the distances long enough to emphasize economy of swimming, as in marathon races, women in fact dominate the competition.

If the differences in both $V_{O_2}/d$ and D cannot be accounted for by the smaller body size of women there must be other factors that assist women during swimming. It is well known that women are less dense than men (Åstrand and Rodahl, 1970), suggesting that body composition may play a role in minimizing the energy cost of swimming in women. Furthermore, Karpovich (1933) suggested a model for understanding the role of leg kicking as a compensatory mechanism for the tendency of almost all individuals' legs to sink in the water when the body is in a horizontal attitude. In this model, Karpovich proposed that the force generated by the leg kick could be divided into a horizontal component, a propulsive force, and a vertical component that compensates for the legs' tendency to sink and that maintains a horizontal attitude. The vertical component of the leg kick requires energy but does not contribute to propulsive force and consequently would lower e. Thus, if women's feet tended to sink with less force than men's, the women would require less vertical force from their leg kicks and would enjoy a considerable savings in energy.

To test this hypothesis, an analysis was performed on body composition and its distribution in 32 men and 16 women who were active in competitive swimming (Pendergast and Craig, 1974; Rennie et al.; Pendergast et al.). The body composition of the subjects was determined from both skinfold and underwater weighing measurements. The distribution of the body composition was determined by two methods. In the first method, the body was strapped to a rigid frame that was submerged 10 cm below the water surface. The frame was supported by a fulcrum placed under the center of air and a strain gauge at the opposite end of the frame. This system allowed the measurement of the tendency of the feet to sink from the horizontal position by determining the force necessary to hold the position of the body horizontal. This sinking force is equal and opposite to the vertical component of the leg kick if the swimmer maintains a horizontal attitude while swimming. In the second method, by weighing the entire body and the mass of body from the center of gravity down the total body density, the density of the body above and below the center of gravity could be determined.

The hypothesis was that women would be less dense in both their upper and lower body segments. Consequently, they would be higher in the water and their feet would tend to sink from a horizontal attitude with less force. The result of this would be less D and higher e at all speeds. The average density of women was significantly less than that of men for both upper and lower body segments (Pendergast and Craig). As a result of lower density, female swimmers were able to swim higher in the water at any lung volume; this tended to reduce the value of D. In addition, the force with which the feet tended to sink was less in women (0.8 kg) than in men (1.6 kg) as a result of lower density of the lower body segments.

The combined effect of the lower densities of upper and lower body segments is a lower D and higher e. The increased e is a result of less energy being wasted to compensate for the tendency of the legs to sink. Although the differences between men and women were great, the range of values for the tendency of the feet to sink was 0.2–1.5 kg for women and 0.4–2.4 kg for men. The variation in these values paralleled variations in the distribution of body composition: most women had lower values than men had.

When compensation was made for the force with which the feet tend to sink, the $V_{O_2}/d$ for men was reduced to 20 liters/km, whereas the women were not assisted when compensated in a similar manner ($V_{O_2}/d$ = 18 liters/km). In fact, when the female subjects' legs were floated and immobilized, they could not maintain a speed that represented only 75% of their $v_{max}$. This suggests that the leg kick provides significant propulsive force for women swimmers.

Theoretically, a swimmer can either let his legs sink in water, thus creating a higher D, or compensate by a facilitated leg kick that would result in a lower e. A decreased e or increased D would result in a higher $V_{O_2}/d$ unless compensated for by a corresponding decrease in D or increase in e. A significantly greater increase in the $V_{O_2}/d$ has been observed when a swimmer does not add sufficient leg kick to offset the effect of his individual lower body density.

It has been suggested (Pendergast, et al.) that the effect of lower body density is dependent only on its absolute value and not on the sex of the subject as a determinate of $V_{O_2}/d$. It was also suggested (Pendergast et al.) that skilled swimmers, regardless of sex, have lower $V_{O_2}/d$ ratios than do their unskilled counterparts with the same density values. Based on the identity of $V_{O_2}/d$ and D/e ratios, multiple linear regression equations for the relationships among e, D, and $V_{O_2}/d$ were computed for men and women competitive and noncompetitive swimmers. The data from this analysis are presented in Table 3.

Both D and e have significant influence in determining $V_{O_2}/d$, but their relative importance varies among men, women, competitive, and noncompetitive swimmers. The D factor seems more influential in competitive women, whereas the e factor assumes greater importance for the noncompetitive women. For competitive men the weighing factors for e and D are similar to those for the noncompetitive group.

Inasmuch as there were no differences in body composition between men or women competitive and noncompetitive swimmers, the lower $V_{O_2}/d$ must have resulted from a lower D for men and women and an improved e in women. These improvements probably result from improved arm strokes used in swimming the front crawl. The reasons for the improved stroke cannot be analyzed with this data. However, the improved stroke is typically characterized by a slower stroke frequency at submaximal speeds and the ability to increase stroke frequency to a high rate to achieve maximum v (Craig and Pendergast, 1974).

If the body composition and its distribution is an important determinant of the energy cost of swimming, boy and girl swimmers, who have similar muscle and fat contents, should expend approximately the same energy to swim a given distance. In a pilot study of 10 swimmers between the ages of 8 and 12 years, $V_{O_2}/d$ was the same for the boys (22 liters/km) as it was for the girls (16 liters/km). The differences between the competitive times of these subjects was a result of their individual metabolic powers. Between the ages of 12 and 16 years, the $\dot{V}_{O_2}$ max per kg body weight was shown by Thorén to increase in boys while decreasing in girls. At first examination, this would suggest a poorer swimming performance for the 12–16 year old girls. Further examina-

Table 3. Multiple linear regression equations for body drag (D) and efficiency (e) as a function of economy ($V_{O_2}/d$), where D is measured in kg, e in percent, and $V_{O_2}/d$ in liters of oxygen per 100 km

| | | |
|---|---|---|
| Competitive | Women | $V_{O_2}d = 31.9 + 6.36\,D - 3.75\,e$ |
| | Men | $V_{O_2}/d = 51.4 + 4.52\,D - 5.04\,e$ |
| Noncompetitive | Women | $V_{O_2}/d = 36.24 + 9.59\,D - 7.15\,e$ |
| | Men | $V_{O_2}/d = 55.5 + 6.43\,D - 7.32\,e$ |

tion reveals that the $\dot{V}_{O_2}$ max of the girls actually increased. This is the important factor in swimming, but body weight increased disproportionally. The disproportionate increase in body weight suggests the addition of fat tissue in this sample of girls and also implies a reduction in the $V_{O_2}/d$ ratio. The observation that both boy and girl swimmers improve their times between the ages of 12 and 16 years is a result of improved $\dot{E}$ in boys and a modest improvement of $\dot{E}$ in girls that is accompanied by a significant decrease in the $V_{O_2}/d$ ratio.

Another biomechanical factor that influences the $V_{O_2}/d$ is stroke selection. Systematic comparisons of the front crawl and breast stroke (Holmér, 1974) and back crawl and breast stroke (Vaudry) have been made. From the data collected, the front crawl seems to be the most economical standard stroke. The front crawl is also the only stroke in which the $V_{O_2}/d$ is constant over a wide range of swimming speeds. The breast stroke has been shown in several studies to be more economical that either the back crawl or butterfly, although the intrasubject variability was very high. Vaudry demonstrated that the breast stroke was no more economical that the back crawl when mean data were considered, but an examination of individual swimmers showed large differences between the two strokes. It seems that the individual subject's technical ability at each stroke is a more important determinant of the $V_{O_2}/d$ than any systematic stroke advantage or disadvantage. It is also apparent that the $V_{O_2}/d$ increases as a function of speed during performance of the breast stroke and butterfly; this emphasizes the need to consider swimming v when making any stroke comparison.

In summary, Equations 1 through 4 provide a basis to analyze swimming performances quantitatively. In a practical sense, the $V_{O_2}/d$ ratio can be measured in any pool and is a useful tool for evaluation of swimming proficiency. However, in order to study the factors that determine the $V_{O_2}/d$, both D and e must be measured. It is important to emphasize that swimming v is determined by two factors: $\dot{E}$, aerobic plus anaerobic power; and the ratio of e and D, technical ability. The wide variability of the D/e ratio suggests that the development of technical ability has the potential to reduce $V_{O_2}/d$ by a factor of four.

In the front crawl, breast stroke, and back crawl, women expend significantly less energy per unit distance than do men, even after corrections are made for body size. This difference is attributable to lower D and greater e values. Female swimmers have lower densities of the upper body, which reduce D, and also for the lower body, which reduce the vertical component of their leg kick and consequently yields greater e. The greater metabolic power of men of all ages is sufficient to more than compensate for the greater $V_{O_2}/d$ observed for men; their competitive times are consequently better.

On the average, the front crawl is the most economical stroke for all individuals. A comparison shows that $V_{O_2}/d$ for other strokes is more dependent on the technical ability of individual swimmers than on any systematic stroke differences. It appears that the $V_{O_2}/d$ for the front crawl is constant over a range of velocities up to 75 and 30% of $v_{max}$ for skilled and unskilled swimmers, respectively. Above this range of v for the front crawl and for the entire range of v for other strokes, $V_{O_2}/d$ increases as a function of v.

## REFERENCES


Adrian, M. J., Singh, M., and Karpovich, P. V. 1966. Energy cost of leg kick, arm stroke, and whole crawl stroke. J. Appl. Physiol. 21:1763–1766.

Alley, L. E. 1952. An analysis of water resistance and propulsion in swimming the crawl stroke. Res. Q. 23:253–270.

Anderson, L. K. 1960. Energy cost of swimming. Acta Circu. Scand. 253(suppl.):169–174.

Åstrand, P.-O., and Rodahl, K. 1970. Textbook of Work Physiology. McGraw Hill Book Company, New York. pp. 545–546.

Counsilman, J. 1955. Forces in swimming two types of crawl stroke. Res. Q. 26(2):127–139.

Craig, A. B., Jr., and Pendergast, D. R. 1974. Relationships of velocity, stroke rate, and stroke distance during freestyle swimming. Physiologist 17(abstr.):305.

Clarys, J. P., Jiskoot, J., Riskey, H., and Brouwer, P. J. 1974. Total resistance in water and its relation to body form. In: R. C. Nelson and C. A. Morehouse (eds.), Biomechanics IV, International Series on Sport Sciences, Vol. 1, pp. 187–196. University Park Press, Baltimore.

di Prampero, P. E., Pendergast, D. R., Wilson, D. R., and Rennie, D. W. 1974. Energetics of swimming in man. J. Appl. Physiol. 37:1–4.

Egolinski, E. A. 1940. Expenditure of energy in competitive swimming. J. Appl. Physiol. (London) 28:700–706.

Hollstrum, and Holgran. 1966. On repeatability of submaximal work tests and the influence of body position on heart rate during exercise at submaximal loads. Scand. J. Clin. Lab. Invest. 18:479–485.

Holmer, I. 1974. Physiology of swimming in man. Acta. Physiol. Scand. (suppl. 407):1–53.

Holmer, I. 1975. Efficiency of breast stroke and freestyle swimming. In: J. P. Clarys and L. Lewille (eds.), Swimming II, International Series on Sport Sciences, Vol. 2, pp. 130–136. University Park Press, Baltimore.

Jiskoot, J., and Clarys, J. P. 1975. Body resistance on and under the water surface. In: J. P. Clarys and L. Lewillie (eds.), Swimming II, International Series on Sport Sciences, Vol. 2, pp. 105–109. University Park Press, Baltimore.

Karpovich, P. V. 1933. Water resistance in swimming. Res. Q. 4:21–28.

Karpovich, P. V. 1939. Mechanical work and efficiency in swimming the crawl and backstroke. Arbeitsphysiologie 10:504–514.

Karpovich, P. V., and Millman, N. 1944. Energy expended in swimming. Am. J. Physiol. 142:140–144.

Key, J. R. 1962. Relationship between load and swim endurance in humans. Res. Q. 33:559–64.

Klissouras, V. 1968. Energy metabolism in swimming the dolphin stroke. Arbeitsphysiologie 25:142–150.

Magel, J. R., and Faulkner, J. A. 1967. Maximal oxygen uptake of college swimmers. J. Appl. Physiol. 22:1929–1938.

McArdle, W. D., Glasser, R. M., and Magel, J. R. 1971. Metabolic and cardiorespiratory response during freestyle swimming and treadmill walking. J. Appl. Physiol. 30:733–738.

Pendergast, D. R., and Craig, A. B., Jr. 1974. Biomechanics of floatation in water. Physiologist 17(abstr.):305.

Pendergast, D. R., di Prampero, P. E., Craig, A. B., Jr., Wilson, D. R., and Rennie, D. W. A quantitative analysis of the front crawl in men and women. In press.

Rennie, D. W., Pendergast, D. R., and di Prampero, P. E. 1974. Energetics of swimming in man. In: J. P. Clarys and L. Lewille (eds.), Swimming II, International Series on Sport Sciences, Vol. 2, pp. 97–104. University Park Press, Baltimore.

Vaudry, S. 1976. A comparison of breast stroke and back crawl in men and women. M. Ed. State University of New York at Buffalo, Buffalo, N.Y.

# The Swimming Flume: Experiences and Applications

**I. Holmér and S. Haglund**

Measurements of a swimmer's movements and propulsion entail complications that have prevented sophisticated physiological and biomechanical studies. Many years ago, Liljestrand and Stenström (1919) and Liljestrand and Lindhard (1919) attempted to measure oxygen uptake and cardiac output during swimming. The measurements were taken from a rowboat pacing the swimmer off the shore of Sweden's western coast. This suggested difficulties in obtaining constant velocity and representative measures of physiological variables. Investigations conducted in a swimming pool in addition to the free water test of Liljestrand and his colleagues included the problem of turns. Many of these problems can be avoided by tethered swimming. However, from a hydromechanical point of view, tethered swimming is different from free swimming. The extent to which this difference influences physiological and biomechanical adjustments to swimming is presently unknown.

In recent years, different devices have facilitated swimming research and have made it possible to simulate almost normal swimming conditions and to reproduce work rate, i. e., swimming velocity, accurately. di Prampero et al. (1974) reported a series of investigations in a 60-m circumference annular pool in which the swimmer was paced by a platform moving at predetermined, constant speed. Clarys (1976) and his coworkers have used a 220-m long ship model basin with a platform setting the velocity of the swimmer. The swimming flume (Åstrand and Englesson, 1972) has been in practical use since 1968. The aim of this chapter is to summarize the experiences gained and to review some results of the research into and applications of the swimming flume.

---

These studies were supported by the Swedish National Association Against Heart and Chest Diseases and the Research Council of the Swedish Sports Federation.

## DESCRIPTION

The swimming flume was first described by Åstrand and Englesson. The construction of the swimming flume is shown in Figure 1. Water is circulated in the basin (1) by two hydrostatically-driven propeller pumps (5) located in the bottom of a 2.5-m wide and 1.25-m deep vertical loop. A 30-watt power pack (6) supplies the propellers of the hydraulic motors with the pressurized oil that rotates the propellers. The front and rear of the basin are fitted with guide vanes (2) that produce a more uniform and near laminar flow in the center part of the test basin where the subject swims. A large inspection window (3) is provided in the side of the test basin. The total water content of the basin is 48 m³.

Water velocity in the flume can be varied between 0 and 2 m/s in intervals of 0.01 m/s. In the velocity range 0.6–1.9 m/s, reproducibility is better than ±0.02 m/s. The velocity is set on a remote control unit (8), with an electronic control device (7) balancing the desired setting and the output of a pulse generator (10) that monitors the rotation speed of the propellers.

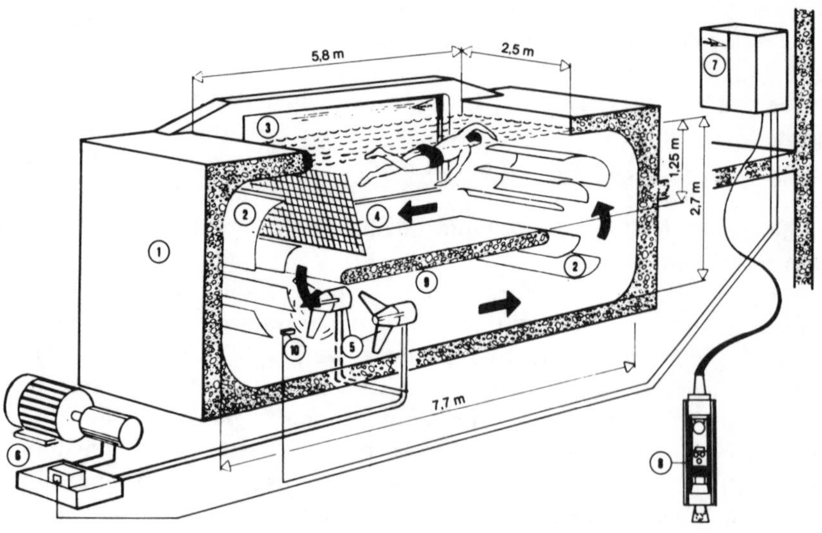


1. Basin
2. Vanes
3. Window
4. Safety net
5. Propeller pumps
6. Hydraulic power pack
7. Electronic control device
8. Remote control
9. Floor of swimming chamber
10. Puls generator

Figure 1. Schematic illustration of swimming flume.

A number of improvements have been made on the swimming flume since 1968. The control equipment utilizes digital instead of analog signals, giving more precise and reliable control. In the first flumes, propeller speed was constant and the change in water speed was achieved by changing the pitch of the propeller. In the present model of the flume, hydraulic transmission is used and water speed is varied by changing the propeller speed (range: 0–265 rpm).

A new driving system provides better control of the water speed and easier montage of the unit. In addition, by lengthening the basin 1 m the flow characteristics at high water velocities have been improved, e.g., "still standing" waves are almost eliminated.

The general opinion among swimmers who have practiced a few times in the swimming flume is that, except for the absence of start and turns, swimming in the flume is in most respects identical to swimming in a pool. The athletes must swim at a constant speed as determined by the water flow rate and consequently cannot vary their pace. Stroke mechanics, as judged by experienced swimming coaches, are not significantly different when compared with those used in pool swimming. Almost identical values for maximal oxygen uptake have been obtained for swimmers swimming in the flume and in a 50-m pool (Holmér, Lundin, and Eriksson, 1974).

## RESEARCH AND APPLICATIONS

Current research in the swimming flume has consisted mainly in physiological and biomechanical studies. A brief review of some of the work done is appropriate within the scope of this presentation. For a more extensive discussion of the results, the reader is referred to the original articles cited in the reference list.

The swimming flume is highly suitable for measurements of the water resistance of the human body in various body positions. However, drag during passive towing of the body through flowing water is not representative of the true resistance a swimmer has to overcome during actual swimming. The concept of active drag is a useful approach for development of a better understanding of the swimmer's propulsive work. Active drag can be calculated using the method described by di Prampero et al. The experimental procedure can be facilitated if conducted in the swimming flume (Figure 2).

During submaximal swimming at a given velocity, the drag of the swimmer is either increased or decreased by adding ($+D_A$) or subtracting ($-D_A$) given loads to or from the swimmer. Average drag during swimming (active drag) is calculated from the relationship between net

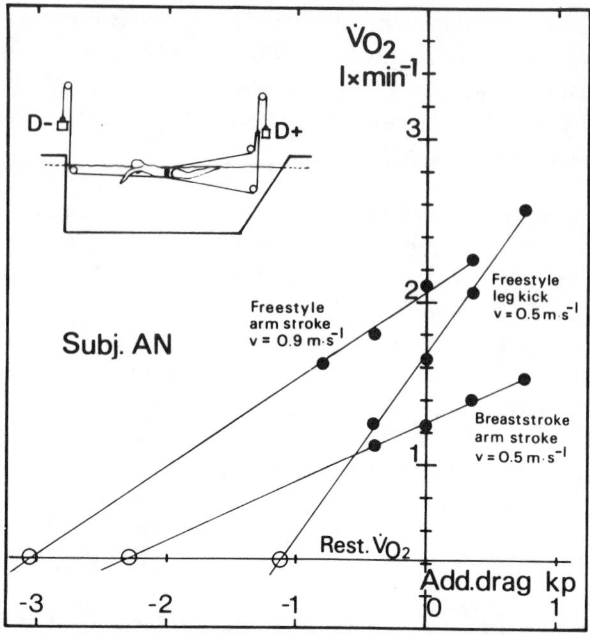


Figure 2. Regression lines of oxygen uptake as a function of added (D+) and subtracted (D−) drag in one subject. The point of intersection with the resting oxygen uptake gives the drag during free swimming. The insert illustrates the experimental set-up. (From Holmér, 1974b).

oxygen uptake measured during steady state and added drag. $D_A$ (Figure 2).

It has been demonstrated that the active drag during freestyle swimming is about 1.5–2 times greater than in passive towing (Holmér, 1974b), a result in accordance with that of di Prampero et al. Relating the value for active drag to the net energy expenditure measured at the same swimming velocity made possible the calculation of propulsive efficiency. Efficiencies were calculated at between 4–6% and 6–7% in breast stroke and freestyle, respectively (Holmér, 1974b). The previously described method gives an indirect estimate of active drag. The need for improved and new research methods for the study of human propulsion in water should be emphasized.

In a series of experiments, the relationship between oxygen uptake and velocity during swimming with different styles was determined. Data were collected for elite swimmers to ensure good stroke technique. As illustrated in Figure 3, the two symmetrical styles of butterfly and breast stroke demand almost twice as much energy at a given submaximal velocity as do the freestyle and backstroke. Furthermore, maximal velocity attained in a 4–5 min swim was significantly higher for the freestyle and backstroke (Holmér, 1974c).

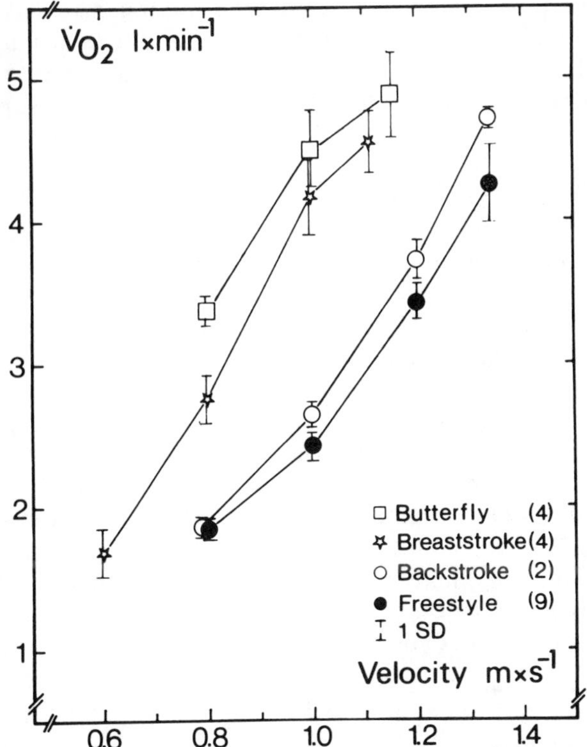


Figure 3. Mean values for oxygen uptake are given in relation to swimming velocity in different styles. The number of swimmers in each category appears in parentheses. (From Holmér, 1974b).

Elite swimmers are distinguished by high maximal aerobic powers. However, in a study of 23 elite swimmers, it was demonstrated that oxygen uptake and heart rate during maximal swimming was significantly lower than during maximal running (Holmér et al., 1974).

It was evident that a more extensive study of cardiorespiratory responses to swimming would be necessary to elucidate the possible explanations for these observed differences between swimming and running. In five subjects, cardiac output was determined by the indicator dilution technique using Cardio-green during submaximal and maximal work in swimming and running (Holmér et al.). The subject swam the breast stroke with a catheter in the femoral artery and vein. The swimming flume made it possible for the swimmer to stay in one well defined spot so that the complicated measuring equipment could be located in the most advantageous position.

In these experiments, it was clearly demonstrated that the swimmers maintained an adequate oxygen saturation of arterial blood despite a tendency to hypoventilation during maximal swimming, as opposed to pronounced hyperventilation during maximal running. Stroke volume was approximately the same during maximal work under both conditions. The reduced oxygen uptake during maximal swimming could be accounted for by a lower cardiac output and a smaller arteriovenous oxygen difference than in maximal running (Holmér et al., 1974).

These experiments included the first invasive determination of cardiac output in man during free swimming. Further investigations are needed for a more general understanding of the circulatory response to swimming.

Figure 4 depicts the maximal oxygen uptake in one famous swimmer, determined in repeated tests throughout his career. Maximal oxygen uptake during running was unchanged, while maximal oxygen uptake during swimming seemed very sensitive to changes in training and performance, judging from swimming results. Sensitivity was even more pronounced in separate arm swimming. This strongly indicates that evaluations of a swimmer's aerobic power should be made during swimming (Holmér, 1974a).

The swimming flume has been used for swimming training. The swimmer is paced by the water flow rate for work bouts of different durations. Feedback is constantly given to the swimmer, because any

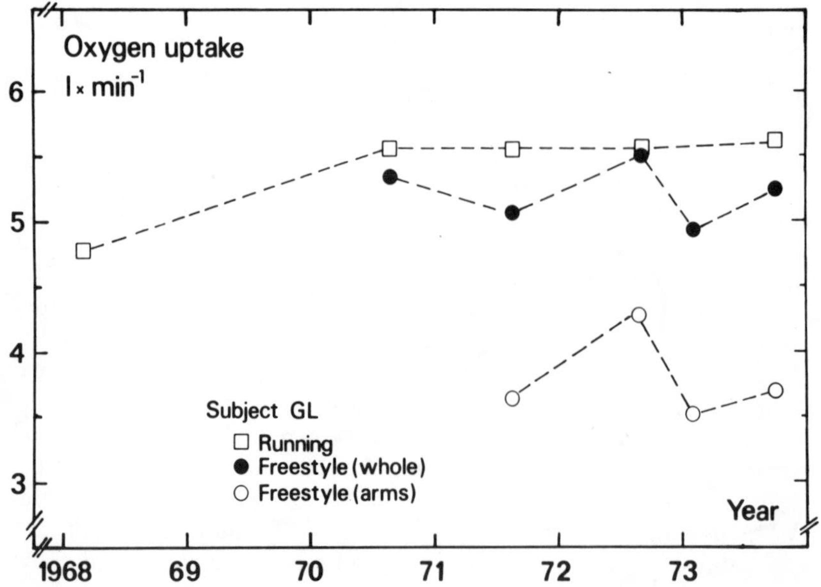


Figure 4. Oxygen uptake during swimming and running at maximal work rates by one world class swimmer over a 6-year period. Data were also obtained during separate arm swimming, with legs supported by a cork plate.

deviation from the desired performance results in an inability to hold a fixed place in respect to the flume.

The flume is also used to teach physical education students swimming technique. With a TV camera and a video tape recorder, the swimmer's movements are recorded and replayed just a few seconds later. Thus the swimmer can almost instantly watch his stroke in slow motion on a TV screen at pool side, and, after instructions from the teacher, can attempt to correct stroke mechanics. This procedure and the making of movie films have been used to analyze stroke techniques of elite swimmers during different periods of swimming training.

In summary, then, the swimming flume has proved to be very useful for swimming research. During free swimming in the flume, complicated measurements on the swimmer can be easily accomplished. It is possible under controlled conditions to analyze physiological adjustments to swimming. Further elucidation of the biomechanical and physiological factors involved in human performance in water is planned with new and improved research methods.

## ACKNOWLEDGMENT

The authors thank the Stenberg-Flygt Co, Solna, Sweden for providing the swimming flume.

## REFERENCES

Åstrand, P.-O., and Englesson, S. 1972. A swimming flume. J. Appl. Physiol. 33:514.

Clarys, J. P. 1976. Onderzoek naar de hydrodynamische en morfologische aspekten van het menselijk lichaam. Vrije universiteit Brussel, Brussels.

di Prampero, P. E., Pendergast, D. R., Wilson, D. W., and Rennie, D. W. 1974. Energetics of swimming in man. J. Appl. Physiol. 37:1–5.

Holmér, I. 1974a. Physiology of swimming man. Acta Physiol. Scand. (suppl. 407).

Holmér, I. 1974b. Propulsive efficiency of breast stroke and freestyle swimming. Eur. J. Appl. Physiol. 33:95–103.

Holmér, I. 1974c. Energy cost of arm stroke, leg kick, and the whole stroke in competitive swimming styles. Eur. J. Appl. Physiol. 33:105–118.

Holmér, I., Lundin, A., and Eriksson, B. O. 1974. Maximum oxygen uptake during swimming and running by elite swimmers. J. Appl. Physiol. 36(6):711–714.

Holmér, I., Stein, E. M., Saltin, B., Ekblom, B., and Åstrand, P.-O. 1974. Hemodynamic and respiratory responses compared in swimming and running. J. Appl. Physiol. 37(1):49–54.

Liljestrand, G., and Lindhard, J. 1919. Concerning the minute volume of the hearts of swimmers. Scand. Arch. Physiol. 39:64–77.

Liljestrand, G., and Stenström, N. 1919. Studies of the physiology of swimmers. Scand. Arch. Physiol. 39:1–63.

# An Experimental Investigation of the Application of Fundamental Hydrodynamics to the Human Body

J. P. Clarys

Most fish and water vertebrates are streamlined and therefore create more frictional resistance and considerably less eddy resistance, as shown in the experiments of Landolt and Börnstein (1955) and Tietjens (1957). The resistance components of such a streamlined body depend on its length/breadth and length/depth relationships. An increase in these relationships increases the body surface and thus increases frictional resistance while eddy resistance decreases (McNeill, 1968).

It is known that the length/thickness ratio is a measure of eddy resistance, while the length/surface area relationship gives an indication of frictional resistance. The slenderness coefficient is a measure of the wavemaking resistance value (Van Lammeren, Troost, and Koning, 1948; Lap, 1954).

By referring to these nondimensional relations, one can obtain a number of dimensional quantities that are basic form elements in the quantitative determination of total drag. These are length, breadth, depth, water displacement, surface area, and the greatest body cross-section.

If streamlined bodies with equal body cross-sections are compared, the resistance is smallest for a length/breadth ratio of two. If these same bodies, but with equal volume, are compared, the smallest resistance is encountered for a length/breadth relation equal to 4.5. These data apply to Reynolds (R) numbers of $\pm 10^7$, but not necessarily to lower R numbers (McNeill, 1968). The Reynolds number is a nondimensional expression of velocity, length, and the dynamic water viscosity coefficient. The Reynolds number may be regarded as a measure of the relative importance of the inertial and viscous forces acting on the water (Gadd, 1963). If the R number is used as a function of the drag coefficient (also a nondimensional relation), one can determine the relative importance of the laminar and/or turbulent flow around the investigated body.

The purpose of this chapter is to investigate the application of a number of these fundamental hydrodynamic principles to the human body, because too many authors may refer to fundamental hydrodynamics in an intuitive and often even in a faulty manner. The question of whether or not the human body is streamlined has been neglected, and, indeed, many previous studies, from Liljestrand and Stenström (1919) and Karpovich (1933) to Klauck and Daniel (1975), used passive drag in a towed prone position as an alternative method of determining the active drag created by the swimming body (Figure 1).

## METHODS AND PROCEDURES

Nine competitive swimmers from the Netherlands and 44 physical education students (control group) submitted to a series of tests using the equipment of the high speed tank in the Netherlands ship model basin. The apparatus, especially the device for measuring the drag forces, was described by Clarys, Jiskoot, and Lewillie (1973), Clarys et al. (1974), Van Manen and Rijken (1975), and Clarys and Jiskoot (1974a, b; 1975). The measuring procedure and final determination of active drag on the swimming body and its difference from passive drag were described by Clarys (1976a, b).

The nondimensional and dimensional data are derived from (and extensively used in) fundamental shipbuilding experiments (Van Lammeren, Troost, and Koning, 1948; Lap, 1954) and dolphin research (Gray, 1936; Gadd, 1963; Kramer, 1965; McNeill; and Lang, 1974). The variables were replaced by anthropometric and body configuration equivalents, as reviewed in Table 1 and mentioned in a drag study of extreme body types (Clarys et al., 1974). The relationship and overall statistics were analyzed with a SPSS computer system (Nie et al., 1975).

## RESULTS AND DISCUSSION

Table 2 shows the mean and standard deviations of the investigated characteristics of both subject groups. The mean passive drag ($D_p$) and active drag ($D_s$) values are expressed as functions of velocity in Figure 1. It must be stated that the application of dimensional and nondimensional data to the determination of hydrodynamic resistance has its origin in the study of harmonic, streamlined, and geometric forms

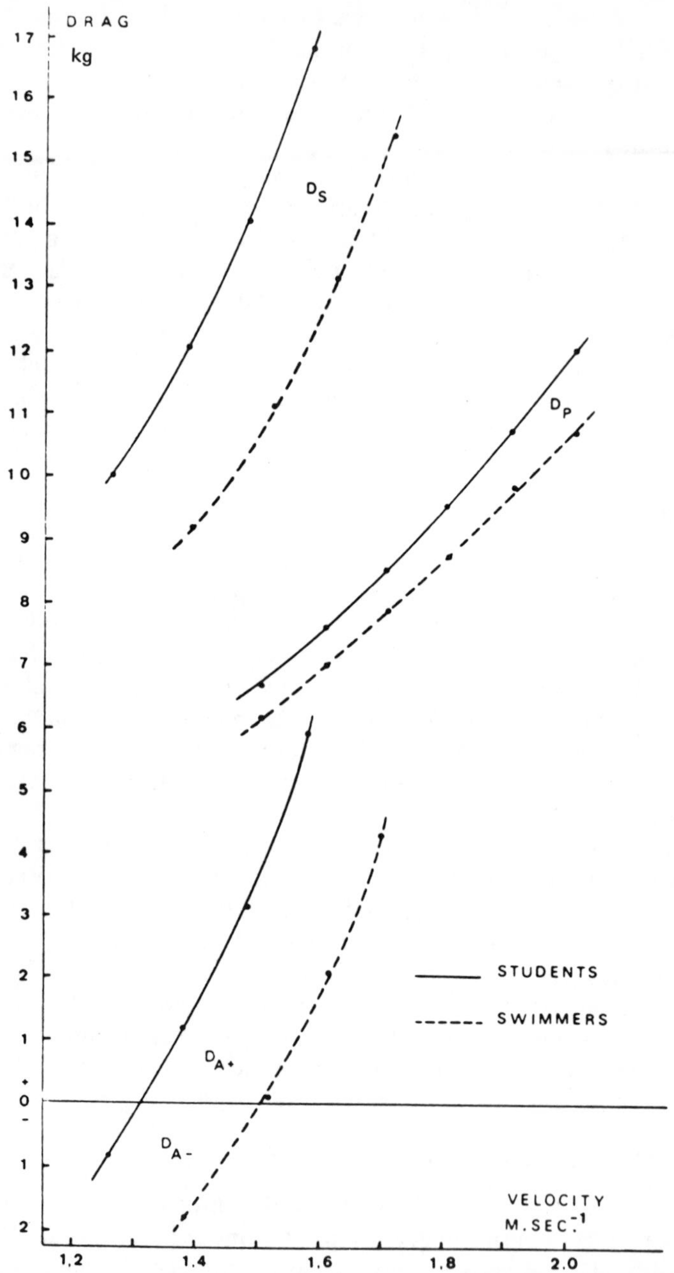


Figure 1. Mean active and passive drag determinations of physical education students and competitive swimmers.

Table 1. Fundamental hydrodynamic relationships and their equivalents for the human body

| Fundamental relationship | Symbols | Human body equivalent |
|---|---|---|
| Length/depth ratio | H/T | Body height/thorax depth |
| Length/breadth ratio | H/B | Body height/acromion breadth |
| Length/thickness ratio | $H^2/\otimes$ | Body height²/greatest body section |
| Length/surface ratio | $H^2/S$ | Body height²/body surface |
| Slenderness coefficient | $H/\Delta^{1/3}$ | Body height/body volume$^{1/3}$ |
| Breadth/depth ratio | B/T | Acromion breadth/thorax depth |
| Reynolds number (R) | $v \times H/\nu$ | Velocity × height/viscosity coefficient |
| Drag coefficient ($C_D$) | $D/0.5 \times d \times \otimes \times v^2$ | Drag/0.5 × density $H_2O$ × greatest body cross-section × velocity² |

(Hertel, 1966). Fish and dolphins seem to fit within such a pattern (Gray, 1936; Gadd, 1963; Kramer, 1965; McNeill, 1968; Jurina, 1972; Lang, 1974).

The question of whether or not the human body is streamlined implies a supplementary problem: Do we consider the human body in a prone position (a passive drag condition) or while swimming, e.g., the

Table 2. Mean dimensional and nondimensional characteristics of competitive swimmers and physical education students

| | Swimmers | | PE students | |
|---|---|---|---|---|
| Variables | $\bar{X}$ | SD | $\bar{X}$ | SD |
| Height (cm) | 183.86 | 8.64 | 180.95 | 6.39 |
| Acromion breadth (cm) | 42.13 | 2.41 | 40.90 | 2.05 |
| Thorax depth (cm) | 20.04 | 1.09 | 20.25 | 1.67 |
| Greatest body cross-section ($cm^2$) | 766.66 | 123.87 | 767.43 | 92.51 |
| Body surface ($m^2$) | 1.677 | 0.158 | 1.665 | 0.118 |
| Body volume (liters) | 67.80 | 8.48 | 68.41 | 7.33 |
| H/T | 8.86 | 0.89 | 8.86 | 0.76 |
| H/B | 4.38 | 0.10 | 4.41 | 0.18 |
| $H^2/\otimes$ | 44.86 | 4.42 | 43.18 | 4.40 |
| $H^2/S$ | 2.00 | 0.10 | 1.94 | 0.09 |
| $H/\Delta^{1/3}$ | 4.55 | 0.07 | 4.49 | 0.12 |
| B/T | 2.10 | 0.18 | 2.04 | 0.17 |

front crawl (an active drag condition). Figure 1 clearly shows the difference between the two types of drag. $D_s$ is twice as great as $D_p$, confirming the findings of di Prampero et al. (1974), Holmér (1974a, b), and Rennie, Pendergast, and di Prampero (1975). It is quite evident that, if the human body is to be streamlined, it must be placed in a prone position.

Gadd (1963) experimented with one subject lying prone in a wind tunnel, head-on to the wind, at a wind speed giving roughly the same Reynolds number as for a man swimming in water. The drag coefficient was about 13 times as great as that on a well streamlined body with the same Reynolds number. These experiments were repeated with all the subjects of this study, but under hydrodynamic circumstances. According to Tietjens (1957), Landolt and Börnstein (1955), and McNeill (1968), the drag coefficient ($C_D$) of a tursiops dolphin varies between ±0.055 and ±0.075. Within the same range of R numbers, the $C_D$ value of the human body varies between 0.58 and 1.041. This is approximately 8–19 times as great as $C_D$ in a streamlined dolphin (Figure 2).

According to theories related to laminar and turbulent flows, the dolphin and the human body both create full turbulent flows (Figure 3). The dolphin, however, possesses a system that reduces this turbulence and increases its laminar flow. This might explain their extremely high swimming velocities (Gray, 1936; Gadd, 1963; Kramer, 1965; McNeill, 1968; Hertel, 1966; and Lang, 1974). The human body does not have such an adaptation; therefore, under all circumstances, the flow around

| | $C_D$ | R NUMBER | R CONSTANT | $C_D$ CONSTANT |
|---|---|---|---|---|
| LAMINAR PROFILE 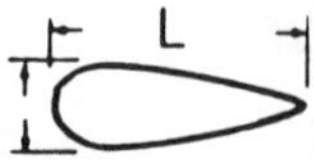 (L) | 0.05 | $10^4 < R < 10^8$ | L | ☒ |
| DOLPHIN TURSIOPS 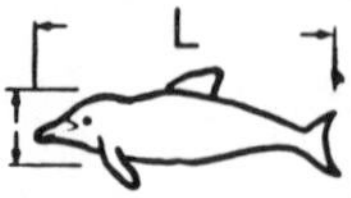 (L) | $0.05 < C_D < 0.08$ | $7.5 \times 10^4 < R < 7.0 \times 10^7$ | L | ☒ |
| HUMAN BODY | $0.58 < C_D < 1.04$ | $6.6 \times 10^5 < R < 3.9 \times 10^6$ | H | ☒ |

Figure 2. Drag coefficients and Reynolds number values.

this body remains fully turbulent. Onoprienko (1967) and Jurina (1972) used the dolphin hypothesis of laminar flow increase and turbulence decrease to explain why women encounter less resistance during swimming than do men. In light of the results of this study, such a statement cannot be considered realistic. The reasons for the women's drag decrease must be attributed to better buoyancy and more rounded forms, which result in a smoother boundary layer transition (Figure 4).

The full turbulent flow of the human body has other consequences as well. It increases the eddy resistance considerably and decreases the frictional resistance. This is confirmed by the significant correlations of $D_p$ with $H^2/\otimes$ and the greatest body cross-section, and by the lack of any relationship of $D_p$ to $H^2/S$ and the surface area. The existing relationship between $D_p$ and the slenderness coefficient also indicates the importance of wavemaking resistance.

Although the form relation values (Table 2) of both physical education students and swimmers are in agreement with similar relationships

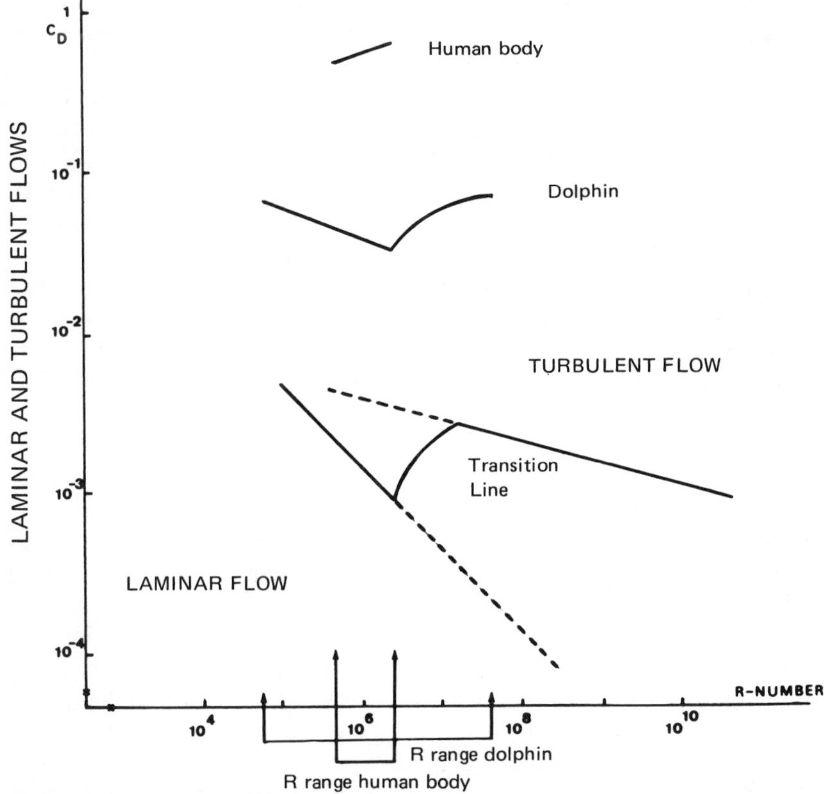


Figure 3. Laminar and turbulent flow areas.

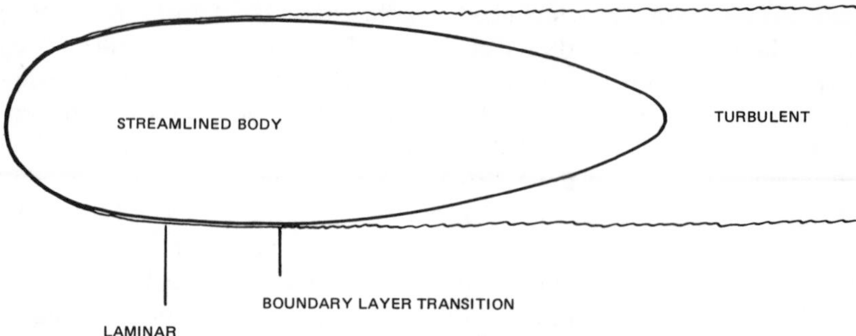


Figure 4. The boundary layer flow around a streamlined body.

to a tursiops dolphin, the human body is far from being streamlined and does not possess the basic hydrodynamic features for efficient progression in water. These results show also that indisputable principles from fundamental hydrodynamics such as drag/surface area and drag/length ratios are not to be applied to the human body. Unfortunately, many authors (Karpovich, 1933; Amar, 1920; Tews, 1941; Onoprienko, 1967; Jurina, 1972; and Zaciorsky and Safarian, 1972) have applied these principles to swimming human beings.

Analysis of the same data, plus active drag determinations (Figure 1) indicates that turbulence, eddy-, and wave-making resistance will increase significantly. Because of the constant body position body configuration changes, none of the fundamental hydrodynamic principles can be applied. Obviously, the basic circumstances for fundamental investigation do not exist, because too many factors cannot be measured. No relationship at all was found between $D_s$ and the form data. Therefore, it is not body configuration that determines active drag; there is sufficient reason to believe that the motor technical aspect of the swimming movement is the dominant influencing factor for drag.

## CONCLUSIONS

Fundamental hydrodynamics is related only to passive drag determination. Not all of the commonly used hydrodynamic principles can be applied on the human body. However, the use of passive drag is not a viable alternative to the use of active drag in studying swimming movements. Fundamental hydrodynamics do not give an exact account of swimming and consequently there seems to be little advantage in attempting to thus apply them. According to Gadd (1963), the sheer difficulties involved in studying this situation in swimming will probably keep the attention of hydrodynamics focused on the subject for a long time to come.

## REFERENCES


Amar, J. 1920. The Human Motor. Routledge and Sons, Ltd., London.

Clarys, J. P. 1976a. Methodology of the determination of active hydrodynamic drag in man. Paper presented at the Premier Congrès de la Société de Biomécanique, June, Lyon.

Clarys, J. P. 1976b. An investigation of hydrodynamic and morphological aspects of the human body. D. Biomedical science dissertation. Vrije Universiteit Brussel, Brussels.

Clarys, J. P., and Jiskoot, J. 1974a. Aspects of resistance of different transcient body positions in swimming. Paper presented at the 3rd Congress on Swimming Medicine, October, Barcelona.

Clarys, J. P., and Jiskoot, J. 1974b. Aspects de la résistance à l'avancement lors de différentes positions du corps chez le nageur. Le travail humain 37:323–324.

Clarys, J. P., and Jiskoot, J. 1975. Total resistance of selected body positions in the front crawl. In: J. P. Clarys and L. Lewillie (eds.), Swimming II, International Series on Sport Sciences, Vol. 2, pp. 110–117. University Park Press, Baltimore.

Clarys, J. P., Jiskoot, J., and Lewillie, L. 1973. A kinematographic, electromyographic, and resistance study of waterpolo and competition front crawl. In: Cerguiglini, Venerando, and Wartenweiler (eds.), Biomechanics III, pp. 446–452. Karger, Basel.

Clarys, J. P., Jiskoot, J., Rijken, H., and Brouwer, P. J. 1974. Total resistance in water and its relation to body form. In: R. Nelson and C. Morehouse (eds.), Biomechanics IV, International Series on Sport Sciences, Vol. 1, pp. 187–196. University Park Press, Baltimore.

di Prampero, P. E., Pendergast, D. R., Wilson, D. W., and Rennie, D. W. 1974. Energetics of swimming in man. J. Appl. Physiol. 37:1–5.

Gadd, G. F. 1963. The hydrodynamics of swimming. New Scientist 19:483–485.

Gray, J. 1936. Studies in animal locomotion. VI. The propulsive power of the dolphin. J. Exp. Biol. 13:192–199.

Hertel, H. 1966. Structure, form, movement. Reinhold Co., New York.

Holmér, I. 1974a. Physiology of swimming man. Acta Physiol. Scand. (suppl. 407).

Holmér, I. 1974b. Energy cost of arm stroke, leg kick, and the whole stroke in competitive swimming studies. Eur. J. Appl. Physiol. 33:105–118.

Jurina, K. 1972. Comparison of swimming in fish and man. (Russian) Theorica Praxe Telesne Vychovy 20:161–166.

Karpovich, P. V. 1933. Water resistance in swimming. Res. Q. 4:21–28.

Klauck, J., and Daniel, K. 1976. The determination of man's drag coefficient and effective propelling force in swimming by means of chronocyclography. In: P. Komi (ed.), Biomechanics V, International Series on Biomechanics V-B, pp. 250–257. University Park Press, Baltimore.

Kramer, M. O. 1965. Hydrodynamics of the dolphin. Adv. Hydrosci. 2:111–130.

Landolt, H., and Börnstein, R. 1955. Values and functions of physics, chemistry, astronomy, geophysics, and technique. Vol. 4, Part 1. Springer-Verlag, Berlin.

Lang, T. G. 1974. Speed, power, and drag measurements of dolphins and porpoises. Paper presented at the Symposium on Swimming and Flying in Nature. Pasadena.

Lap, A. J. W. 1954. Fundamentals of ship resistance and propulsion. Nat. Shipbuilding Progress. Rotterdam. Report 129a NSMB

Liljestrand, G., and Stenström, N. 1919. Studies on swimming physiology. Scand. Arch. Physiol. 39:1–63.

McNeill, A. R., 1968. Animal Mechanics. Sidwich and Jackson, London.

Nie, N. H., Hull, C. H., Jenkins, J. G., Steinbrenner, K., and Bent, D. H. 1975. Statistical Package for the Social Sciences. McGraw-Hill Book Company, New York.

Onoprienko, B. I. 1967. Influence of hydrodynamical data on the hydrodynamics of the swimmer. (Russian) Theorica Praxe Telesne Vychovy 4:47–53.

Rennie, D. W., Pendergast, D. R., and di Prampero, P. E. 1975. Energetics of swimming in man. In: J. P. Clarys and L. Lewillie (eds.), Swimming II, International Series on Sport Sciences, Vol. 2, pp. 97–104. University Park Press, Baltimore.

Tews, R. W. J. 1941. The relationship of propulsive force and external resistance to speed in swimming. Masters thesis, State University of Iowa, Iowa City.

Tietjens, O. G. 1957. Applied Hydro- and Aerodynamics. Dover Books, New York.

Van Lammeren, W. P. A., Troost, L., and Koning, J. G. 1948. Resistance, Propulsion, and Steering of Ships. Technical Publ. Co. H. Stam, Amsterdam.

Van Manen, J. D., and Rijken, H. 1975. Dynamic measurement techniques on swimming bodies at the Netherlands Ship Model Basin. In: J. P. Clarys and L. Lewillie (eds.), Swimming II, International Series on Sport Sciences, Vol. 2, pp. 70–79. University Park Press, Baltimore.

Zaciorsky, V. M., and Safarian, I. G. 1972. Study of factors for the determination of maximal velocity in the front crawl. Theorie und Praxis der Körper Kultur 8:695–709.

# Water Resistance in Relation to Body Size

**M. Miyashita and T. Tsunoda**

Because measurement of the water resistance of a self-propelled human body is extremely difficult, water resistance has been determined for swimmers in the static position (Counsilman, 1955; Clarys, Jiskoot, and Lewillie, 1973). Faulkner (1968) compared the exponential relationships between velocity and drag as determined by different investigators. However, few data are available that relate the velocity/drag relationship to body size other than in one study by Karpovich (1933). Based on the exponential relationship between water resistance (R) and water velocity (V), i.e., $R = kV^2$, Karpovich determined the constants (k) in relation to body surface area (2.23 to 1.77 and 1.77 to 1.53 $m^2$, respectively).

Recently, the number of younger swimmers has increased. Because the body surface areas of younger swimmers are usually less than 1.50 $m^2$, the present study was designed to determine the water resistance of the human body in the static position for swimmers of various body sizes, and to verify the relationship between water resistance and body size.

## METHOD

To determine the drag of the human body, a swimming flume was used that had been originally constructed for the analysis of models of nets and other fishing units. The inside dimensions of the measuring section were 8 m in length, 3 m in width, and 1.2 m in water depth (water capacity: approximately 300 tons). The speed control impeller (4-blade assembly type) was set for circulating water, and the velocity of water flow through the channel could be varied from 0 to 2.5 m/sec. An arched slope was used as a wave absorber.

One end of a cord (about 2 m in length) was attached to a load cell; the other end was held in the hands of the swimmer lying in the water. The load cell (measuring range: 0–50 kg) was fixed at the edge of the flume ahead of the swimmer. The tension of the cord was recorded by a penwriting oscillograph through the load cell, which was calibrated with a known weight before and after the measurements.

The subjects were 10 male and 8 female Japanese swimmers, and 2 male Caucasian swimmers, aged 9–38 years. Their physical characteristics are shown in Table 1.

The drag in two static prone positions with the head under and above water was measured at several velocities (range: 0.4–1.8 m/sec). The former was a position with face down, arms extended and parallel, legs straight and together, and with the head held underwater. The latter was the same position except the face was up and the head was held above water so that the water level was approximately across the mouth.

The bathing suits were of the type usually used in competitive swimming. The measurements were performed on July 30 and September 1 and 2 in 1975 at Hakodate Seimo Sengu Co., Ltd., in Hokkaido, Japan. The temperature of water in the flume was 23–24°C.

## RESULTS

### Relationship between water resistance and water velocity

In the field of hydrodynamics, it is generally understood that the water resistance offered to an object moving through water is proportional to the square of the velocity of water flow. The formula for resistance is: $R = C \times dL^2V^2/2$, where R represents the water resistance, V the velocity of water flow, d the density of the fluid, L the length of an object moving through water, and C the constant for each object. This formula is applicable when an object moving through water maintains a uniform position and shape. In this experiment, however, the object, a human body, was not solid. Consequently, it must be assumed that the water resistance offered to a human body is affected by other factors. It was assumed therefore that the water resistance was proportional to a function of the water velocity, i.e., $R = aV^b$ (a and b are the constants). The regression equations between resistance and velocity were assessed by using the method of least squares for Japanese male and female swimmers, respectively. The results were as follows:

1. male—prone position with the head under water
   $R = 2.49\ V^{1.91}$ (N = 10)
2. male—prone position with the head above water
   $R = 5.39\ V^{1.18}$ (N = 7)

Table 1. Physical characteristics and water resistance of subjects

| | Physical characteristics | | | | | Water resistance (kg) | | | | | |
|---|---|---|---|---|---|---|---|---|---|---|---|
| | | | | | Body surface | Head above water[a] | | | Head under water[a] | | |
| | Subject | Age (years) | Height (cm) | Weight (kg) | area ($m^2$) | V = 0.8 | V = 1.2 | V = 1.6 | V = 0.8 | V = 1.2 | V = 1.6 |
| Male | A.S. | 10 | 130.0 | 27.0 | 1.00 | 1.50 | 2.55 | — | 3.23 | 4.85 | — |
| | T.K. | 16 | 176.0 | 69.8 | 1.87 | 2.00 | 3.43 | 6.44 | 3.72 | 4.18 | 7.93 |
| | C.K.[b] | 17 | 170.4 | 63.0 | 1.75 | 1.87 | 4.42 | 5.95 | 4.44 | 6.77 | 9.89 |
| | C.S. | 17 | 174.7 | 64.0 | 1.79 | 2.00 | 5.44 | 7.81 | 3.15 | 6.44 | 11.59 |
| | S.I. | 17 | 177.2 | 64.0 | 1.81 | 2.42 | 4.47 | 7.61 | 3.86 | 8.01 | 12.85 |
| | S.N. | 18 | 169.3 | 86.0 | 1.98 | 1.38 | 3.08 | 5.10 | 5.22 | 8.45 | 12.41 |
| | N.T.[b] | 24 | 173.1 | 68.6 | 1.83 | 1.63 | 3.03 | 4.98 | 3.86 | 5.24 | 8.36 |
| | T.T. | 32 | 168.9 | 61.5 | 1.72 | 1.56 | 2.98 | 5.53 | — | — | — |
| | K.S. | 35 | 170.0 | 62.0 | 1.73 | 1.12 | 2.72 | 5.53 | — | — | — |
| | M.M. | 38 | 163.4 | 67.5 | 1.75 | 1.45 | 3.40 | 6.75 | — | — | — |
| | J.N.[c] | 19 | 196.6 | 85.0 | 2.20 | 1.00 | 2.46 | 5.40 | 1.72 | 6.43 | 8.86 |
| | J.M.[c] | 20 | 193.4 | 88.5 | 2.21 | 2.00 | 3.43 | 6.89 | 2.74 | 5.40 | 9.43 |
| | Correlation coefficient between body surface area and water resistance | | | | | 0.021 N.S. | 0.089 N.S. | −0.089 N.S. | −0.183 N.S. | 0.265 N.S. | −0.251 N.S. |
| | | | | | | V = 0.6 | V = 1.0 | V = 1.2 | V = 0.6 | V = 1.0 | V = 1.2 |
| Female | T.K. | 9 | 137.5 | 29.0 | 1.05 | 0.34 | 1.53 | 2.38 | 1.53 | 3.92 | 4.22 |
| | M.N. | 11 | 147.2 | 40.0 | 1.26 | 0.37 | 1.29 | 2.04 | 1.28 | 3.09 | 4.74 |
| | Y.M. | 11 | 144.7 | 43.0 | 1.28 | 0.51 | 1.62 | 2.30 | 2.21 | 4.98 | 6.02 |
| | N.O. | 12 | 155.8 | 40.5 | 1.32 | 0.51 | 1.79 | 2.23 | 1.45 | 3.88 | 4.34 |
| | C.K. | 13 | 157.3 | 58.5 | 1.55 | 0.51 | 1.70 | 2.55 | 1.87 | 4.67 | 5.95 |
| | Y.H.[b] | 17 | 159.9 | 47.7 | 1.44 | 0.92 | 2.00 | 2.29 | 2.03 | 3.95 | 5.44 |
| | K.B. | 17 | 165.6 | 56.4 | 1.59 | 1.12 | 2.78 | 2.95 | 2.75 | 5.41 | 7.10 |
| | M.O. | 18 | 161.4 | 55.5 | 1.55 | 1.52 | 3.43 | 4.04 | 3.58 | 5.87 | 7.81 |
| | Correlation coefficient between body surface area and water resistance | | | | | 0.725 *[d] | 0.687 N.S. | 0.578 N.S. | 0.661 N.S. | 0.641 N.S. | 0.795 * |

[a] V = water velocity in m/sec
[b] Japanese record holder in 1976
[c] World record holder in 1976
[d] (*) = $P < 0.05$, by t-test

3. female—prone position with the head under water

$$R = 1.81\ V^{2.37} \qquad (N = 8)$$

4. female—prone position with the head above water

$$R = 4.29\ V^{1.63} \qquad (N = 8)$$

where R is water resistance in kg and V is water velocity in m/sec.

The water resistance with the head above water was definitely greater in both sexes than that with the head underwater for a given water velocity. The water resistance of female swimmers was slightly less than that of male swimmers in the same position (Figure 1).

For both sexes, the regression curve for the position with the head above water was more linear than that with the head underwater. This indicates that the water resistance in prone position with the head above water is relatively greater at lower velocities.

## Individual differences in water resistance

Large individual differences in water resistance were seen at the same water velocity. The ranges of water resistance are shown in Table 2 for the two prone positions in relation to velocity and sex. The range of water resistance with the head underwater was less than that with the head above water at the same velocity, and both ranges became wider as velocity increased.

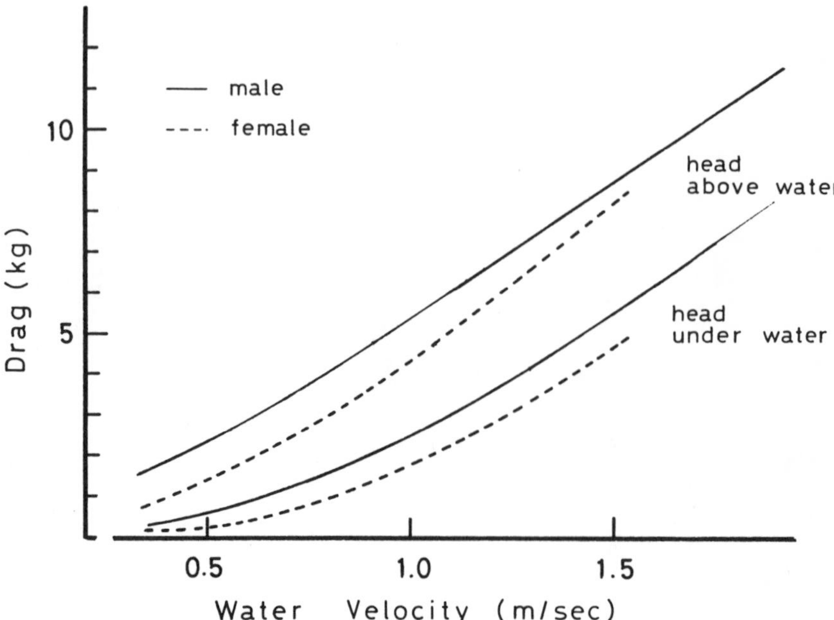


Figure 1. Relationships between water resistance and water velocity.

Table 2. Ranges of water resistance (kg)

| Conditions | | Velocities (m/sec) 0.4 | 0.6 | 0.8 | 1.0 | 1.2 | 1.4 | 1.6 | 1.8 |
|---|---|---|---|---|---|---|---|---|---|
| Male, head under | range | — | 0.36 | 1.42 | 2.06 | 2.98 | 3.33 | 2.83 | 1.74 |
| water | (N) | — | (3) | (12) | (12) | (12) | (11) | (11) | (3) |
| Male, head above | range | — | 0.87 | 3.50 | 3.88 | 4.27 | 5.47 | 4.92 | 3.11 |
| water | (N) | — | (3) | (9) | (9) | (9) | (8) | (8) | (3) |
| Female, head under | range | 0.36 | 1.18 | 1.83 | 2.14 | 2.00 | 2.68 | — | — |
| water | (N) | (4) | (8) | (8) | (8) | (8) | (4) | — | — |
| Female, head above | range | 1.19 | 2.30 | 2.40 | 2.77 | 3.60 | 3.34 | — | — |
| water | (N) | (4) | (8) | (8) | (8) | (8) | (4) | — | — |

## Relationship between water resistance and body surface area

The wet surface area and the surface condition of the swimmer are important factors that affect water resistance. In evaluating the surface conditions for swimmers of each sex, the wet surface area was considered the more important. In the present study, assuming that the wet surface area was approximately equal to the body surface area, the relationship between water resistance and body surface area was assessed for each sex and including all subjects. The following formulas were used for determination of body surface area (BSA):

$$BSA = 72.46 \times W^{0.425} \times H^{0.725} \text{ for males}$$
$$BSA = 70.49 \times W^{0.425} \times H^{0.725} \text{ for females}$$

where W is body weight in kg and H is body height in cm. The results showed no significant correlation between the water resistance and the body surface area except in a few instances (Table 1).

## DISCUSSION

Water resistance determined by towing the swimmer is not the same as resistance to a self-propelled swimmer moving through water. However, Faulkner (1966) stated that the formulas presented by Karpovich provided a reasonably accurate estimate of resistance throughout the usual range of swimming velocities. Therefore, in the present study, the authors used the similar method to determine the water resistance on the swimmers of various body types of both sexes.

The relationships between water resistance and water velocity obtained in the present study coincide well with data previously reported (Karpovich; Alley, 1952; Counsilman; Clarys, Jiskoot, and Lewillie). It was found that the higher head position creates significantly greater resistance. A definite difference in water resistance was also found between the two types of body position, and the lower the water velocity was, the larger was the difference. For instance, for male swimmers the water resistance with the head above water was greater by approximately 3.6 times at a velocity of 0.4 m/sec, 2.2 times at 1.0 m/sec, and 1.5 times at 1.6 m/sec than that with the head underwater. This tendency might have been attributable to the fact that it was difficult for the swimmer to maintain uniform position at lower water velocities. In other words, in order to maintain counterbalance, the legs sank the most when the swimmer assumed the prone position with the head above the water moving at lower velocities. At higher velocities, the water flow may lift the legs.

The reason the water resistance of female swimmers is slightly less than that of males might be explained by the significant, sexually linked difference in body density: the smaller the body density, the greater the influence of the lift. In Japanese young adults, the mean value of body density is 1.0487 g/ml for ordinary females and 1.0696 g/ml for males ($P < 0.01$, by t-test) (Kitagawa, Miyashita, and Yamamoto, 1977).

The main purpose of this study was to verify the relationship between water resistance and body size. Although the subjects employed in the present study showed a wide range of body surface

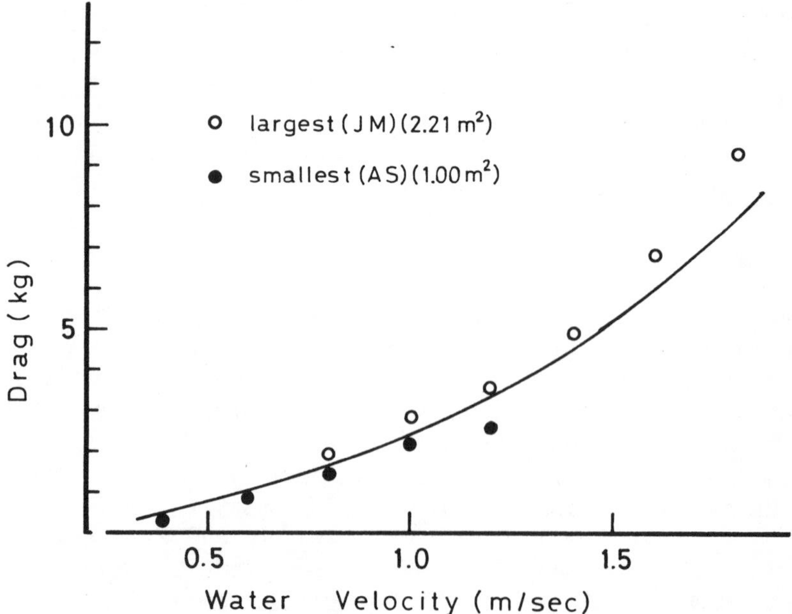


Figure 2. Comparison of water resistance between the largest and the smallest of the subject swimmers in the prone position with heads under water.

areas (1.00 $m^2$–2.21$m^2$), the correlation between water resistance and body surface area was low when evaluated under the same conditions of water velocity, body position, and sex. For instance, the water resistance of the largest Caucasian swimmer (Subject J.M.) increased with water velocity in a manner parallel to that of the smallest Japanese swimmer (Subject A.S.) (Figure 2). It was difficult to explain the lack of effect of body size on the water resistance because so many complicated factors affect the water resistance (i.e., velocity, position, body type, body density, body surface condition, wet surface area, etc). One possible explanation is that, in the present study, each swimmer was asked to maintain a static position throughout the experiment. However, control of the body in water is very difficult and this ability must be developed by long and hard practice. Younger, smaller Japanese swimmers seemed to be unable to keep their body positions uniform. Consequently, their body positions changed more than did those of the larger, highly trained Caucasian swimmers, who were able to control their positions as effectively as possible. As a result, the water resistance was found to be the same in the present study for both small Japanese and large Caucasians.

## REFERENCES

Alley, L. E. 1952. An analysis of water resistance and propulsion in swimming the crawl stroke. Res. Q. 23:253–270.

Clarys, J. P., Jiskoot, J., and Lewillie, L. 1973. A cinematographic, electromyographic, and resistance study of water polo and competition front crawl. In: S.Cerquiglini, A.Venerando, and J. Wartenweiler (eds.), Biomechanics III. Medicine and Sport Series, Vol. 8, pp. 446–452. Karger, Basel.

Counsilman, J. 1955. Forces in swimming two types of crawl stroke. Res. Quart. 26:127–139.

Faulkner, J. A. 1966. Physiology of swimming. Res. Q. 37:41–54.

Faulkner, J. A. 1968. Physiology of swimming and diving. In: H.B. Falls (ed.), Exercise Physiology, pp. 415–446. Academic Press, New York.

Karpovich, P. W. 1933. Water resistance in swimming. Res. Q. 4:21–28.

Kitagawa, K., Miyashita, M., and Yamamoto, K. 1977. Maximal oxygen uptake, body composition, and running performance in Japanese young adults of both sexes. Jap. J. Phys. Educ. 21:335–340.

# Extreme Velocities of a Swimming Cycle as a Technique Criterion

**S. Kornecki and T. Bober**

The objective estimation of most sport techniques can be performed using biomechanical criteria. These criteria should take into consideration not only those parts of the movement pattern that determine the efficiency and economy of sport techniques but also the specific character of the environment in which the sportsman is participating. The influence of the environment is particularly important for swimmers because of the high density of the medium and the close relationship between swimming velocity and hydrodynamic resistance. Therefore, variations of velocity within the stroke cycle are undesirable because they demand that the swimmer overcome the forces of inertia as well as hydrodynamic resistance. Fluctuation of speed within the stroke cycle is especially high for butterfly swimmers (Molinskij, 1961; Kornecki and Reiter, 1975).

A biomechanical criterion was established that allows for variations in the swimmer's velocity. This criterion assumes that swimming techniques are more effective, and more economical in terms of motion, if the difference between instantaneous and mean velocities within the stroke cycle is minimal. Mathematically this criterion can be expressed by the Economy Index (EI):

$$EI = \frac{\frac{v_{max\ c}}{v_{mean\ c}} - 1}{v_{mean\ d}} \times 100 \quad (\rightarrow \min)$$

where:

$v_{max\ c}$ = maximum velocity within the stroke cycle,

$v_{mean\ c} = \frac{1}{t_c} \int_0^{t} c\ v\ dt$ = mean velocity within the stroke cycle

$t_c$ = duration of the stroke cycle

$v_{mean\ d}$ = mean velocity at a given distance

Thus EI is the ratio of relative deviations between maximum and mean velocities within the stroke cycle to the mean velocity at a given distance.

The purposes of this study were: to verify the above mentioned criterion by finding the relationship between the index EI and the time that is necessary to cover a given distance using one butterfly stroke; and to analyze the swimmer's movements and their relationship to changes in the EI. This analysis deals with the swimmer's velocity changes and the trajectories of selected points of the swimmer's body.

## MATERIALS AND METHODS

Twenty-two of the best Polish butterfly swimmers were tested. The general characteristics of the swimmers involved are shown in Table 1. In order to find the terms that express the index of the given criterion, it was necessary to obtain the velocity and displacement patterns of a swimming cycle. Obtaining these patterns required the use of a speedometer synchronized in time with a cyclophotographic technique (Figure 1). Both of these techniques have previously been used in testing swimmers who covered 20 m at maximum speed.

In the butterfly stroke, most of the swimmers' movements took place in the sagittal plane. The important parts of the body were the hands, feet, and hips. To photograph their trajectories in a given plane, light bulbs were fixed on the left ankle, on the hip (greater trochanter), and on the hand. An Exakta IIb camera with a Flectagon lens was positioned in a waterproof box. The camera was set up in the middle of the swimming pool, 4 m from the swimmer's path. From this position the distance covered in three swimming cycles was within the optical field of the camera. Black and white film (speed: 27 DIN (ASA 400)) was used. The pool was kept dark and the swimmers were able to monitor their positions by the use of additional bulbs at the side of the pool.

Table 1. General characteristics of the swimmers (N = 22)

| Measurements | Unit | Mean | SD | Min-max |
|---|---|---|---|---|
| Best result | s | 65.3 | 3.7 | 59.8 – 75 |
| Age | years | 18.4 | 2.8 | 15 – 27 |
| Practice | years | 9.4 | 2.8 | 4 – 15 |
| Height | cm | 179.2 | 5.5 | 169 – 189.6 |
| Weight | kg | 71.4 | 7.3 | 51 – 82 |
| Body area | $m^2$ | 1.89 | 0.12 | 1.56 – 2.07 |
| Arm circumference | cm | 29.6 | 2.3 | 26 – 33 |
| Chest circumference | cm | 103.4 | 4.1 | 91 – 109 |

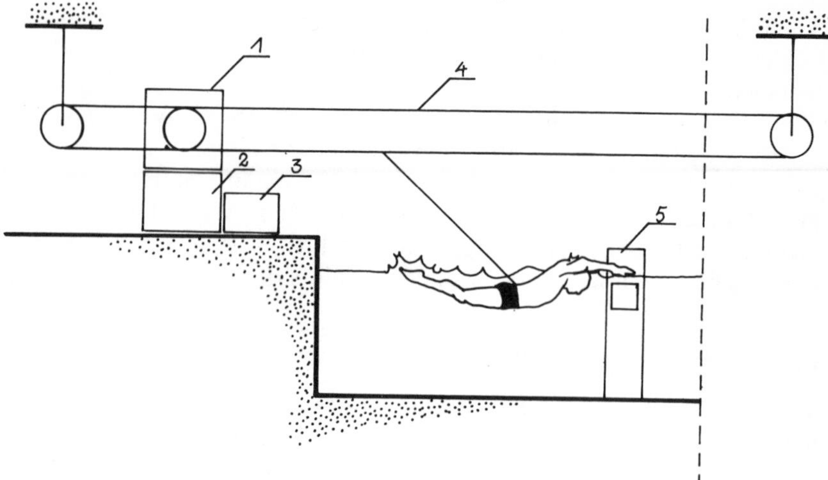


Figure 1. Schematic representation of the measuring system: 1 speedometer, 2 recorder, 3 power supply, 4 transmission system, 5 container with camera.

Before each test, a photograph of the underwater reference system was taken to determine the scale of the picture. A photoelectric speedometer (Bober and Czabański, 1975), with linear characteristics up to 4.2 m/s, and a TSS 101 recorder were used to record the swimming speed as a function of time. A test of the procedures used in the measuring system indicated that maximum error was 6.3%, resulting mainly from mechanical parts of the system.

## RESULTS

The speedograms for the total distance and the cyclophotograms of three succeeding swimming cycles were obtained (Figure 2). The trajectories of the chosen points on each swimmer's body were redrawn on graph paper using a scale of 1:10. The synchronization with time made it possible to choose one cycle on the cyclophotograph and to match it with the corresponding one on the speedograph. The mean $v_{mean\ c}$, maximum $v_{max\ e}$, and minimum $v_{min\ e}$ velocities and the duration ($t_c$) and frequency ($f_c$) of the swimming cycle were calculated. It was also possible to distinguish such phases of the cycle as the duration of the backward push of arms ($t_2$) and the duration of the recovery phase of the arms (when the arms were out of the water) ($t_4$), (Figure 2). The coefficient of resistance for men (Cx) according to Onoprijenko (1969) was calculated using the equation, $Cx = 0.079/Re^{0.2}$.

Comparison of the synchronized speedogram with the cyclophotogram made it possible to divide the cycle into phases and to make some

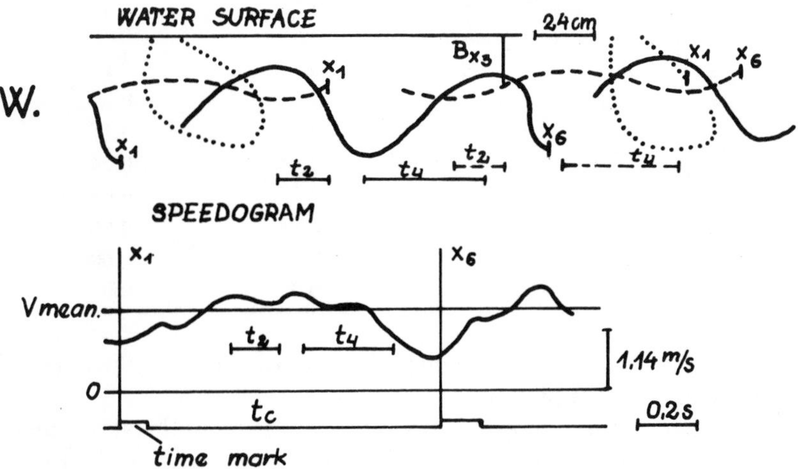


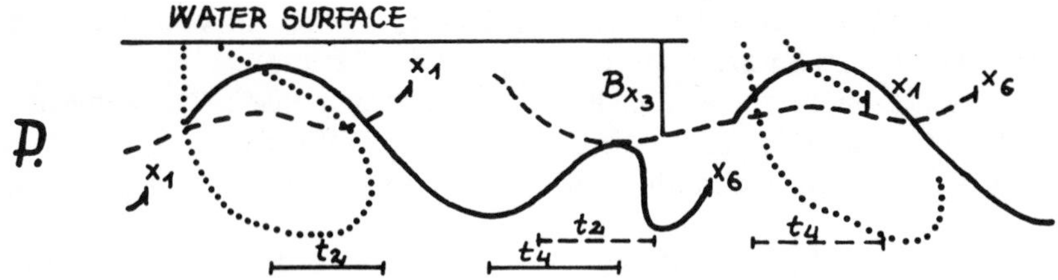


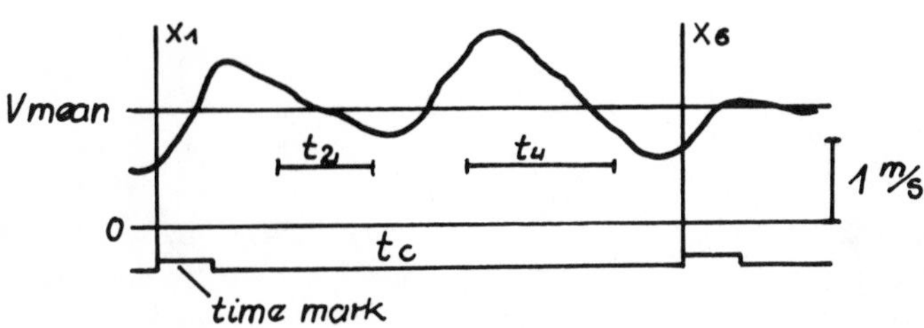


Figure 2. Cyclophotograms of the displacement patterns in the sagittal planes and speedograms of two selected competitors.

Table 2. Kinematic parameters of the swimming cycle

| Parameters | Units | Mean | SD |
|---|---|---|---|
| $v_{mean}$ | m/s | 1.51 | 0.1 |
| $v_{max}$ | m/s | 2.17 | 0.15 |
| $v_{min}$ | m/s | 0.72 | 0.27 |
| $t_c$ | s | 1.2 | 0.09 |
| $T_{rf}$ | s | 0.59 | 0.11 |
| $t_2$ | s | 0.18 | 0.04 |
| $t_4$ | s | 0.32 | 0.05 |
| $f_c$ | liters/s | 0.84 | 0.06 |
| Cx | | 0.041 | 0.0005 |
| Bx3 | m | 0.25 | 0.07 |

additional measurements of the displacement pattern, e.g., the range of the movement of the hip (Bx3).

The mean values and standard deviations (SD) of the above mentioned parameters are shown in Table 2. The mean value of the Economy Index for the tested swimmers was 28.1 and the SD was 9.9. These results showed a statistically significant positive correlation coefficient between EI and time for the tested distance ($r = 0.50$). The EI was later correlated with the kinematic factors of the movement pattern and the chosen anthropometric parameters (Table 3).

According to the established criterion, a decrease in the numerical value of EI corresponds to an increase in the efficiency and economy of the swimming technique. The data in Table 3 show that, with the

Table 3. Correlation coefficients between Economy Index and kinematic parameters of the stroke cycle and body circumferences

| Parameters | EI (r)[a] |
|---|---|
| $v_{mean}$ | −0.68 |
| $v_{max}$ | 0.7 |
| $v_{min}$ | −0.46 |
| $t_c$ | 0.68 |
| $t_2$ | 0.51 |
| $t_4$ | 0.46 |
| $f_c$ | −0.66 |
| Cx | 0.49 |
| Bx3 | 0.44 |
| Arm circumference | −0.54 |
| Chest circumference | −0.62 |

[a] Significant at 0.05 level, $r > 0.42$

decrease in EI, the following parameters also increased: mean and minimum velocities within the stroke cycle, frequency of the stroke cycle, and chest and arm circumferences. At the same time, such parameters as duration of the cycle ($t_c$), duration of the push back phase ($t_2$), duration of the recovery phase of the arms ($t_4$), and resistance coefficient (Cx) also decreased. Some measurements of the displacement of the body parts in relation to the water's surface were taken from cyclophotograms. Hip movements in relation to the EI were the most interesting. A significant correlation ($r = 0.44$) was found between EI and the submersion range of the hips at the end of the push back phase.

## INTERPRETATIONS

Speedographic and cyclographic techniques presented in this chapter confirm the importance of movement economy to a swimming technique. The increase in efficiency resulting from economy of efforts is also important. An essential relationship was found between the criterion of movement economy, as expressed by oscillations of instantaneous velocities inside the stroke cycle, and swimming speed. These results support existing opinions that movement economy is an essential indicator of correct technique.

According to the obtained results, the efficiency and economy of technique can be characterized by: shortened duration of the stroke cycle, the push back phase, and the arms' recovery phase; high minimum velocity within the stroke cycle; and a relatively small range of hip movement throughout the stroke cycle.

## REFERENCES

Bober, T., and Czabański, B. 1975. Changes in breaststroke techniques under different speed conditions. In: J. P. Clarys and L. Lewillie (eds.), Swimming II, International Series on Sport Sciences, Vol. 2, pp. 188–193. University Park Press, Baltimore.

Kornecki, S., and Reiter, A. 1975. Criterion of the effect of the swimming technique. Sport Wyczynowy 7:25–28.

Molinskij, K. K. 1961. Speedography as a method of investigation in swimming. Teoria i Praktika Fiziczeskoj Kultury 7:537–539.

Onoprijenko, B. I. 1969. Nomograms for the qualification of water resistance. Teoria i Praktika Fiziczeskoj Kultury 8:5–7.

# Lightstreak Photography: A Simple Method for Recording Movement Patterns

**K. Reischle**

The principal purpose of this study was to conduct an objective analysis of movement skills with the aid of an economical biomechanical method. By means of the lightstreak method, an attempt was made to analyze the typical level of motor skill in swimming and to record directly the momentary effective stroke length for swimming the crawl, backstroke, and butterfly. Brown and Counsilman, (1970), Clarys, Jiskoot and Lewillie, (1973), and Hoecke and Gruendler, (1975) have previously examined movement patterns in swimming by the lightstreak method.

## METHODS

The backstroke, crawl, and butterfly swimming styles were tested by two methods: the usual lightstreak method, and a modified lightstreak method. In the second method, the lightstreak is treated with a modification of an electric resistor. The 2.4-volt bulbs were attached to wrist and ankle, and a rechargeable Ni-Cd battery (Varta 2.4-volt) served as a power source. The batteries were made watertight by embedding them in a polycasting resin. By means of a bulb at the hip that flashed during the pull/push phase, the momentary effective stroke length was recorded (Figure 1). The electric circuit consisted of one Varta 6-volt Ni-Cd battery, one transistor, one electric resistor, and electrodes of copper, at the swimmer's palm. Because of the continuous change in resistance at the copper electrodes while the hand was plunged into the water and brought to the surface again, the bulb that was fastened to the hip was switched on and off (Figures 2 and 3).

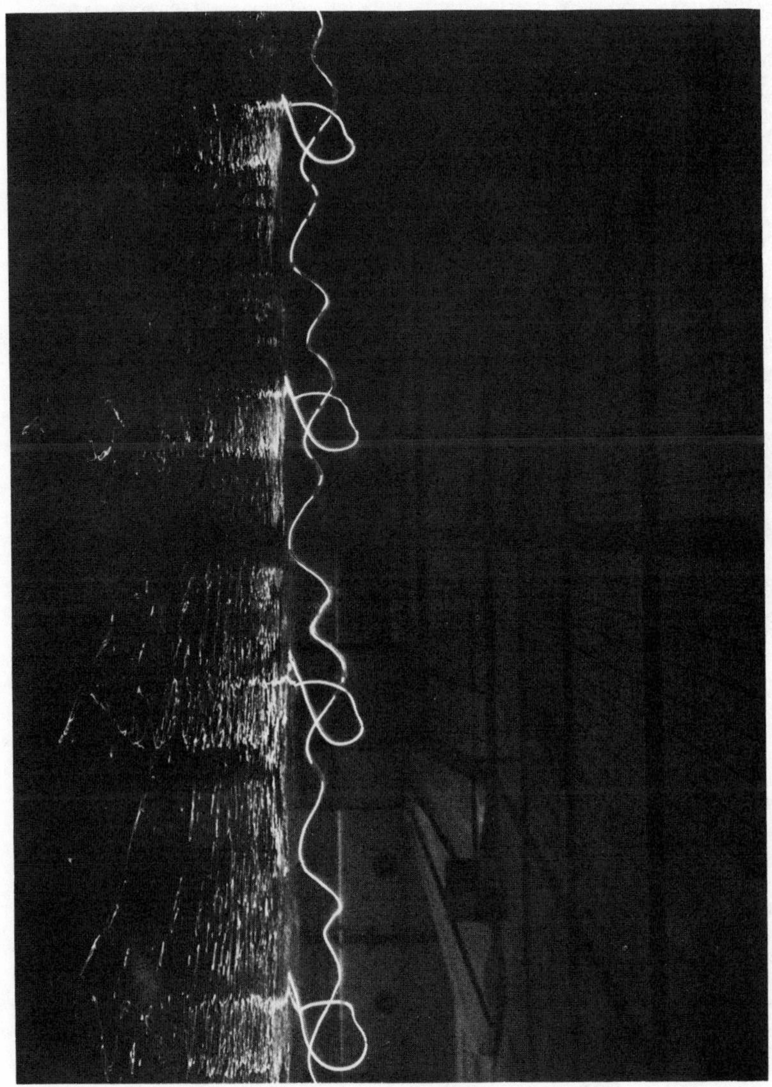

Figure 1. These light streaks were made with the crawl stroke (pull and kick phases).

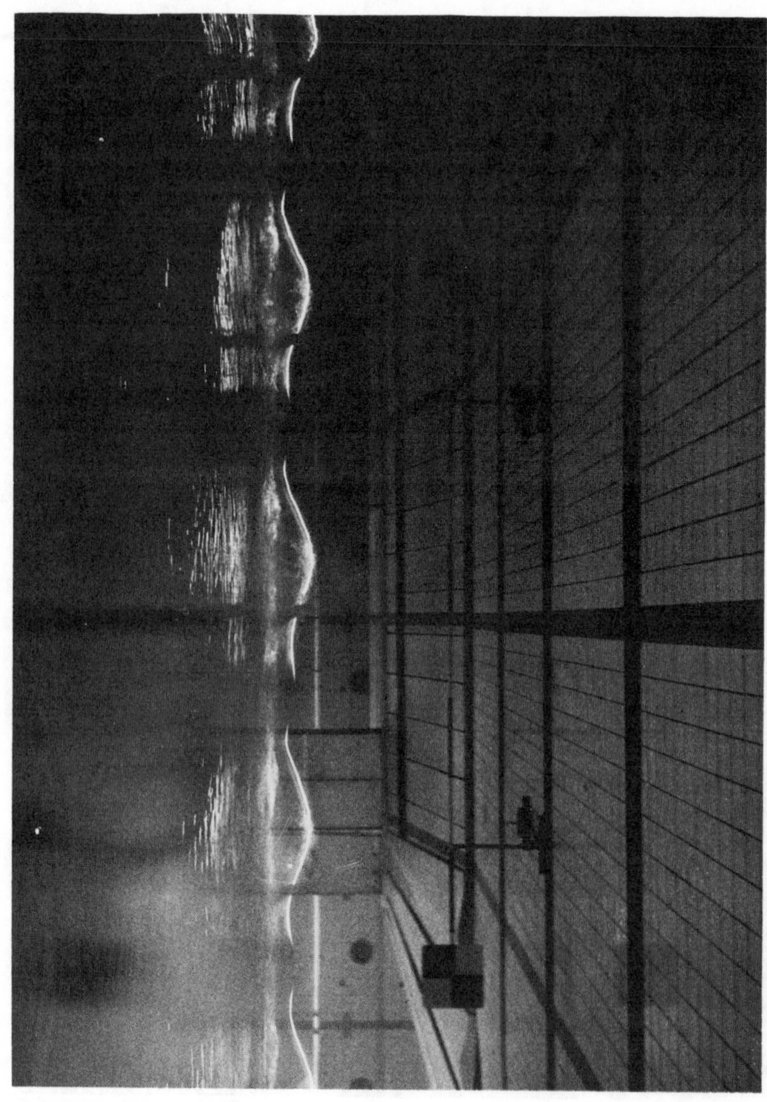

Figure 2. These tracings show the hip distance covered in one stroke.

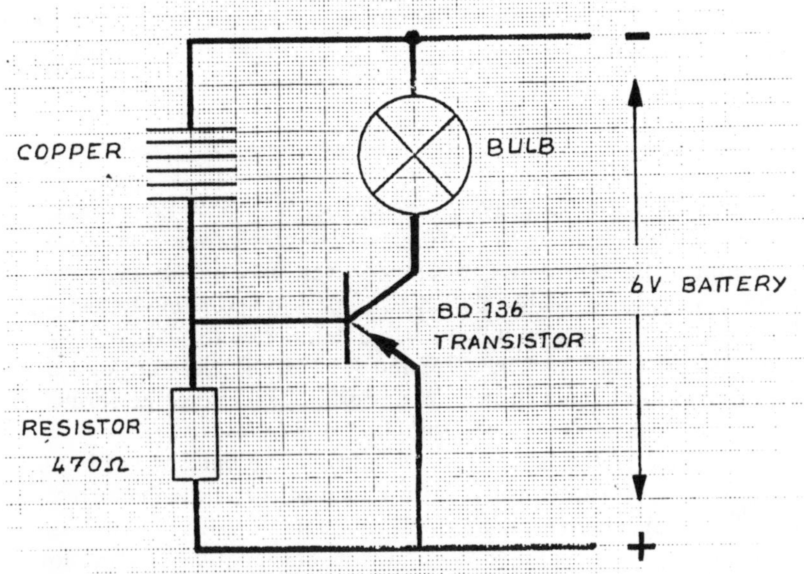


Figure 3. Electric circuit used in the modified lightstreak method.

The tracings were recorded by an underwater camera (Nikonos III). This camera employed a lens that was adjusted for underwater conditions. While the camera was working, the shutter opened for 3–6 sec at *f*/11. The Kodak Tri-X Pan (27 DIN or ASA 400) film proved satisfactory for filming in underwater conditions. The distance from the camera to the plane of motion was 8.75 m, the lens axis was per-

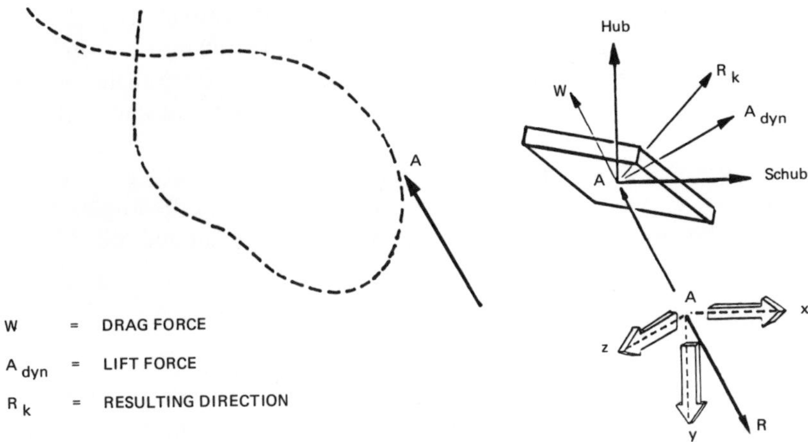


Figure 4. Components of lift and drag forces on the hand.

pendicular to the direction of swimming, and a reference scale was attached in the plane of motion. The subjects swam at maximum speed and stroke frequency was ascertained by means of a frequency meter.

## RESULTS

The analysis of the light rays gave significant information about propulsion during swimming (Counsilman, 1971): the propulsion results as a reaction to lift and water resistance (Reischle, 1976). Light traces of the movements of highly skilled swimmers support this statement in two ways. First, the arm pull showed a distinctive forward/downward phase (Barthels and Adrian, 1975) and second, the kick, during execution of the crawl, backstroke, or butterfly, was never performed in opposition to the direction of swimming (Figure 4).

By means of the lightstreak method, stroke defects can be diagnosed objectively. Defects in performance of the butterfly stroke, for instance, might include kicking defects such as active flexion of the shank, defects in the pulling phase such as missing the forward/downward phase because of submerging of the arm after recovery, or coordination defects such as the use of one kick per arm pull or two kicks in the forward/downward phase.

The record of the stroke length provides information about the relationship among stroke length, stroke frequency, and swimming velocity. For this purpose, the stroke lengths as well as the stroke frequencies were plotted on a coordinate system with hyperbolic branches (Figure 5). One hyperbolic branch corresponded, therefore, to a certain swimming velocity ($v_{max}$ m/min), which can be obtained by means of various stroke frequencies and stroke lengths. The hyperbolic branches were constructed according to the equation $lv_{max}/f = l_e$, where $l_e$ is the effective stroke length, $lv_{max}$ is m/min at $v_{max}$, and f is the stroke frequency. The point of the coordinates for a faster swimmer is always to the right of the hyperbolic branch that can be fixed by the point of the coordinates for a slower swimmer.

Thirty physical education students (Group 2) and 40 highly skilled swimmers (Group 1) were tested by means of the modified lightstreak method. The interpretation of the test results is summarized in Table 1.

## DISCUSSION

Some aspects of swimming technique problems can be solved by use of the lightstreak method described in this article because this method provides information on the influence of training methods on movement patterns, success or failure as the result of different teaching methods, e.g., part-whole versus whole method, and consequences of

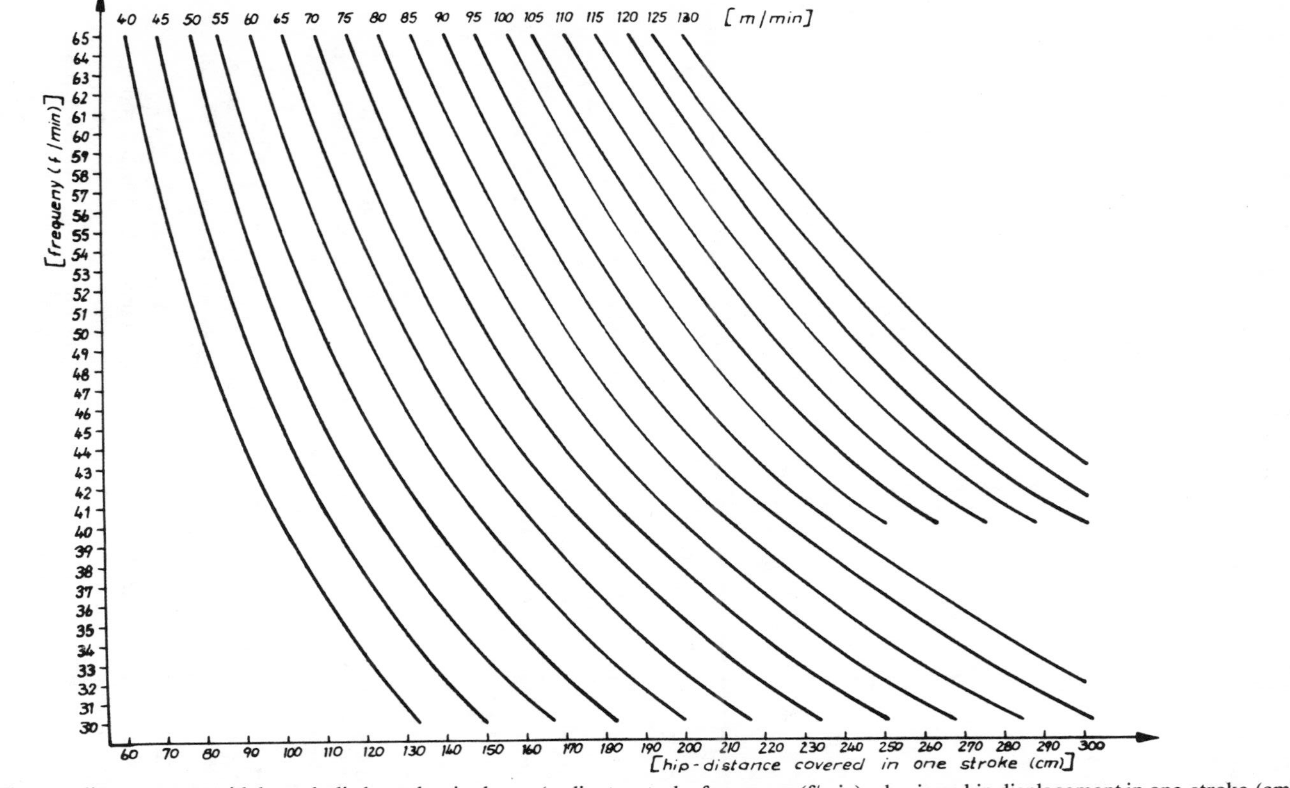


Figure 5. The coordinate system with hyperbolic branches is shown (ordinate: stroke frequency (f/min); abscissa: hip displacement in one stroke (cm)).

Table 1. Differences in mean performances between highly skilled swimmers (Group 1) and physical education students (Group 2), including stroke frequencies DF (butterfly), KF (crawl), and RF (backstroke), and hip displacements per stroke for butterfly (DZR), crawl (KZR), and backstroke (RZR)

| Variable | | Number of cases | Mean | | t-ratio |
|---|---|---|---|---|---|
| DF | | | | | |
| | Group 1 | 42 | 54.0714 | (f/min) | 7.59[a] |
| | Group 2 | 30 | 40.5333 | (f/min) | |
| DZR | | | | | |
| | Group 1 | 42 | 171.3095 | (cm) | 2.17[a] |
| | Group 2 | 30 | 134.6667 | (cm) | |
| RF | | | | | |
| | Group 1 | 38 | 37.2899 | (f/min) | 0.92 |
| | Group 2 | 27 | 36.0741 | (f/min) | |
| RZR | | | | | |
| | Group 1 | 38 | 207.6842 | (cm) | 8.75[a] |
| | Group 2 | 27 | 159.1111 | (cm) | |
| KF | | | | | |
| | Group 1 | 37 | 49.9189 | (f/min) | 6.77[a] |
| | Group 2 | 33 | 41.2424 | (f/min) | |
| KZR | | | | | |
| | Group 1 | 37 | 173.5459 | (cm) | 3.45[a] |
| | Group 2 | 33 | 152.2424 | (cm) | |

[a] Significant at >0.05 level of probability

peripheral and central fatigue on swimming technique compared with physiological parameters.

## REFERENCES

Barthels, K. M., and Adrian, M. J. 1975. Three-dimensional spatial hand patterns of skilled butterfly swimmers. In: J. P. Clarys and L. Lewillie (eds.), Swimming II, International Series on Sport Sciences, Vol. 2, pp. 154-160. University Park Press, Baltimore.

Brown, R. M., and Counsilman, J. E. 1970. The role of lift in propelling the swimmer. In: J. M. Cooper (ed.), Selected Topics in Biomechanics. Proceedings of the CIC symposium on Biomechanics, pp. 179-188. Athletic Institute, Chicago.

Clarys, J. P., Jiskoot, J., and Lewillie, L. 1973. Use of the lightstreak method in the biomechanical analysis of different swimming styles. Kinanthropologie 5.

Counsilman, J. E. 1971. Application of Bernoulli's principle to human propulsion in water. In: J. P. Clarys and L. Lewillie (eds.), Biomechanics in Swimming, pp. 59-71. Universite Libre de Bruxelles, Brussels.

Hoecke, G., and Gruendler, G. 1975. Use of light trace photography in teaching swimming. In: J. P. Clarys and L. Lewillie (eds.), Swimming II, International Series on Sport Sciences, Vol. 2., pp. 194-206. University Park Press, Baltimore.

Reischle, K. 1976. Problem of propulsion in swimming. Leistungssport 1:4.

# Survey of Instructor Profiles and Leadership Needs in Swimming Programs in Canada

**J. V. Daniel, J. Zeigler, and M. J. Tropea**

## BACKGROUND

The Canadian Red Cross began its Water Safety Service in 1945. The objectives were, and are, to reduce suffering caused by drowning and water accidents, to encourage the development of ideal aquatic facilities, and to improve health through promotion of aquatic programs.

To meet these objectives today, the Service provides standardized courses in aquatic programs, a leadership training program in cooperation with the Royal Life Saving Society of Canada (RLSSC), and support materials and technical assistance for aquatic personnel in the field.

The present organization and content of the combined RC/RLSSC Instructor Course is similar to the one originally designed in the mid-1940s to train generalists who operated as instructors, lifeguards, and organizers at the natural waterfronts and outdoor pools that accounted, until recently, for the great majority of swimming instruction sites in Canada.

This pattern of a predominantly outdoor summer program served by a young high school or university student generalist remained relatively stable until about 1960, when the trend toward building indoor swimming pools increased at a rapid rate. This increase in indoor facilities and thus the much greater opportunity for Canadians to receive swimming instruction entailed a proliferation of aquatic activities and precipitated the development of more specialized programs with more specialized leadership needs.

At least two problems related to leadership training in the Red Cross have emerged. First, a considerable proportion of indoor pool time is during school hours when the traditional instructor, typically a student, is not available. Thus, one need is a broader base from which instructor candidates could be drawn, i.e., housewives, teachers, etc. Secondly, few or no instructor preparation programs are available at present for some of the more specialized courses offered, i.e., pre-school, adapted for the handicapped, fitness, etc.

In light of these problems, reinforced by numerous and increasing requests from divisions, it became apparent that an evaluation of the leadership training program of the Canadian Red Cross Water Safety Service was needed. Within the total leadership program, the combined RC/RLSSC instructor training program would of necessity be a major element.

In light of increasing public awareness of aquatic activities, increasing availability of facilities, and changing and more sophisticated needs, the question was: What requirements and expectations of aquatic personnel throughout the country will better serve these trends and how should these be reflected in the leadership training program of the Canadian Red Cross?

### Working Hypothesis

The Resource and Development Committee (RDC) of the Canadian Red Cross Water Safety Services, after considerable preliminary work, set the following working hypothesis: Specialized and differentiated needs within the broad spectrum of swimming activities require a leadership training program that meets these new needs more effectively by providing a more varied and flexible training program from which candidates and instructors might choose a core and/or other appropriate additional experiences that are more directly related to their special interests and the special needs they serve.

### Limitations

In addition to the limitations inherent in any survey, this study was limited in that the data were collected by the divisions in the field and not by the survey team. Therefore, it was not certain that forms were received by all personnel or that identical instructions were given for completing the survey forms.

## METHOD

### Population

Canada is a very large and diverse country comprised of ten provinces and two territories. The ten divisions of the Canadian Red Cross Water

Safety Service correspond to the ten provinces; the Yukon territory is included with British Columbia, and the Northwest territories with the province of Alberta. To generate a picture of the national leadership needs, as well as local and regional differences, the survey was conducted through all ten divisions and the armed services. Survey forms were distributed to the above divisions which in turn distributed and collected the forms from the aquatic personnel within the respective divisions.

Three groups of personnel were asked to respond to the survey: aquatic program directors were asked to fill out forms detailing programming of their facilities, describing personnel working in their programs, and evaluating their RC/RLSSC instructors' effectiveness; instructor course conductors were asked to evaluate the RC/RLSSC instructor courses with respect to a number of factors assumed to influence instructor effectiveness; and certified RC/RLSSC instructors with 2 or more years of experience were asked to evaluate the training they had received in light of the responsibilities and demands typically placed upon them.

### Survey Forms

The survey forms consisted of six parts. The first part dealt with the rationale for the study and with instructions for the completion of the subsequent forms. The second part, Form 1, dealt with the instructor profile; the third, Form 2, dealt with representative weekly facility timetables; the fourth, Form 3.1, dealt with questions to be answered by aquatic program directors; the fifth, Form 3.2, dealt with questions to be answered by instructor course conductors; and the sixth, Form 3.3, dealt with questions to be answered by RC/RLSSC instructors. The survey forms were made available through the office of the Canadian Red Cross Society.

### Timetable

Survey forms were distributed to the divisions and the armed forces in the spring of 1976, and the data were collected by October 1976. The project report was submitted to the Resource and Development Committee in January 1977.

### Analysis of Data

Data were summarized and analyzed by the descriptive method, using tables and summary lists of subjective comments. These appear in detail in the original report. This chapter will present the findings in a condensed form.

## FINDINGS AND INTERPRETATIONS

The data collected represented responses from over 300 different program facilities (waterfronts and indoor and outdoor pools) and are presented in Table 1.

Each facility in turn represented the responses of a number of aquatic personnel (directors, course conductors, and instructors). A small program facility employed five to ten instructors, while the larger facilities required 25 or more instructors. The number of survey forms received by the investigators was thus considerable.

The data received provided information in three areas: instructor profiles, use of facilities, and subjective comments from program directors, instructor course conductors, and RC/RLSSC instructors.

### Instructor Profile

In its briefest form this information can be summarized nationally as follows. The typical swimming instructor was female, held joint RC/RLSSC Instructor Certification (range= 83–100%), was 17–20 years of age (armed forces excepted), was almost always paid, had fewer than 3 years of experience, and taught classes of 6–10 students, with 11–15 being the next most prevalent class size. These generalizations represent the majority of cases; variations from these typical situations appear in the original report.

### Use of Facilities

Aquatic program directors submitted information on the use of facilities under subcategories of swimming activities. These are summarized as national averages in Table 2.

One interesting finding from Table 2 was the considerable amount of time devoted to free swimming (38.6%). The relatively significant proportion of time spent on competitive swimming was also noteworthy (8.4%). Although the ranges in the categories represent considerable diversity, the extremes were isolated often and for good reasons (e.g., upper frequency range of scuba diving by armed forces). The results were therefore quite consistent in their emphases on specific swimming activities.

From this account of facility use, it was found that, in addition to the more specialized activities, the RC/RLSSC instructor spent giving preschool, beginner, advanced, and lifesaving instruction for an average of about 28% of the total facilities time. Of this instruction, more than half was spent with preschoolers and beginners. If the advanced groups (Red Cross Junior, Intermediate, and Senior) were broken down into Juniors and others, the time spent by instructors on beginners including preschoolers and Juniors—beginners moving into the first level of swimming—was approximately 20%. Considering that

Table 1. Number of facilities responding, by division

| Division | Facilities responding (N) |
| --- | --- |
| BC/Yukon | 45 |
| Alberta/NWT | 17 |
| Saskatchewan | 21 |
| Manitoba | 13 |
| Ontario | 161 |
| Prince Edward Island | 2 |
| Nova Scotia/New Bruswick[a] | 9 |
| Newfoundland | 8 |
| Armed services | 17 |
| Quebec[b] | — |
| Total[b] | 293+ |

[a] Data were mixed on receipt, thus summed by investigators.
[b] Data submitted in summary form did not include this figure.

Table 2. Facilities use by swimming activity (national average)

| Category | Average facility use (% of total time) | Range | Divisions reporting (N) |
| --- | --- | --- | --- |
| Preschool | 5.7 | 2.5 – 10.2 | all |
| Beginners | 9.0 | 5.6 – 11.5 | all |
| Advanced (Red Cross jr, intermed, and sr) | 8.6 | 4.8 – 11.0 | all |
| Lifesaving (all RLSSC levels) | 4.7 | 3.5 – 5.8 | all |
| Leader/inservice (Red Cross leader and inservice for aquatic personnel) | 3.0 | 1.0 – 5.5 | 6 |
| Free (no scheduled activity) | 38.6 | 25.6 – 47.0 | all |
| Adapted (blind, retarded, etc.) | 1.1 | 0.1 – 3.8 | 8 |
| Skin/scuba diving | 1.3 | 0.1 – 4.8 | 8 |
| Diving | 0.8 | 0.1 – 2.0 | 7 |
| Waterpolo | 1.2 | 0.4 – 2.6 | 7 |
| Synchronized | 1.6 | 0.4 – 3.0 | 9 |
| Competitive | 8.4 | 2.9 – 26.0 | all |
| Adult | 5.0 | 3.2 – 7.5 | 8 |
| Fitness | 1.4 | 0.3 – 2.1 | 5 |
| Others | 9.6 | 0.7 – 34.7 | 6 |

about half of the total available time was spent in free swimming and an undefined other category, the time spent in teaching at introductory levels became even more significant.

### Subjective Comments

Survey Forms 3.1, 3.2, and 3.3 provided aquatic personnel with the opportunity to express their views on the present instructor training program, its congruency with expectations and needs in the field, and with the general effectiveness of instructors in their jobs.

Two overriding impressions appeared. Those responding were generally satisfied with the training the instructors were receiving, and the suggestions made were of a positive and constructive nature. In addition, the needs, expectations, and requirements expressed throughout the country were very consistent. These findings are summarized in a list of suggestions made most consistently for improving the Instructor Course:

1. Give more practice in teaching real learners rather than peers
2. Place greater emphasis on how to correct stroke faults effectively
3. Devote greater attention to evaluation standards
4. Extend course time to include apprenticeship
5. Spend less time on development of personal skills
6. Spend less time on review of prerequisites and skills
7. Place greater emphasis on how and what to teach at various age and skill levels
8. Devote more time to teaching the RLSSC program
9. Make provision for a mechanism for becoming more specialized in various specialized program areas: adapted, synchronized swimming, waterpolo, and fitness
10. Present fewer boring lectures
11. Provide precourse experiences for course candidates
12. Develop public relations strategies
13. Give instruction in natural site and pool maintenance
14. Use long-term lesson and program planning
15. Institute tougher pass/fail standards for instructors

## CONCLUSIONS AND RECOMMENDATIONS

The results from three major sources of information—instructor profiles, use of swimming facilities for different programs, and subjective comments on the effectiveness of instructor training from aquatic program directors, instructor course conductors and certified RC/RLSSC instructors—point with considerable confidence toward a number of elements that call for modification of the present Instructor Training Program.

These elements relate essentially to two broad issues. One issue deals with what should be taught and what type of instruction is needed most (i.e., teaching introductory levels of swimming). The other deals with whether graduates from basic instructor courses should be capable of teaching a large number of subspecialties or whether they should have the opportunity to pick up knowledge and skills specific to a specialty they choose. The questions of the pool from which the candidates for instructor training are drawn relates significantly to both issues. For example, if one needs instructors for daytime instruction of beginners or preschool children, possibly the best source of instructor candidates is among housewives. Is it then necessary to expose them to an extensive training program with difficult prerequisites to graduate an instructor who can teach every level up to and including lifesaving and other specialties?

In conclusion, it seems warranted to suggest that the Instructor Training Program needs modification to reflect more clearly role definition and, possibly, role differentiation. If the present 40-hr time limit of instructor training is retained, role definition will have to reflect fewer and therefore more carefully selected priority elements in the basic or core instructor program. The survey results suggest that these priority elements should be oriented toward the fundamentals of the learning/teaching environment and to the lower levels of swimming instruction. Alternatively, extending the time limit would permit inclusion of a greater number of elements and a more sophisticated instructor training program that would result in instructor competencies with greater adaptability and more flexible service potential.

A third alternative would be to design a leadership training program which would satisfy both—a program with a core to train instructors for the most pressing needs within the existing time limit, plus additional instructor training packages that would satisfy various special needs. These additions would depend on the particular needs and could be pre- or postcore experiences.

The decision concerning which alternative to follow is an organizational one, but it seems that, based on the information from the survey and the short life of an instructor in actual service, the alternative of a flexible, adaptable, multimodular and special needs oriented leadership program is most logical. The working hypothesis set by the Resource and Development Committee for the survey study thus seems tenable.

## REFERENCE

Special subcommittee of the Resource and Development Committee of the Canadian Red Cross Water Safety Service. 1977. Project report, National leadership survey summary. The Canadian Red Cross Society Water Safety Service, Toronto, Ontario, Canada.